ONE BODY

NOTRE DAME STUDIES IN ETHICS AND CULTURE

series editor, David Solomon

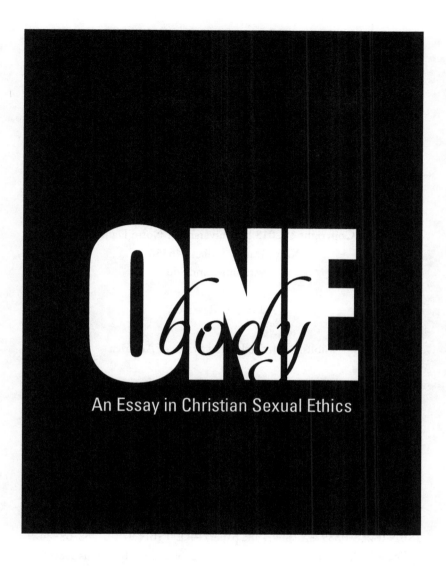

ONE *body*

An Essay in Christian Sexual Ethics

ALEXANDER R. PRUSS

University of Notre Dame Press

Notre Dame, Indiana

Library of Congress Cataloging-in-Publication Data

Pruss, Alexander R.
One body : an essay in Christian sexual ethics / Alexander R. Pruss.
    p.   cm. — (Notre Dame studies in ethics and culture)
Includes bibliographical references and index.
ISBN 978-0-268-03897-7 (pbk. : alk. paper) —
ISBN 0-268-03897-X (pbk. : alk. paper) — E-ISBN 978-0-268-08984-9
1. Sex—Religious aspects—Christianity. 2. Sex role—Religious aspects—
Christianity. 3. Sexual ethics. 4. Christian ethics.   I. Title.
BT708.P75   2012
241'.66—dc23
2012036268

Ad maiorem Dei gloriam

Contents

Acknowledgments

I would like to thank David Alexander, Michael Almeida, Michael Beaty, Ron Belgau, Todd Buras, Sarah Coakley, Mike Darcy, Stephen Evans, Ted Furton, Richard Gale, Sherif Girgis, Alfonso Gomez-Lobo, Luke Gormally, Germain Grisez, David Jeffrey, Christian Jenner, Daniel Johnson, Christopher Kaczor, Mark Lance, Patrick Lee, Ron Lee, James Lennox, David Manley, Richard Manning, Lawrence Masek, Anthony McCarthy, Mark Murphy, Adam Pelser, Amy Pruss, Richard Sisca, Abigail Tardiff, Nicholas Teh, Eric Telfer, two anonymous readers, the students in my Philosophy of Love and Sex classes at Georgetown and Baylor, and various commenters on my own blog (http://AlexanderPruss.blogspot.com) and on the former RightReason blog, for encouragement, discussion, disagreement, comments, and/or suggestions concerning various parts of this project.

Particular thanks are due to Emily Glass, who has stylistically improved just about every page of this book, and has gone over and above the call of duty by contributing important philosophical comments as well. I take full responsibility for the remaining infelicities, some of which are no doubt due to my not following her advice at every point.

Much of this book was written while I was at Georgetown University, and I am grateful to Georgetown University for summer research support.

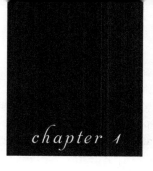

Introduction

Therefore a man leaves his father and his mother and cleaves to

his wife, and they become one flesh. (Gen. 1:24)

1. PROBLEM AND METHOD

Many of the great controversies within Western Christianity in the latter half of the twentieth century and the beginning of the twenty-first have been over sexuality. And while Christianity entered the twentieth century with agreement on a reasonably clear set of rules of sexual conduct, the level of theoretical elaboration of these rules was relatively low, as compared to, say, the amount of theoretical work on the Sacraments or the doctrines of the Creed—despite some notable exceptions such as reflection on the relationship between marriage and celibacy. The reason for this underdevelopment was a relative lack of controversy within the Christian community about much of sexual ethics. Groups outside of mainstream Christianity, like the Albigensians, had widely different sexual ethics, but this did not pose a particularly strong challenge to the dominant lines of the tradition. Within mainstream Christianity, there were particular disagreements on issues such as divorce, but in practice, these appeared to have concerned relatively rare special cases. Typically, it is when significant disagreement begins that the theoretical background for a doctrine begins to be worked out in earnest.

The twentieth century, on the other hand, saw a number of attempts to build a theoretical foundation for sexual ethics. The surface difference between these attempts is in the way they addressed controversies over which of the traditional "rules" are objectively valid. But disagreement over these rules does sometimes mask an agreement over methodology. A dominant methodological approach has been to distance oneself from biological considerations, such as those connected with reproduction, and to focus on us as persons instead, looking at the interaction between our subjectivity and our sexuality, and focusing on human dignity and the need not to trample on the autonomy of others. And yet an approach like this has led to widely different results, even within a single denomination—producing on the one hand Karol Wojtyła's personalist defense of traditional norms,[1] and on the other hand the American Catholic Theological Association's rather more revisionary approach.[2]

The purpose of this book is to defend a particular, coherent Christian sexual ethic. This ethic is influenced by both "personalist" approaches and older, more biologically-oriented "Thomistic" ones, and will be developed by starting with some central Christian claims about sexuality and showing the normative consequences of these claims.[3] The approach is both theological and philosophical. For although the central claims can be accepted on the basis of revelation, they are also independently plausible, and can be studied through philosophical methods. Comprehensive engagement with the voluminous literature on sexuality in ethics and moral theology is not the purpose of this book, but rather the development and defense of a particular line of thought.

While I shall cite scripture and the Christian tradition, the central argumentative line of this book does not assume divine inspiration of all the texts of scripture. Thus, I shall not be arguing that normative issues of homosexuality are settled by famously controversial Pauline passages such as 1 Corinthians 6:9–10. Rather, I will

2

argue that deeper and more general New Testament principles of independent philosophical plausibility settle the issue. Thus the argument should appeal to readers who either accept the philosophical plausibility of the principles I will invoke or who believe that, at least, basic principles found in the New Testament are inspired.

2. SCRIPTURE, TRADITION, AND SEMINAL TEXTS

A central part of our approach to scripture will be to take seminal biblical texts to be true in a deep way. Seminal texts lay down the theoretical foundation for a major area of biblically grounded theology. A text is seminal either because scripture itself grounds discussion on a topical area in the text or because the Christian tradition finds the text central to its thinking about the issue (or both). While the context of a text must never be neglected, a seminal text can have a message that transcends the context. A seminal text continually bears fruit on reflection, leading to profound and sometimes surprising conclusions.

A theology on which a seminal text has a trivial interpretation is unfaithful to Christianity: it makes shallow what the lived religion sees as deep. Consider, for instance, an interpretation of the text "God is love" (1 John 4:8 and 16) that simply says God loves some people very much. The universal is made parochial. The mysterious is rendered unpuzzling. Not only is metaphysical discussion about how God could be identical with one of his properties forestalled, but the text no longer inspires one to sacrifice oneself for *every* human being in need.

Or consider God's self-description in Exodus 3:14 as "I am who I am." This is echoed by the fourth evangelist's Jesus saying "I am," and "I am" was a divine name in Judaism. Eastern Orthodox icons put *ho ōn* on the halo of Christ, the "who is" of the Septuagint translation of this text. The translators of the Syriac Peshitta Old Testament find the text so mysterious that instead of translating it, they simply copy out the Hebrew *"ehyeh asher ehyeh"* in Syriac characters. Grammatically, the Hebrew is compatible with a multitude of interpretations, *ehyeh* being the incompletive first person singular form of *hyh*, "to be"

3

or "to become," and therefore capable of meaning "I (now) am," "I will be," "I (timelessly) am," and so on. One grammatically permissible interpretation would cut off the host of meanings and not render the text as implying anything about God's own nature, but as saying simply "I will be (for you) what I will be (for you)," i.e., "I am not telling you what I'm going to do for you—it'll be a surprise." But such an interpretation would be shallow. To think that although the Christian community has found great profundity in the text, the text itself lacks that profundity appears implausible given the Holy Spirit's guidance of the Christian community (John 16:13).

A seminal text is typically true in multiple ways, and was quite possibly intended as such by the author. Thus, that God is love can be read as simply saying that God does good things for everyone. But it can also be read as revealing to us something about the nature of God, as indeed 1 John 4:9 makes clear by distinguishing the love of God from its manifestation. Or consider the richness of the first verse of the Gospel of John. The text no doubt uses *logos* in a way intended to connect somehow with first-century Neoplatonism. In Greek, *logos* could mean "word," "discourse," "account," "argument," or "reason." At the same time, the notion of the "word of God" has a rich history in the Hebrew scriptures, and Philo connects the *logos* with Neoplatonic themes. Much of the diversity in meanings is, no doubt, intended by the author of the prologue of John.

A theological methodology based on seminal texts is, however, obviously open to abuse. If a text is so rich, it is probably at least somewhat ambiguous and the exegete might well insert an interpretation completely alien to the intentions of the author. As a check against this, the interpretation should be compatible with the ways in which the text has been fruitful, and should even explain some of that fecundity. When the text is used, say, by scripture to ground some practical conclusion, the interpretation of the text should make that practical conclusion plausible. Thus, the sixth chapter of 1 Corinthians uses the claim that sexual union results in two people becoming one flesh as the grounds for a prohibition on visiting prostitutes. Prima facie, the argument seems question-begging or, at best, ad hominem, since someone who does not think prostitution immoral should not feel revulsion at the thought of being united with a prostitute. If an inter-pretation of the "one flesh" text makes this into a better argument, then this speaks in favor of that interpretation.

Additionally, I shall assume that those basic principles which are not only contained within a single seminal text, but which suffuse the New Testament, are true, such as the principle that love is the basis of the moral law.

Someone who thinks that *all* texts of scripture are true and deep will, of course, a fortiori have no disagreement with my methodology. But my approach is intended to appeal to readers with a wider range of theological positions on questions of inspiration. It should not be plausible for a Christian of whatever stripe to say that Christianity gets wrong *basic* principles concerning sexuality. It is clear, I think, both biblically and phenomenologically, that sexual behavior should be a particularly deep and intimate expression of love. Yet Christianity, at base, is a revealed religion of love. The duty to love is the center of Christian ethics. Sexual love is one of the central forms of love in human life. If Christianity is essentially the revelation of love—both of God's love for us and of what our love for each other should be like—then Christianity, as a whole, would be an implausible religion if it got wrong basic principles in the sexual sphere. Note, however, that saying Christianity is right on the basic principles does not pre-judge the question of whether it got the *application* of these principles right.

I shall also take other statements of scripture and of the Christian tradition in general to have epistemic weight, albeit my arguments do not require the infallibility of either.

3. SEX

It is experientially and sociologically clear that sexual behavior is a very important facet of human life. Any analysis of eros that rendered it something unimportant and trivial would be its own refutation. But if we can give a unified and coherent account of sexual love, based on plausible principles, making clear why sexual love is something that matters, and doing justice to many of our conflicting intuitions, then this account should have some plausibility. The method of Aristotle in his *Nicomachean Ethics* was to take our mutually incoherent ethical intuitions and provide a coherent and unified account that did as much justice to them as possible. Once we have done likewise, the resulting account is likely true.

There is a basic split in the way most of us think about sex. On the one hand, we think it is an "animal thing to do," an area for instinct, an area where our rational self is laid to rest and primal urges move us. But on the other hand, we think of it as an avenue for profound interpersonal union, a setting in which one can *know* the other person as a person. All accounts of sexual ethics can be situated as attempts to come down on one side of the split or the other, or else as attempts to reconcile the two. I shall argue for such a reconciliation. The biological nature of the sexual act makes it fit for interpersonal union, and the specific kind of interpersonal union in which sexuality results requires this biological nature. It is in and through a profound biological union that interpersonal union occurs, and it is this fact that makes sexual love unique among human loves. There is a union of persons because there is a union as "one body."

None of what I have said so far is especially controversial on its own. What will be controversial is the particular way in which I shall analyze the union as "one body" and the implications of this analysis. Yet I shall argue that an account like the one I propose is necessary if we are to do justice to the seminal text from Genesis cited at the beginning of this chapter.

4. WHAT IS TO COME

I will begin by a brief discussion of the nature of love in general, focusing on the phenomenon of "forms of love." Love comes in many varieties: filial, parental, fraternal, erotic, friendly, companionate, charitable, and so on. We call them all "love" and the Greek scriptures use the word *agapê* for all of them. This textual claim is controversial but will be defended (see section 2 of the next chapter). Thus love in each of its forms is in some way the same, and yet the forms are different. Moreover, love becomes distorted when we get the form wrong—for instance, by standing in a relation of eros to one's parent. I shall discuss how this distortion works and why it constitutes a failure of love. Because this is a book of Christian ethics, a failure of love shall always be taken as a moral wrong. Conversely, I believe that every moral wrongness is constituted by a failure of love, though I shall try to minimize use of this more controversial claim.

Next, I will argue for the meaningfulness of sexuality. How we act sexually with our bodies matters in a way in which it does not matter how exactly we shake hands. We will discuss the notion of union as one flesh, both exegetically and philosophically, and examine an account of how union as one flesh can be related to interpersonal union. This builds on the earlier discussion of love and is the argumentative center of the book.

All this will have concrete applications. Not all possible sexual activity is appropriate in light of the nature of erotic love. This will take us through discussions of masturbation, homosexuality, and contraception, as well as consideration of the settings in which different varieties of erotic love are appropriate. Hence, we will discuss premarital sex, the nature of marriage, the morality of adultery, and the morality and possibility of divorce and remarriage. Throughout, it will be argued that seeing sexuality as a union as one body, called for by love, has substantial practical implications. Finally, I will discuss noncoital forms of reproduction, and end on a brief discussion of celibacy.

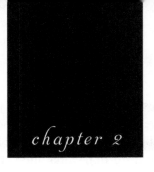

chapter 2

Love and Its Forms

This is my commandment, that you love [agapate] one another as

I have loved [ēgapēsa] you. Greater love has no man than this, that

a man lay down his life for his friends. (John 15:12–13)

1. THE NEW TESTAMENT AND *AGAPĒ*

The central ethical concept in the New Testament is love. Usually, the Greek word is *agapē* or a related verb, which is typically taken by interpreters to indicate a selfless charity, while occasionally a version of *philia* is used, a word whose classical Greek meaning was the love in a friendship. The New Testament does not contrast *agapē* and *philia*, although typically when a command to love is given, the language of *agapē* is used. However, this difference in usage does not appear to mark a difference in meaning. Thus, at John 3:35 we read that "the Father loves [*agapai*] the Son, and has given all things into his hand," while at 5:20 we are told that "the Father loves [*philei*] the Son, and shows him all that he himself is doing." Similarly, at Luke 11:43 the accusation is made to the Pharisees: "you love [*agapate*] the best seat in the synagogues and salutations in market places," while at

20:46 we are warned of the scribes "who … love [*philountôn*] saluta-tions in the market places and the best seats in the synagogues and the places of honor at feasts." There does not appear to be reason to trans-late the two words differently into English.

What, then, are *agapê* and *philia*? The ethics of the New Testa-ment is centered on the duty to love. This implies that *agapê* cannot indicate a loving feeling or emotion. For, first of all, feelings do not seem to be subject to direct control. While we can cause feelings in ourselves indirectly—say, rouse ourselves to feel indignation by dwell-ing on the wrongs someone has done—we cannot do so immediately and we cannot do so always, whereas we are always obliged to love.

Secondly, feelings of affection are transitory. They disappear while one sleeps, and yet no one would say: "My wife does not love me, for she is asleep." But more seriously, love according to the New Testament is best exhibited in situations of great distress, the para-digm being Christ's passion. In these situations, one may be unable to feel anything other than suffering even as one is engaging in a para-digmatic act of love, as in the case of Christ's cry of abandonment[1] on the Cross (Mark 15:34, Matt. 27:46). As Kierkegaard notes, "Christ's love was not intense feeling, a full heart, etc.; it was rather the work of love, which is his life."[2]

Finally, feelings do not have the close connection to action that love has in the New Testament, indicated most clearly by the text at the head of this chapter. A feeling need not be acted on, but can be ignored by force of will. The basic claim of New Testament ethics is that love is sufficient for fulfilling the moral law.[3] We are not told that what would be sufficient is love *and* an absence of any emotion that counters it or thwarts its expression. It is taken for granted that love expresses itself and is sufficient, in and of itself. As Augustine put it, "Love, and do what thou wilt."[4] This does not rule out the possibility that a love might be unsatisfactory and distorted, as in the case of the love of money, but if so, then this unsatisfactoriness will be due to a failure by love's own standards, rather than due to the presence of something outside the love. We will examine such failures shortly.

Neither do we want to say that *agapê* is a *disposition* or *tendency* to feel an emotion or an attitude. Such a dispositional account of love would explain why the woman who is asleep can be said to love her husband, for she has a disposition to feel a particular emotion under appropriate circumstances. Likewise, such a view might handle the case of great distress, for the person who is suffering could still have a disposition to feel a more positive emotion under less distressing circumstances. However, *dispositions* and *attitudes* are even less under direct volitional control than feelings are, and their connection with action is still not such as to *guarantee* right action.

The parable of the Good Samaritan is supposed to present us with a paradigmatic instance of love of neighbor. Emotion is mentioned only once, at the very beginning, when we are told that when the Samaritan saw the wounded man, "he had compassion" (Luke 10:33). If love were a feeling, however, it would be something different from compassion, and even though the parable is about love of neighbor, love as a feeling never occurs in the parable itself; indeed the word "love" never occurs (either as *agapê* or *philia*). Instead, after telling the parable, Christ asks who was neighbor to the wounded man and is told: "The one who showed mercy on him" (Luke 10:37). The words "who showed mercy," or more literally "who did mercy [*ho poiêsas to eleos*]," suggest that action is at least a central component of love.

An interesting and perhaps significant linguistic fact is that the verbal form of *agapê* occurs in the aorist tense on a number of occasions in the New Testament. The aorist is a "punctual" tense: it indicates a single temporally isolated event or act. It is an odd tense to use to describe an emotional disposition or attitude, since such endure over time. In John 5:12, Christ says to love—*agapate*, subjunctive second person plural—one another as he loved—*êgapêsa*, aorist—them. Christ's paradigmatic love is thought of here as a single act.

This could still be read consistently with seeing *agapê* as an emotional disposition or attitude, provided that we took the aorist to indicate a flare-up of this disposition or perhaps its initiation, "falling in love." This might prima facie explain John 5:12 as well as some other texts like Mark 10:21. It is nigh impossible to read John 13:1 in such a way, however: "having loved [aorist] his own who were in the world, he loved [aorist] them to the end." Likewise, John 12:41–42 does not appear to indicate a flare-up or the start of love when it talks of those who did not confess Christ because "they loved [aorist] the praise of men more than the praise of God."

The use of the aorist suggests that we can see *agapê* not just as an enduring attitude, but also as closely associated with a particular *act* of will, an act of will bound up with an action: "Christ loved [aorist] the church and gave [aorist] himself up for her" (Eph. 5:25). On this interpretation, we can very naturally see the non-aorist uses of *agapê* as implying a disposition, not to an emotion, but to *acts* of love, and the aorist versions as expressing the activation of this disposition.

Or consider the double use of the aorist in John 15:9: "As the Father has loved me [aorist], so have I loved [aorist] you; abide in my love." The first "loved" seems to indicate a transcendent act of love between the Father and the Son, perhaps even the generation of the Son. There does not appear to be any other tense that would adequately express this love. And then Christ's act of love toward us mirrors this love. Since the impending passion gives context to the whole discourse, it appears that Christ's sacrifice on the cross is seen as parallel to a mysterious transcendent act of love. By entering into this passion, by abiding in Christ's love, we are drawn up into this.

If the aorist is to be understood as above, the connection between *agapê* and action is very close. *Agapê* is concentrated in an action. But actions are the expression of one's will. It is plausible to define *agapê* as including a determination of one's will in favor of the beloved. It is not possible, then, for love to fail to result in good action on behalf of another, because, by definition, if one does not will the good, one does not love, with an exception when the action is bad on extrinsic grounds—say, when one accidentally gives the wrong medication.

2. IS *AGAPÊ* A FORM OF LOVE?

Since the classic study of Nygren,[5] a fairly common reading of the New Testament sees *agapê* as a form or kind of love, distinguished from and privileged over other forms of love. While *erôs* is a form of love that aims to possess the beloved for oneself, and *philia* is a form of love that seeks to form equal and reciprocal friendly relationships, *agapê* is allegedly a selfless willing of the good for the other with no thought of reciprocation. While the connection we saw between *agapê* and action may make this view plausible, such a reduction of *agapê* to selfless benevolence is mistaken, both as to the Greek and as to the content. *Agapê* is not a form of love. It simply *is* love, capable of taking on many forms depending on what is appropriate in the relationship.

Linguistically, forms of the verb *agapao,* the verb behind the abstract noun *agapê,* are used in the New Testament for every kind of love, including the love we are commanded to have for our neighbor and our enemies (e.g., Mark 12:31 and Matt. 5:44), the love between spouses (e.g., Eph. 5:25), the love of God for us (e.g., John 3:16), our love for God (e.g., Mark 12:30), and, as we saw, love for the best seats in synagogues and for salutations (Luke 11:43). The range of the verb is at least as great as the range of the English "to love." In the Septuagint Greek translation of the Old Testament, forms of *agapao* appear to be freely used anywhere where the English "to love" or the Hebrew "*ahav*" might be used. This specifically includes cases where the love is erotic in content, as in the Song of Songs:

> Sustain me with raisins, refresh me with apples; for I am sick with love [*agapês*]. (2:5)
> I adjure you, O daughters of Jerusalem, by the gazelles or the hinds of the field, that you stir not up nor awaken love [*agapên*] until it please. (2:7)
> Many waters cannot quench love [*agapên*], neither can floods drown it. If a man offered for love [*agapêi*] all the wealth of his house, it would be utterly scorned. (8:7)

In fact, the word is even used in cases that are more like lust than love, including Amnon's desire for Tamar (2 Sam. 13:9), whom he eventually rapes.

Biblical Greek does not, thus, use *agapê* to indicate a particular form of love. Every love is *agapê*. But we know from our own experience that there *are* different forms of love, such as romantic, filial, or friendly. These, then, must be seen as forms of *agapê*, rather than as relations standing over and against *agapê*. *Agapê* is not a form of love, but love itself.

What appears to be a driving force behind the desire to see *agapê* as a particular form of love is the idea that *agapê* is selfless generosity and hence does not seek reciprocation in the way that paradigmatic cases of romantic or friendly love do. But this is mistaken on both theological and philosophical grounds.

Theologically, one of the two main examples of *agapê* is God's gracious love of us. But God's sanctifying gift to us, the gift of his love, is precisely the ability to reciprocate that love of his. In the Incarnation, God became like us, in part that we might be able to love him not just as God but as a brother, and this is the ultimate instance of the equalizing tendency in love noted by Aristotle[6] and Cicero.[7] God seeks to be loved and praised, of course, not in order to fill some deficiency in himself but for our sake. One of the prefaces to the Roman Liturgy of the Mass says: "You have no need of our praise, yet our desire to thank you is itself your gift." God does desire reciprocation—but for our own sake.

The second, and ultimately the deeper, of the two main examples of *agapê* is the love between the persons of the Trinity. But this love is essentially reciprocal: the Father loves the Son and the Son reciprocates this love. In Western reflection, the Holy Spirit is often seen as the very love that proceeds from the Father *and* the Son. The love and its reciprocation are one and the same bilateral relationship.

Likewise, our *agapê* must include a unitive aspect when directed at people, because this is what the people we love need, and love's union with a fellow human being is only fully complete with reciprocation. In his encyclical *Deus Caritas Est*, Pope Benedict XVI directs this challenge to the staff of humanitarian organizations: "[W]hile professional competence is a primary, fundamental requirement, it is not of itself sufficient. We are dealing with human beings, and human beings always need something more than technically proper care. They need humanity. They need heartfelt concern."[8] This heartfelt concern arises from an "encounter with God in Christ which awakens their love and opens their spirits to others."[9]

One's spirit is opened to a unitive reaching out for communion with others, and this unitive aspect of *agapê* helps one avoid the danger of helping another out of superiority (a "white man's burden")—a form of "help" that demeans the recipient in a way contrary to our basic human fellowship. It can be humiliating to be the recipient of "charity" in the cold and narrow sense. But it does not demean us to receive gifts from someone seeking loving communion with us, someone who makes him or herself vulnerable to our rejection of that offer of communion. It is this aim at reciprocation, for Christian brotherhood (and hence a component of evangelization is appropriately present), and for communion with another that makes *agapê* the opposite of the attitude that C. S. Lewis describes where "spiteful people will pretend to be loving us with Charity precisely because they know it will wound us."[10]

Thus the very seeking for reciprocation that was supposed to be alien to *agapê* is crucial to it, and considerations of reciprocation are not a ground for distinguishing *agapê* from allegedly separate loves. But we should still consider another seminal text: "[*agapê*] *ou zetei ta heautês*"—"[love] does not seek the things that are its own" (1 Cor. 13:15). Grammatically, the "its" in "the things that are *its* own" refers unambiguously back to "love": love does not seek the things that belong to love. If one thinks that reciprocation and a relationship are things that belong to love, then one might conclude that love does not seek them.

However, this is neither the only reading of the text nor the most natural one. First observe that the claim about love not seeking its own is found among other statements about what love does and does not do—love rejoices together in the truth but does not reckon wrongs, for instance. But these claims all seem to involve a metonymy. For it is not the *love* that rejoices in the truth and does not reckon wrong, but the *lover*, insofar as he or she loves. Insofar as one loves, one rejoices in the truth, and insofar as one reckons wrongs, thus far one does not love. But if "*agapê*" as subject of the sentences stands metonymously for the lover as informed by love, we should likewise metonymously read *ta heautês* as the things that belong *to the lover*. Thus, we are told that *the lover*, as a lover, is not self-seeking.

One may, however, continue to maintain that aiming at a return of love and for a union with the beloved would be self-centered. But that, surely, is a mistake. For the lover is focused on the appreciated beloved, and it is on account of the beloved that the lover is drawn there. The lover seeks union, but seeks a union that is essentially a joint good. This joint good is good not only for the lover but also for the beloved, and insofar as this is love and not, say, lust, it is sought as a joint good. Thus, the lover does not seek his or her own good, but the joint good of lover and beloved. Humility does require that in a human relationship one acknowledge the good to oneself (lest one set oneself up as superior), but this good is not a self-centered good. This will become particularly clear in section 6 below, where we will see that a central aspect of the union is found precisely in seeing things through the beloved's point of view and in willing the beloved's good "from the inside," as it were. If that is what union is, it is surely not a self-centered good. Of course, it *might* be sought for one's own sake, but the true lover does not do that. As Nozick wrote, "There is a difference between wanting to hug someone and using them as an opportunity for yourself to become a hugger."[11] We do not love in order to be lovers, but because of the fascination of the beloved.

The idea that *agapê* is not self-seeking does, however, rule out an account on which I seek the good of the beloved simply because *my* well-being extends in some way to include the beloved.[12] The good of the beloved moves the lover, not just because it is the lover's good.

There may also be more than one sense in which *agapê* literally does not seek itself. 1 Corinthians 13 is a seminal text in the Christian tradition. It is plausible that it has multiple levels of meaning. While the most obvious reading is metonymous, with the lover not seeking the lover's own, there are ways in which we can also read the love as literally not seeking *its own*. These ways highlight what one might call "the humility of love."

One way love is humble is that the actions of love are not focused on *agapê* itself (we shall discuss a different aspect of love's humility in section 5 below). There would be something odd about a parent explaining why he stayed up the night with a sick child by saying: "I love my son." Surely the better justification would be the simpler: "He is my son." The latter justification puts the parent in a less grammatically prominent spot ("my" instead of "I"), and shows that the focus is on the son. Most importantly, however, the use of "I love my son" as a justification would suggest that if one did not love him, the main reason to stay up the night would be missing. But the main reason to stay up the night is that he is one's son. That he is one's son is also a reason to love him as one's son, and that one loves him may provide one with a *further* reason to stay up with him. However, the main reason for staying up is not that one loves him; rather, the love, expressed in the staying up, is a response to a reason that one would have independently of the love. Thus, in an important sense, the parent acts lovingly—acts in a way that is at least partly constitutive of love—without acting *on account of* love. Love's actions are not focused on love but on the beloved as seen in the context of a particular relationship.

However, to explain why we made some sacrifice for someone to whom we had no blood ties, we might well say, "I love him." Nonetheless, I suggest, this may be an imperfection—it may be a case of seeking one's own. Why not instead act on account of the value of the other person in the context of the relationship? It is true that love may be a central part of that relationship, but I want to suggest that love is not the part of the relationship that actually does the work of justifying the sacrifice. For suppose that I stopped loving my friend. Would that *in itself* take away my obligation to stand by him in his time of need? Certainly not. The *commitment* I had implicitly or explicitly undertaken while loving him, a commitment that made it appropriate for him to *expect* help from me, is sufficient for the justification. If I need to advert to my own love, then something has gone wrong.

Besides, there would a circularity in appealing to one's own present love to justify one's basic willingness to engage in loving actions for the beloved. For if one were not willing to do loving actions for the other, then one would not be loving the other, and hence a total failure to will to do loving actions for the other would not be a *violation* of love, for there would be no love there to be violated. Of course, such a failure might well be a violation of one's *duty* to love the person (whether arising out of personal commitment, or a general duty to love everyone or some specific duty like those we have to our relatives), but that is a different issue. It is not love, then, that justifies the general willingness to act lovingly, but the value of the other and the kind of relationship that one stands in to the other *apart from* the fact of love.

This argument could, to some extent, be countered by allowing that *past* love justifies present willingness to engage in loving actions. At the same time, a part of the relationship as it presently exists may be the fact of *having loved*. Thus, *having loved* may justify present loving actions. But, still, present *agapê* is not focused on present *agapê*—it is too busy looking at the fascinating beloved in the context of the relationship. This is one way *agapê* is self-effacing, humble.

There is, however, a special puzzle in the case of love of oneself. The command in Leviticus (19:18) to love one's neighbor as oneself is a seminal text, including in the New Testament which quotes it frequently (Matt. 5:43, 19:19, 22:39, Mark 12:31–33, Luke 10:27, Rom. 13:9, Gal. 5:14, James 2:8; all these verses use a form of the verb *agapao*). But how can love of oneself not be self-seeking? One answer to the puzzle could be that Paul is giving us a general quality of love: love focuses us on the beloved. In the special case where the beloved is oneself, this calls for a focus on self. This focus on self is not the result of a general quality of love, but of the particularity of the beloved in this form of love. However there may be deeper ways to understand how a love of oneself can be non-self-seeking, and we will discuss those in section 9 below.

And there is another serious difficulty for the above understanding of *agapê* as comprising all loves. It threatens to undercut the distinction between natural and supernatural love. In 1 John, we find a very close connection between love for others (everyone? fellow Christians?), love for God, and knowledge of God. To love and know God in the Christian sense surely requires grace—it is something supernatural, a way of living in the Holy Spirit. The *agapê* for others, then, had better be supernatural, too, since "love is of God, and he who loves is born of God and knows God" (1 John 4:7). But the erotic *agapê* spoken of in the Septuagint Song of Songs is surely not something like that—surely it can easily coexist with a disregard for God.

Though an extended account of the relationship between love of God and love of neighbor is beyond the scope of the book, two brief answers to this difficulty can be given here. The first is to read the claims in 1 John as giving "insofar" conditions. Insofar as one loves one's neighbor, thus far one knows and loves God. Thus, the person who erotically loves another, insofar as this is love (rather than, say, lust or vanity), is knowing and loving God. But it may be that this love is far from perfect and complete, and hence the knowledge and love of God is correspondingly imperfect and incomplete. Insofar as the love of neighbor is merely a natural human response, thus far the correlated knowledge and love of God is merely a natural human response—an implicit recognition and appreciation of the one who made the beloved neighbor.

A second answer is that there is indeed a distinction to be made between a supernatural *agapê* and a natural *agapê*. All love involves appreciation and a tendency to union. But in supernatural *agapê*, we recognize the neighbor as someone created and loved by the triune God. In appreciating that neighbor, we appreciate the Trinity who created him, an appreciation only possible in grace. Moreover, in willing the good to the neighbor, we can be acting in friendship to God. For if x has a love of friendship for y, then benefits and harms to y are, in an important sense, benefits and harms to x, so that since God has a love of friendship to our neighbor, we live out our love for the triune God by doing good to the neighbor, since we cannot directly do good to God.[13] In a trinitarian context, all of these things are possible only by grace, since it is only by grace that we can believe in God as triune. However, there is an important way in which the supernatural *agapê* is simply love, though informed by and appreciative of dimensions of our neighbor we need grace to know about and appreciate—namely, our neighbor as related to the Trinity. By grace, a new form of union becomes additionally possible—it is now possible to be brothers and sisters in Christ, fellow members of the body of Christ.

Is the supernatural *agapê* on this reading an additional form of love? I think not. Rather, it is a qualitatively new deepening of the different forms of natural love. In supernatural *agapê* one does not cease to appreciate one's mother as a mother, but one comes to appreciate her as created and loved by a triune God. Moreover, one does not merely appreciate a general human createdness and being-loved in her. For God does not merely create and love her as a human being, but God also created her to be one's mother and loves her as the mother that she is. Thus, the features that are distinctive of the particular forms of love are deepened by supernatural *agapē*, though the commonalities are deepened likewise.[14]

3. THE ETHICS OF LOVE

Love does no wrong to a neighbor; therefore love is the
fulfilling [plērōma] of the law. (Rom. 13:10)

The New Testament presents an ethics where love is central. There are at least three ways of understanding this. On a weak version of the ethics of love, love is the central virtue, but not necessarily the only one, and considerations of love are always the most important, but not the only ones, in decision-making. It is always wrong to be unloving, i.e., to act in ways actually opposed to love, but no claim is made that the lovingness of an action is sufficient or necessary for the action to be virtuous. But there is more than this to the New Testament ethics of love. For not only are we sometimes told that the commandments of love are of central importance (e.g., Mark 12:31), but we are also told that the whole of the law is fulfilled in love (e.g., Rom. 13:10, Gal. 5:14).

What I shall refer to as "the ethics of love" is more than just the above weak ethics of love, but includes the additional claim that, necessarily, we are obliged to love everyone, and to love everyone appropriately, and that if we do so, then we will fulfill all our moral obligations and have all the virtues. The word "appropriately" may seem to smuggle in a moral constraint exterior to love, but I do not mean the word in this sense. Rather, I shall say that a love is *appropriate,* provided that it loves the beloved *as the beloved is.* Thus, loving my daughter as if she were God would be an inappropriate love, since I would not be loving her as the creature of God that she is; likewise, loving God as my daughter would be inappropriate. But to love God as God and my daughter as my daughter is appropriate.

In an inappropriate love, I love someone as other than what he or she is. In some sense, then, I am loving someone nonexistent. To love my daughter as if she were God would be to love my-daughter-who-is-God. But my-daughter-who-is-God is a nonexistent entity—I have no divine daughter. In this love I would shortchange God, by denying him the exclusive love I owe him, and I would shortchange my daughter by failing to love her as a creature of God. It might be thought that in loving someone as *more* than she is I would not do her any wrong, but that is not so, since there are goods that are appropriate to one person but not to another. If I love my daughter as God, it makes no sense to feed or teach her, say.

Note that the appropriateness must take account not only of who the beloved is in him or herself, but who the beloved is in relation to the lover. Thus, Abraham loves Isaac *as his son*, and not just *as Isaac*. To misunderstand the beloved's relation to the lover is just as much to love someone who does not exist.

The ethics of love is compatible with the claim that there are virtues that cannot be reduced to love, as long as these are virtues that must exist in anyone who loves everyone appropriately. For instance, it might be that courage is a virtue distinct from love, but that everyone who loves appropriately must first be courageous, in order, for instance, to be able to face the unknown challenges that love may set. An unloving action is an action opposed to love, and hence wrong. But the ethics of love, as I define it, is compatible with the claim that an action might be nonloving, i.e., neither opposed to nor flowing out of love, and yet positively morally good. Thus, a day of mountain climbing might be a good thing—an exercise of courage—without being an act of love.[15]

A nontheological reason to think that the ethics of love is true is that a central aspect of loving someone is willing that good things should happen to him or her, and not willing that bad things should happen to him or her. Moreover, if the love is appropriate, the particular kinds of good things that one wills to the person shall be ones that are appropriate to who he or she is. If one is willing good things to everyone, then it seems as if the only way a wrong can arise would be when one's willing of a good to one person conflicts with the willing of a good to another, in a way that wrongs one of the two.

Now, indeed, many think that there could be such a conflict. People can wrong strangers, seemingly out of love of those close to them. However, I claim that when one wrongs one person out of love for another whom one is striving to benefit, then one has an inappropriate love for at least one of the parties. For if one appropriately loves the person whom one wrongs, then one loves him or her for being a fellow person having the dignity of personhood, just as the party whom one is trying to benefit has the dignity of personhood. And it is a dubious benefit that one's alleged beneficiary gains at the expense of the victim. For to be the recipient of ill-gotten gains is a harm—one is at least in danger of being placed in debt to the victim. An appropriate love will not make one's beloved the recipient of ill-gotten gains, since an appropriate love will recognize the beloved as a member of society interconnected with the victim of the action. Thus, an appropriate love for both parties will not benefit one at the expense of a wrong to the other.

Nor will an appropriate love bestow a harm thinking it to be a benefit. For if we love someone, then the things we bestow on our beloved are seen as goods for the beloved. One is loving the beloved as someone benefited by these items. But if our beloved is not, in fact, benefited by the goods, then we are not loving our beloved as our beloved is. We are loving our beloved as our beloved is not, and hence loving inappropriately. Of course, we will not be culpable if the mistake is innocent.

If we have duties to nonpersons—say, to dogs and trees—the ethics of love will have to be extended from a love of everyone to a love of everything. I have no problem in principle with such an extension, but for simplicity will assume we only have duties to persons. The extension would not affect my arguments, especially since any wrong to a nonperson is also a wrong against the Creator, who is also a person (or, more precisely, three persons). Thus, I shall assume that while loving everyone, we do not do wrong. Every wrongdoing implies a failure of love for someone.

The ethics of love is indeed a consequence of the teaching of the New Testament. One might refer to what I have described here as the "moderate ethics of love," as opposed to the weak form that we have already seen and the strong form I will present shortly. Throughout the book, I assume at least the weak ethics of love, and I assume that love is the central virtue and that unloving actions are always wrong, but some of the arguments require the moderate ethics of love.

Occasionally, however, it is worth thinking about matters from the point of view of an even stronger, but still I believe true, position: the *strong* ethics of love. On the strong ethics of love, there is ultimately only one virtue, love. What we call "the virtues," such as courage and faith, are particular aspects of love. Thus, faith is a species of trust, and trust is the living out of a particular kind of appreciation of a person (for instance, appreciation of the person's truthfulness); in the case of supernatural faith, this person is Christ. And courage is love in respect of its firmness in the face of danger. On the strong ethics of love, an action is morally good to the extent that it is loving. Wrong actions are unloving, morally neutral actions are neither loving nor unloving, right actions are loving, and supererogatory actions are loving actions whose omission would not be unloving.

The crucial difference between the moderate and strong views is with the attitude toward nonloving actions, or actions not insofar as they are loving. On the strong view, these are judged to have no moral value. As far as the moderate view goes, they may or may not have moral value. The stronger views imply the weaker. And all views agree that no unloving action is right.

Paul's paean to love in 1 Corinthians 13 implies that without love, nothing has moral value. This, however, is compatible with the claim that, say, courage might have moral value *in the presence of love,* a value not reducible to that of the love. Nonetheless, the strong ethics of love seems to be the best way to explain why it is that love is necessary and sufficient for the fulfilling of the moral law. There is a plausibility in thinking that to act well, we simply need to be acting in appropriate response to goods around us. But the appropriate response to the good is surely to love it, or to love its potential recipients as such, and all else seems to be the working out of the love.

4. GOODWILL, APPRECIATION, AND UNION

We have already seen that New Testament *agapê* cannot just be a feeling. It is connected to action in such a way that having love for God and neighbor guarantees right action. If it guarantees right action, and if right action proceeds from our will, then love must, at least in part, reside in the will, and must be something for which we are responsible rather than something that happens to us, though of course the ultimate source of supernatural, Christian love must be grace.

This suggests that we should have as part of our concept of love the idea that to love someone is to will a good to the beloved for the beloved's sake. But there is more to love than that. For in addition to willing a good to the beloved, one also appreciates the beloved and seeks union with the beloved. We can, thus, look at love as containing at least three aspects: willing a good to the beloved, appreciating the beloved, and seeking union with the beloved.

The willing, appreciating, and seeking union are intertwined. As we can learn from St. Thomas Aquinas,[16] by willing a good to the beloved for the beloved's sake, one is already united with the beloved in will, since the beloved also wills what is good for him or herself. Likewise, in willing a good to someone, one is appreciating the beloved as the sort of being to whom it is appropriate to will goods. Thus, willing a good to the beloved implies at least some appreciation and union. Similarly, sufficient appreciation of a person will make it clear to us that it is no less appropriate to bestow goods on this person than on ourselves, and a full appreciation will surely involve the recognition of this in one's acts of will. Moreover, appreciation of a person naturally leads to one's aiming at union, while in union the other person's good becomes to some extent one's own. Finally, if one aims at a union intimate enough that one should treat good and bad things befalling the beloved as good and bad things befalling oneself, then one will naturally will goods to the beloved, just as one wills them to oneself, and in doing so, one will appreciate the other as a being to whom it is worthwhile to will benefits.

It is tempting to define love as a determination of will that involves goodwill, appreciation, and union, or perhaps to tack some other features onto the definition. Unfortunately, such a definition leaves out the unity between these features. Love is not experienced as three or more features, but as a single thing. A desire to give a definition of love should abate somewhat when we reflect that not everything can be defined without circularity or vicious regress. Moreover, since God is love, at least the *perfect* instance of love cannot be comprehended by us. Yet, one might think that a definition of love would make clear what a perfect instance of love is like and how the less perfect ones approximate it.

We might even see a trinitarian aspect to the above threefold model of love, much as Augustine saw trinitarian aspects to many facets of human life.[17] The Father eternally wills the Son's existence, and *bestows* on him all that he himself has, as the Gospel of John says many times. The Son *appreciates* the Father, eternally glorifying him by this appreciation. The Holy Spirit, at the same time, is traditionally seen as love's *union* between the Father and the Son. If indeed this is the right way to see things, then the difficulty in seeing exactly how the three features of love are interrelated and united is no surprise, for love mirrors the Trinity.

At the same time, even though love is not a feeling, it can be argued, following Aquinas, that it gives rise to feelings, perhaps indeed all feelings: "Love is the *source* of all the emotions. For joy and desire are only of a good that is loved; fear and sorrow are only of evil that is contrary to the beloved good; and from these all the other emotions arise."[18] Thus, even if we do not see love as a feeling, we can do some justice to the widespread conviction that it is such. Love naturally gives rise to closely related feelings. If I appreciate the beloved as good, my appreciation naturally tends toward positive feelings about the beloved, but it is well-known that such positive feelings are no guarantee of loving action.

But the appreciation can also exist without the feelings: we would not say that a person who undergoes torture to save a friend from the torture fails to appreciate her friend, even if the torture swamps her feelings. Appreciation is akin to knowledge in that it can be both active (or occurrent), as on the rare occasion when I am thinking that 2+2=4, and quiescent as the rest of the time when I know that 2+2=4 but am not actively thinking about it.

The connection between appreciation and knowledge is closer than that, however. Augustine famously said that one cannot love what one does not know.[19] This is not entirely correct: it might be enough to *believe* that the beloved exists and has certain qualities. If I lovingly appreciate someone, I appreciate the beloved for some quality that I take the beloved to have. However, in an ideal case, this will be a quality that the person in fact has and that I know the person to have. Moreover, the appreciation of the value of the beloved itself is, in ideal cases, a kind of knowledge. And it is not just a knowledge *that* the beloved is good, but a knowledge of the particular ways in which the beloved is good. For what Aristotle says about honor applies just as much to love, especially in its appreciative aspect:

> [H]onour too one should give to one's parents as one does to the gods, but not any and every honour; for one should not give the same honour to one's father and one's mother, nor again should one give them the honour due to a wise man or to a general, but the honour due to a father, or again to a mother. To all older persons, too, one should give honour appropriate to their age, by rising to receive them and finding seats for them and so on; while to comrades and brothers one should allow freedom of speech and common use of all things. To kinsmen, too, and fellow-tribesmen and fellow-citizens and to every other class one should always try to assign what is appropriate, and to compare the claims of each class with respect to nearness of relation and to excellence or usefulness.[20]

The adage that love is blind would be a tragedy if true. For if one loves, one wants to know more about the beloved, in order to have more to love in the beloved. It is true that, as a matter of fact, people "in love" frequently are blind to aspects of the beloved. But note two points about this. First, insofar as they are blind, they may be failing to appreciate the beloved as the beloved is, and hence failing in the appreciative aspect of love. Second, a certain charitable "blindness" to bad characteristics may in fact be an appropriate way of seeing what is really there. For there is good reason for a theist to think that evil, as such, is always a lack. If it were not a lack, if it were something positive, then like everything in existence, it would be sustained by God, whereas God would not sustain evil, as such, in existence. If this is correct, then when we see what is truly *there* in someone we love, we will not see the evils, since they literally do not exist. At the same time, we may well see that there are ways in which the beloved could be better, which potential for greater goodness is actually a good feature of the beloved, a feature worthy of appreciation.

Knowledge is connected with each of the three characteristic features of love we have been discussing. We have just seen this in the case of appreciation. In willing a good to someone, too, we have a twofold role for knowledge. We want to ensure that the good is indeed good for the beloved. Moreover, if we want the bestowing of the good to be an expression of love, we need to ensure that the good is appropriate to the particular relationship. Finally, it is plausible that the best ways of being united with someone are all going to involve consciousness of union. We are rational beings, and hence it is appropriate for the union at which we aim in love to be one of which we are conscious. That is why an anonymous benefactor's relationship with an anonymous recipient of benefits is not the ideal example of *agapê*.

Observe that except perhaps for the case of the widow's mite (Mark 12:41–44), the main illustrations of *agapê* in the New Testament are of the non-anonymous variety. And if we look at the widow as giving a gift to God, then she, too, knows something about the recipient, and God knows her. It is true that Christ counsels that charitable donations not be public, lest they become occasions for vanity. But it is not obvious that this means that the giver needs to hide from the *recipient*, and certainly it does not mean that the recipient needs to be hidden from the giver. If the giver deeply loves the recipient, the giver will strive to appreciate the recipient as more than just a "needy anonymous person," and will strive to be united with the recipient.

Thinking about the unitive aspect of love makes clear one difference between an ethics of love and a consequentialist ethics of maximizing total human well-being. For while the nature of love calls on us to do good to others, it does not merely call for us to bring it about that good things happen to our neighbor, but to act lovingly toward our neighbor. This is compatible with acting in ways that produce suboptimal results for those we love. Suppose an eccentric billionaire writes up a legal contract where he binds himself to give a certain destitute stranger a million dollars if I spit in the stranger's face and then spend two minutes verbally abusing and denying the worth of this stranger, before telling him what this is all about. It could turn out that, all things considered, it would be better for the stranger to suffer this and to get a million dollars than to get neither, and the stranger may resent my opting not to do this. (The judgment that it is better to abuse this stranger depends on details about the stranger's psychology; to know that this is so, one would have to know that the stranger would not become a worse person due to this abuse, would not be driven to suicide, and so on; let us assume this.) But even so, it would be an unloving action to disparage the intrinsic worth of another person, an action that is directly contrary to loving union with our neighbor and contrary to our duty to love that neighbor. In such a case, love does not allow us to act in the way that will in fact maximize the stranger's good.

It is essential that one refrain from acting in ways *opposed* to love, either by directly setting out to inflict inappropriate harm on the other—since insofar as I do so, my will is opposed to the will of the other (assuming all people will their own appropriate good)—or by doing things that are, in and of themselves, opposed to the real union that love seeks, such as the verbal abuse in the previous example.

5. LOVE'S FORMS AND LOVE'S HUMILITY

We apply the word "love" to a variety of cases. We talk of the love between father and son, husband and wife, sister and sister, friend and friend, anonymous benefactor and anonymous beneficiary, companion and companion, and so on, even including one's love for oneself, though most of my discussion will concern love of another. We may think it stretches language a little to talk, as Aristotle would, of the love (*philia*) between business associates ("friendship of utility" being the Aristotelian term), but a relationship of working together for a common cause does not seem very distant from love.

I have suggested that it is plausible on theological grounds to take the same thing to be present in all of these cases of love. Moreover, the three characteristic features of love—goodwill, appreciation, and a striving for union—are all present in these relationships, but in different ways. In some cases, for instance, the union is confined to willing the same thing as the other, as in the case of the benefactor and beneficiary who do not know each other. In others, the union seems the predominant feature, as in the case of husband and wife. But the difference between the forms of love is not simply in the balance of love's characteristic features. The love between two close friends could be just as unitive as that between husband and wife, but the two loves are and should be different in kind. In general, it is not so much the degree of union that distinguishes the loves, as the kind of union.

For a moment, let me raise what seems a different topic: Is love static? If I begin to love someone in a particular way, does love require me to keep on loving *in the same way*? Clearly not. There is, rather, a tendency in love itself to improve the love, so as to love the beloved in a better, more appropriate way. The balance of the characteristic features of love and of the ways in which they are expressed in the relationship could be inappropriate. Thus, it would be inappropriate for a parent to insist on the wrong kind or degree of union with a child, say, a union that fails to allow for an appropriate independence, especially if the child is an adult. And if the parent insisted on the inappropriate union, the parent would not be faithful to love.

This suggests that there ought to be a responsiveness in the relationship to what is appropriate to the relationship and to the persons involved. Moreover, on the strong ethics of love, all moral failure is a failure of love. Thus, at least if the strong ethics of love is correct, it must be an innate part of the nature of love that it be responsive to the situation. Each form of human love, thus, potentially calls us to another form, should the beloved change. And that is a part of the connection between love and knowledge: in love we need to figure out *how* to love the particular person in the particular kind of relationship. I used the strong ethics of love to argue for this conclusion, but I think the conclusion is independently plausible.

If the duty to love is what grounds all obligations, the call for a more appropriate love must be grounded in the nature of love itself. This gives an additional argument for seeing all the forms of love as, at base, the same. For each form of love, we have seen, carries with it an obligation to make the love appropriate, changing its form as appropriate. If the nature of love calls for us to make the love take an appropriate form, then the form that the relationship should take is determined, at least in part, by facts outside the love itself. And this is how it must be since we need to appreciate the beloved as the beloved *really* is, to bestow things on the beloved that will *really* benefit him or her, and to unite with the beloved in reality. Thus, the characteristics of the beloved should have a role in determining the form of love.

But likewise, one's own characteristics and one's relation to the beloved should have such a role. Here, in order to avoid circularity, "one's relation" must be a relation that is logically distinct from love: thus, the genetic and/or educative relation between parent and child is logically distinct from love and makes some forms of love appropriate and others not.

It is the unitive aspect of love which most clearly implies that love's form will need to be appropriate not just to the features of the beloved but also to the features of the lover and the features of the relation between them. For it is plain that the kind of union that is appropriate between oneself and the beloved depends in part on one's own characteristics. Thus, if one is ignorant of French, a verbally communicative union with someone who speaks only French is not presently possible. And if neither party is even capable of learning a new language, then those forms of love, such as certain kinds of friendship, that call for verbal communication appear inappropriate.

This shows another way in which love does not seek its own. A particular form of love, insofar as it is a form of *love*, does not seek its own as the form that it is, since it is open to turning into another form of love should either the beloved or one's knowledge of the beloved change. The primary focus of the lover is on the beloved, though not in the abstract but as seen from a particular point of view, a point of view that must be open to reevaluation, at least for a non-omniscient lover. This primary focus on the other combined with the awareness of fallibility makes for humility, a submission to the situation and above all to the reality of the beloved.

In *The Four Loves*, C. S. Lewis paints the unforgettable image of Mrs. Fidget, who would stay up late for her children, keep dinner for them, make things for them, and otherwise force them to be the recipients of her "generosity," no matter how old they were and no matter how much they begged her not to. On one reading, she was selfless, at least insofar as did not seek her own. But she did seek *her love's own*. She had a love that insisted on seeing the beloved as absolutely dependent on herself, and she loved the beloved in accordance with that conception. Mrs. Fidget's love was not humble. And to that extent, it was not faithful to itself, and was indeed a distortion of love. We can even say that, insofar as she treated those who were not dependent as dependent, she did not love *them* but fictions she put in their place. If one is to stay a lover of one person without coming bit-by-bit to love instead a fiction of one's creation, one's love cannot be seeking its own, but must remain focused on the beloved, open to change in the beloved and in one's knowledge of the beloved.

Seeing love as humble and other-seeking, then, allows one to see an objectivity and absoluteness in the duties of love. Our love is humble insofar as it is a response to reality. The central salient part of that reality is the beloved. But that is not all. We also need to humbly, i.e., realistically, examine ourselves and our relationship with the other, and there is an objectivity here. The nature of love calls on us to respond to reality, and this need to respond to reality is what makes the duties of love not be subjective. If, on the other hand, the duties in love were entirely subjective, there would be nothing to listen to, no reality to be responsive to, since what we perceived as a duty in love would by definition be that duty. The other-focus of love then goes hand-in-hand with a rejection of a relativistic approach to ethics.

"Love, and do what thou wilt" is not an invitation to license but to acting in light of objective facts, facts that may force us to reevaluate just about every concrete aspect of the form that our love for someone takes.

6. FORMAL AND REAL UNION

According to Aquinas, a love that appreciates the other for his or her own sake always involves "ecstasy" and mutual "indwelling." The lover enters within the beloved both by will and by intellect. The lover enters the beloved by intellect, because the lover strives to understand the beloved from the inside, seeing the beloved's goals and nature from the beloved's own point of view. In love, this understanding leads to willing the other's good, and not just the abstract good of the other, but the other's particular good as it is found in the goals that the other pursues. Thus, the lover leaves him or herself and lives outside of him or herself; this is *ek-stasis*.[21] The beloved comes to be in the lover's mind, because the lover thinks about the beloved, but at the same time the lover is in the beloved because "the lover is not satisfied with a superficial apprehension of the beloved, but strives to gain an intimate knowledge of everything pertaining to the beloved, so as to penetrate into his very soul." In the lover's will, goods and bads happening to the beloved are treated as happening to the lover, and the beloved's will is treated as if it were the lover's own. Thus it is as if the beloved were in the lover by means of will. Moreover the lover acts for the sake of the beloved as if the beloved were him or herself, and so the beloved comes to be in the lover.[22] Simply by loving someone, one dwells inside the person intellectually and in will, and the beloved dwells in one's intellect and will. Even unreciprocated love involves this fourfold indwelling union of lover with beloved.

Indeed as soon as one has recognized the beloved as a human person, one already has some intellectual grasp of the beloved and his or her motivations, and, to some extent, can see things from his or her point of view. For by recognizing the beloved as a person, one recognizes that the beloved *has* a point of view, and by recognizing the beloved as a *human*, one realizes what certain central aspects of this point of view must be. After all, every human, Aquinas insists, appreciates certain goods, such as life and community, simply by virtue of being human.

There is thus a union in love, even in unreciprocated love, as soon as the beloved is recognized as a human person. This union should increase as one gains knowledge of the beloved, since one will better understand the beloved's point of view, both gaining an understanding of what is particularly good or bad for this particular beloved, as well as deepening, through the example provided by the beloved, one's understanding of the general features of every human being. Moreover, one's will is united with the beloved's in willing the beloved's good. Thus there is a union that is had simply in virtue of loving. Without it, we can say there is no love. Aquinas calls this union "formal union."

But in addition to the formal union that is always found in love, there is what Aquinas calls "real union." This is the particular form of togetherness to which one is called by the nature of a given form of love. With a colleague, it may be exhibited, say, in cooperating on curriculum development; with a casual friend, in going to the movies together; with a spouse, in intercourse, verbal or sexual.

But love and formal union can exist without any reciprocation, physical presence, or real union. I can love someone halfway around the world, with whom I will never have any contact, simply because I have read something about this person. (Such a love need not be entirely cheap; it might, for instance, include a *commitment* in favor of this person.) But we know that when we love, we are not satisfied with absence, even though we can love just as truly *in absentia*. Absence makes the heart fonder, but it does so precisely by making the lover long for presence. This is another way of seeing that love is not about its own growth: while absence makes love grow, what the lover desires is not absence, but presence. Formal union can be had even with those who are completely absent (note that absence is not just a physical distance; there is a sense in which a comatose beloved is largely absent), but love impels us toward *real* union.

An important aspect of real union is the reciprocation of love. For insofar as two people love each other, recognize each other as loving each other, and love each other in part for loving each other, they are achieving an additional union through their *shared* activity. Aquinas listed four modes of union in unreciprocated love, and reciprocation adds at least four more.

7. CONSUMMATION

A relationship of love between people is something continually developing. But we do not generally act to achieve the impossible, unless we wrongly think it is possible. A genuine form of love needs to call for a union that is in an appropriate sense *attainable,* if it is something that the lover is to try to achieve. Granted, perhaps love may impel one toward an asymptotic approach to some unattainable state, but then it is the approach rather than the state that love calls on one to achieve. Trying to achieve an impossible goal—say, to draw a square circle—is not something that love, given its focus on reality, calls for.

Now, it seems that formal union is already achieved at any time love is there, though it can always be deepened, and love does call one to such continual deepening. This deepening has a natural goal, which is to make the things one appreciates and believes about the beloved match reality, and to cover all of those aspects of the beloved that are relevant to the relationship.

Real union is something that may be entirely absent from a relationship, and it is the form of real union sought that appears to be the primary distinguishing factor between different forms of love. Love makes one pursue real union. Real union, thus, has to be attainable.

Now it may be that for some forms of love, real union cannot be achieved *in this life.* If these forms of love are genuine and nondefective, it follows that there is an afterlife in which the real union can be achieved. However, in any case, romantic love is not one of these forms, because romantic love is about this-worldly, fleshly union. The appreciation of the body is essential to romantic love, and it is generally acknowledged by Christians that most of the specific commitments of romantic love end with the death of the body—thus, one may remarry after the spouse's death.

Therefore the real union that corresponds to romantic love must be something attainable in this life. We can now introduce the notion of the *consummation* of a form of love, as a real union that attains those aspects of the union that are distinctive to that form of love. A consummation, thus, underscores the particular *form* of the love. It need not completely fulfill love's unitive longings, because these longings tend to go beyond one's specific to the particular *form* of love. Arguably, intellectual and emotional sharing is something toward which every human love tends, but this general kind of sharing will not be a part of the consummation of a particular human love. On the other hand, two academics may consummate their collegiality by submitting a joint paper. In paradigmatic cases, we can expect that a consummation will be a joint *activity*. Thus, it is the joint submission that consummates the love rather than the paper getting accepted. (In fact, they might find a rejection quite emotionally unitive.)

In some loves, consummation is sharply delineated—thus, the consummation of the teammate union between pitcher and catcher is found when the pitcher throws the ball and the catcher follows the ball mentally and physically. But some loves can be consummated by a variety of actions. Thus, parent-child love may be consummated in any joint activity that distinctively exhibits the child's dependence on the parent and the parent's activity to bring the child to maturity— such as the parent's feeding the hungry baby, the parent's telling a story and the child's listening to it, or the parent's sending the child forth either from the womb to the outside world, or from the family home to the larger world. Each of these activities consummates a particular subform of parent-child love.

Note, too, that as these examples show, a consummation can be repeated and can be had multiple times with different meanings, while yet each time summing up the distinctiveness of the kind of relationship.

Consummation is important, but need not be the most important thing about the relationship. Thus, while the essence of the parent-child relationship requires that the child learn from the parent, sometimes the sentiment that the parent learned more than the child did might be true. Or it might be that a parent literally sacrifices his or her life for the child, or vice versa. Such sacrifice is not distinctive to parent-child love—it can occur between strangers—but when it occurs, it is likely to be the most significant point in the relationship. But even though consummation need not be the most important part of a relationship, love does seek it.

In consummation, love is fulfilled with respect to the particular form it has taken. That does not mean that full union is achieved in every other respect. Two colleagues can consummate their academic relationship by jointly writing and submitting a paper, but they might still be rude to each other. The unitive aspect of love is only fulfilled when the consummation is tied to all the generic aspects of interpersonal union, such as emotional, intellectual, and spiritual union. One may not be emotionally sharing while jointly working out the details of a mathematics paper on the symmetrization of functions on graphs, but the joint work can still support and partially express certain emotional commonalities and a spiritual recognition of mathematics as, say, a science of abstract ideas in the mind of God.

Consummation expresses the *form* of love, but the most important thing about a form of love is not that it is of a particular form, but that it is *love, agapê*. As already noted, sacrificing one's life, while not specific to any form of love, is a better expression of love than any individual instance of one of these kinds of consummation of particular loves.[23] But even if the form is not the most important thing, nonetheless, to love someone as she is requires that the love have an appropriate *form* and that one's actions be true to that form. Hence, consummation is indeed of significant importance. The form of a love is not something tacked on as an afterthought—it is the particular way of expressing the general aspirations of love.

8. REASONS AND UNCONDITIONALITY

What justifies our choice of whom to love? What reasons could we give for loving those whom we love? The "Aristotelian" answer, inspired by the account of friendship in the *Nicomachean Ethics,* takes the reasons for love to be good features of the beloved, so that the beloved is loved because of his or her possession of these good features, say, virtue or pleasantness. In Aristotle's own account, were these features to disappear, it would become appropriate to terminate the love, after a decent interval during which the beloved has a chance to reform.[24] An Aristotelian who believes that love should be less conditional might also modify the account by allowing historical facts about the beloved, such as the facts that the beloved was once loved by one or used to be virtuous, to play a role in justifying the continuation of love.

On the opposite side is a particularist account, on which the person is loved as a particular individual, independently of any qualities. The staunchest adherent of this view was Søren Kierkegaard, in the case of romantic love. (What I say does not apply to Kierkegaard's view of charity.) One of the central features of Kierkegaard's work is the parallel between faith and love. Now Kierkegaard took faith to be independent of reasons, indeed endangered by the presence of reasons:

> It is possible to talk half humorously about reasons: So, at long last you want to have a few reasons. I am happy to oblige. Do you want to have 3 or 5 or 7? How many do you want? But I can say nothing higher than this: *I* believe. This is the positive saturation point, just as when a lover says: She is the one I love, and he says nothing about loving her more than others love their beloveds, and nothing about reasons.[25]
>
> "[R]easons" in connection with faith are a subtraction. I believe— not one word more—is the maximum; if I have seventeen reasons, my faith is less, and still less if I have eighteen.[26]

There are arguments in favor of both the Aristotelian and Kierkegaardian accounts of love. The strength of a Kierkegaardian account of love as independent of reasons is that if the love is for a reason, then it appears to be conditional. This is even true if the reason is a historical one, say, when one loves someone for past virtue. Such a reason would seem to allow for an unconditional love, given that the past cannot change. But this is not exactly right. For while the past cannot change, our *beliefs* about the past can, and that introduces a conditionality. A love dependent on my beliefs about history does not seem to be unconditional—I might have good reason to change my mind about that history—while a truly unconditional love would be one that could have no good reason to terminate as long as my beloved continued to exist.

At the same time, the Aristotelian account seems true to much of the experience of love. The lover appreciates the beloved for various qualities. "You do not have lovable qualities, but I still love you" is not a particularly endearing remark, and we have already cited C. S. Lewis's remark about the way one can wound by saying that one loves someone out of "charity." On the Kierkegaardian view, one loves the other person for the other's unrepeatable identity, for being the particular individual that he or she is. But the worry now is that being the particular individual that he or she is does not say anything about the beloved, since everyone is a particular, unrepeatable individual.

However, Kierkegaardian love is not even based on the general quality of uniqueness, but rather on the particular identity of the beloved; this particular identity abstracts from all of the beloved's actual qualities. It does not contain the beloved's wit, intelligence, beauty, or individual goodness. It does not contain that endearing dimpled chin, that peculiar tone of voice when tired, or that generous impulse so often given in to. For all of these things can come and go. The beloved is loved as what philosophers call "a bare particular," an individual thing conceived simply as an individual with its own identity and with nothing else. This does not do justice to the way love is actually experienced.

It is worth noting that any criticism that Kierkegaardian love is covertly based on the general quality of uniqueness would be off base. For the beloved is not loved because she is *a* particular individual, but because she is *this* particular individual. Nonetheless, the criticism that the view is still based on a quality of the beloved can be made to stick. For either the love is based on a choice or it is something that simply happens. Given Kierkegaard's view that faith is based on a choice,[27] the first option is exegetically correct. Now, if based on a choice, the love is grounded in a quality of the beloved, namely, *his or her having been chosen by the lover.* This recenters the love on the lover rather than on the beloved, since the quality is one that depends not on what the beloved is like but on what the lover is like. Thus, the love *is* based on a quality. We can now understand the choice in two different ways. If it is a choice that one keeps on remaking as one goes through life, and one loves the beloved on account of that choice, this love is the most fragile, most conditional of all loves. And hence the Kierkegaardian account does not do justice to the love. On the other hand, if the choice is made once for all time, then the love is based on a historical quality of the beloved, namely, that the beloved is someone that one had chosen to love. And hence the love is still conditional. Suppose one found out, or thought one had found out, that one never really *chose* to love one's beloved, but that the love was simply something that had *happened* to one. On this account one would no longer have a subjective reason to continue loving. Nor is it a very far-fetched hypothesis that one didn't choose to love but love simply happened to one. Note, also, how poorly an account grounded in choice would work for many nonromantic loves, like that between parents and children (though very likely Kierkegaard intended his account to be restricted to romantic love).

Suppose, on the other hand, that Kierkegaardian love is not a choice, but simply something that happens. Then the love is grounded in chance external circumstance. And that seems the poorest grounding of all. One's love has no reason at all, not even one's choice. It has fallen upon one, like the flu or a sudden feeling of joy. This is compatible with unconditionality, for it might be that one has a moral duty to preserve a love forever once it has befallen one—after all, there is an element of chance in parent-child love, in that the parent did not choose to have *this* child, and may not have chosen to have a child at all, but still ought to love this child. But a chance-based account does not appear compatible with our nature as rational choosers given that love is tied to action, and it is certainly no compliment to be loved in this way. Worst of all, if love is simply something that happens to one, it can surely disappear just as easily for no reason at all. Thus there is no reason for chance-based love to last.

Of course, a theist will insist that there is no such thing as chance: divine providence is involved in everything. In such a case, the account becomes more plausible, but only because it ceases to be particularist. The love is then based on the beloved's having been chosen for one by God. This *is* a significant quality. It does yield unconditionality if one thinks that, necessarily, anyone whom one loves has been chosen for one by God and hence one must persevere in love. But most problematically, it gives an excuse whenever we do not find ourselves loving a stranger whom we should love: "I just don't love this person and never have. If God wanted me to love this person, he would have in his providence arranged for me to begin to love this person."

The Kierkegaardian view, thus, does not do justice to love. But the Aristotelian view, it seems, does not make unconditional love possible, and an account of love should leave open the possibility of unconditional love. There is, however, a solution to the conundrum. The Aristotelian account makes unconditional love possible if the reason for loving a person is a quality of the beloved that could not disappear and about which quality we could not find out we were wrong (except perhaps in a way that implied the beloved person never existed). Being *this* particular person, as on the Kierkegaardian account, is indeed a quality that the person could not lack, but as we have seen this is problematic as a ground for love. But there is another such quality: *being a person.* Arguably, one cannot cease to be a person without ceasing to exist. Moreover, if one found out that one's beloved was not a person—say, if a woman found that the man she thought she loved was but a mannequin in a window—one would thereby have discovered that the beloved *person* never existed.

There is a philosophical difficulty with this account. Some philosophers think that human beings who lack certain mental capacities, like those between conception and about a year of age, or those suffering from a mentally debilitating disease like Alzheimer's, are not persons. If so, then a love conditioned on the beloved being a person seems unacceptably conditional. It implies that one might reasonably cease to love one's wife when she got Alzheimer's, which seems to be quite unfair to the notion of the love as unconditional. I think, however, that this conclusion is a reductio ad absurdum of the position that human beings lacking certain mental capacities are not persons. Love ought to endure under those circumstances, and hence such human beings are persons.

However, even those who think such humans are not persons can accept one of two modified versions of the above account. The first version says that the quality on which love is based is *humanity*. This does introduce some conditionality, in that should we find out that the person we have loved and with whom we have shared many experiences, is in fact an alien or an angel, the love could permissibly terminate. This meager amount of conditionality may not be problematic. Or, more daringly, we could say that we love beings because of their having existence. This is particularly plausible on a theistic view, on which, necessarily, any being that has existence either is God or participates in God. Or, finally, one might simply love creatures for being created by God.

To proceed further, we need to clarify what unconditional love is. One sense of "unconditional" is negative: there are no conditions on account of which one is loving the beloved. This negative sense, however, denies the truism that if someone loves you unconditionally, you can count on his or her love. A love that comes about for no reason at all might, as already noted, equally well disappear for no reason.

Let us, then, hold on to the truism. An unconditional love is one you can count on, no matter what. On the face of it, this makes unconditional love something humanly unattainable. For in our earthly lives, brainwashing and sin are always possible: the continuation of love is never completely certain. There is no present state of earthly love that guarantees a future continuation. It is plainly a myth, though a not uncommon one, that the way two people love each other at the beginning of their relationship determines the future course of the relationship.

The unattainability objection to the possibility of unconditional love understands an unconditional love as one that is certain to last. This would mean that if I said that I love my children unconditionally, I would be presumptuously asserting that my future love will last forever. But we need to distinguish two senses of the claim that one "can count on" the loving continuing. In one sense, something can be counted on provided that you have epistemic certainty of its truth. But there is another sense: we can read "can count on" as "have the *right* to count on," in the way that you have the right to count on people to keep their promises to you. But you only have the *right,* in the relevant sense, to count on my doing something if I owe it to you to do it.[28] Having the right to count on someone to do something is correlated with an obligation on the part of that person. Thus, unconditional love is a present love that the lover is obligated to persevere in no matter what (even if the beloved should no longer desire that perseverance—this is important in the case of children, who have the right to count on their parents loving them even at times when the children might say that they don't care about the parents' love).

The obligation to persevere, however, is not enough to make a love unconditional. All parents have the obligation to love their children no matter what, but not all love their children unconditionally. Thus, to say that a love is unconditional if and only if that the obligation to continue loving is certain to be kept would be to make unconditional love unattainable in our earthly lives. But to say that a love is unconditional simply providing that there is an obligation to continue loving, whether or not the lover accepts the obligation, would also not be enough. We need something in between. The notion of *commitment* gives us what we need. An unconditional commitment to a moral obligation is an unreserved acceptance of the obligation. Such an acceptance does not make *certain* the fulfillment of the obligation—we do sometimes wrongfully go back on our commitments, after all—but it does set one on the path to fulfillment, and gives others reason to think we will fulfill the commitment. It is worth noting here that probably only an obligation can be accepted unconditionally, unreservedly, because we are unable to predict the future with great certainty, and anything other than a moral obligation may be something that one day we might have a reason to go against.

Unconditional love, thus, includes an obligation and an unreserved acceptance of the obligation. Sometimes the two seem to be disjointed. Thus, what generates the obligation to love my children is simply, and always, the fact that they are my children, and I have this obligation whether or not I accept it. At times, however, there is a closer relationship between the two aspects. Thus, while uttering one's marriage vows, one is both generating the unconditional obligation of future love and accepting that obligation. Of course, if Christianity is right that one always owes love to everyone, then even in marriage, the obligation precedes the acceptance. However, even so, the marriage vows generate an *additional* duty to love the spouse, and this additional duty is closely tied with its acceptance.

Unconditional love, thus, should be understood as unconditionally *committed* love, and if I am right that what justifies unconditional love is a general feature everybody shares, then it follows that everybody is unconditionally lovable.

In fact, although we shall not need this claim for the rest of the book, something stronger may follow: namely, that everyone *ought to* be loved unconditionally. If so, then we have an argument for the central proposition of Christian ethics, the duty to love everyone. The argument starts by arguing that unconditional love must be based on a feature that everyone shares and proceeds to the claim that this love is not only permitted but is actually required, since the appropriate response to any feature that makes someone unconditionally lovable is unconditional love.

We have already seen that unconditional love is closely tied to an obligation to persevere in love. However, we have also encountered the possibility that the obligation may be freely generated by the lover, say by uttering vows. Let us explore this possibility. Perhaps the primary ways of generating new obligations to others is through promises, explicit and implicit. But a promise made to someone ceases to be binding when the person to whom it is made releases one. Thus an unconditional obligation cannot be generated by a promise, and a love conditional on the beloved's wanting to be loved is still objectionably conditional. My children have the right to count on my loving them even at times when they might not want me to love them. And even a promise to God only generates a conditional obligation, since God could always release one from that promise, maybe through the authority of the Church (as is Catholic canonical practice in the case of nonmarital vows) or maybe by sending one a prophet.

It may be that there are ways of generating obligations that are absolutely indissoluble. Two kinds of examples appear possible here. One way is by a natural event, such as a conception—by conceiving a child a couple generates an unconditional obligation to that child. The other way is by some kind of super-promise, or covenant, that is indissoluble. There are two difficulties with such suggestions as the basis of unconditional love.

The first difficulty is that in each case the love would still seem to be conditional on a belief that such a special natural event or super-promise took place. Now if I had an unconditional commitment to maintain my belief that such a thing took place, then the fact that the love depended on the belief would not make my commitment any less unconditional. A Christian might have an unconditional commitment to believe that everyone is created by God, and thereby the commitment to love people on account of their having been created by God would be an unconditional commitment. However, it is not clear that one has the right to any unconditional commitment to a belief that some special natural event or super-promise took place in one's life. In fact, it is not clear that one has the right to *any* unconditional commitments to belief, other than in cases of things that are self-evident or indubitable or a part of faith. The morality of belief may well require open-mindedness about things other than those that are self-evident, indubitable, or a part of faith.

The second difficulty is as follows. It ought to be possible to choose to love various people unconditionally, if everyone is unconditionally lovable. But covenants are hard to find. Marriage is one of the few examples we can find of an almost indissoluble covenant between human beings, and even marriage is dissoluble by death if there is no more marriage in the afterlife (Mark 12:25). We do not have the ability to make a lifelong indissoluble covenant between friends, apart from the case of marriage. And yet, everyone is unconditionally lovable. Likewise, the natural events that generate unconditional obligations are limited in kind. Conceiving or being conceived are one example. Adopting or being adopted may be another. Other examples are hard to find. Of course, some readers may simply accept the conclusion that we cannot generate the obligations needed for unconditional love except in a very few cases, but if one sees unconditional love as an ideal for friendship, then this will not do.

If we reject the idea of the obligation to love being entirely created, we must suppose the obligation is always already there. But if one ought to love everyone, then the urgency of questions about reasons to love or about the disagreement between the Aristotelians and the Kierkegaardians, seems to disappear.

However, with this disappearance, it appears we are no longer faithful to a basic intuition that lovers love their beloveds not just for being persons, but for particular ways of exhibiting personhood: for a dimple, a tone of voice, or a particular kind of wisdom. But we now have ingredients in our account of love that allow us to be faithful to this intuition as well.

For even given an unconditional commitment to love, the exact *form* of the love should not be something to which I am unconditionally committed. If the form of the love were also unconditional, the love would be rigid and could not be appropriately responsive to the beloved. If a friend is being stifled by my company and I am unable to become less stifling to her, I may need to leave her company and love her in a different way. If a man finds out that the woman he loves romantically, and to whom he has promised undying, unconditional love, is in fact his long-lost sister, then the duty to love her forever remains—but now he must love her as a sister. The dynamism of love, thus, implies that the *form* of love for another human being must always be conditional.

The same is true in the case of love for God. Even if one thinks, with Kierkegaard[29] and the First Vatican Council,[30] that one can be absolutely and unconditionally committed to faith, one should acknowledge that although someone's conception in faith of God may be correct, his or her love will probably not do full justice to that conception. Moreover, what form of love is appropriate depends not just on the intrinsic qualities of the beloved, but also on what the beloved is in relation to the lover. Since we change and are not liable to understand ourselves correctly in relation to God, our love for God, too, should have this dynamism.

The dynamism of love is like the dynamism in our beliefs. Our beliefs answer to reality. So long as there is any possibility that reality might not be as we think it to be, we need a commitment to change our beliefs to fit reality. Love likewise should respond to the reality of the beloved.

Note that this provides an argument for the claim that one and the same love can take multiple forms. For unconditionally committed love can surely be appropriate, at least sometimes. Unconditionally committed love will go on forever as long as the lover does not fall short of the commitment. But even when without any shortfall in the duty to love, the lover may have to change the form of his or her love, for instance, because the beloved has changed or because the lover has been innocently mistaken about the beloved. An unconditionally committed love must be capable of surviving these changes. But if it is, then a love can survive changes of form.

The reason for loving someone then, is the same for all people, while the reason for having a particular form of love differs from case to case. Indeed, sometimes this reason may include an element of Kierkegaardian choice—for instance, that the beloved is someone with whom I have chosen to start a family is surely relevant to the sort of love I should have for her—and the reason for love will also include Aristotelian ingredients. Likewise, someone's wit should not be *the* reason for loving her, since a sufficient reason is already present in the fact that she is a person (or a creature of God, and so forth). But it can be a reason for loving her *in the way I do.*

Once we see that the momentous question whether or not to love someone at all does not ride on his or her qualities, but should always be answered affirmatively, we have much more freedom to allow various ingredients such as our own choice, chance, providential circumstance, and the endearing qualities of the beloved to enter into the justification of the form of love, and to provide additional reasons for the love. The wife can say that she loves her husband for his wit, meaning that because of his wit she loves him in the particular way that she does, and maybe also that his wit constitutes an additional reason for love. The exact role played by the qualities of the beloved depends on the form of love in question, and may also differ from case to case. At the same time, the qualities that determine the form of love may pale in importance when compared to personhood or being a creature of God, the quality that justifies our loving the beloved at all.

9. LOVE OF ONESELF AND SELF-SEEKING

Recall the puzzle about how Paul's observation (1 Cor. 13:15) that *agapê* does not seek its own applies to *agapê* for oneself. One solution offered already was that Paul was simply making a general point about the nature of love—love as such is not focused on self. But of course a particular form of love, namely self-love, is focused on self.

But there are two deeper solutions available. The first notes, with Aristotle and (in different terminology) Jesus, that the virtuous life is our paramount good. In genuine love of oneself, one seeks what is good for oneself. But what is good for oneself is the life of virtue, and central to such a life is care for others. Thus, genuine self-love requires us to pursue the good of others, and in pursuing the good of others we promote our own good.

For a complementary but more speculative response to the puzzle, recall that we saw that we need to distinguish the reasons for loving someone from the reasons for having a particular form of love for someone. The reasons I have for loving need not vary from beloved to beloved. My son, my daughter, my wife, my sister, my father, my friend, and my enemy is each a human being created in the image and likeness of God, and this always calls out for a response of love. So I can love each of my neighbors for the very same reason. But the different forms that the love should take are each justified by different reasons. I love my son with a paternal love that includes a certain kind of authority because he is my son and because he is young. I love my friend with a friendly love perhaps because of our shared history of companionship.

Aristotle in *Nicomachean Ethics* IX.4 observes that good people have the same kinds of reasons for loving themselves as they do for loving others: namely, they can love themselves for their character. At the same time, Aristotle seems to think that thoroughly corrupt individuals have no reason to love themselves, and indeed do not love themselves. Aristotle was wrong in thinking that there was no reason to love the thoroughly corrupt—they, too, are people—but the idea that virtuous persons love themselves for the same reason that they love others is compelling.

This then suggests another way in which well-ordered love of oneself is not self-seeking. When Francis virtuously loves himself, i.e., Francis, he does not love Francis because Francis is *himself*, but he loves Francis because Francis is a human being in the image and likeness of God. Or, at least, he does not *primarily* love Francis for being himself, but primarily loves him for the attributes that Francis shares with all other humans. Virtuous people love their neighbors as they love themselves. Conversely, they love themselves as they love their neighbors, namely, for the same reason. And in this sense the love is not self-seeking, since although the beloved is oneself, the beloved is loved primarily for reasons for which one loves one's neighbor rather than for being oneself.

At the same time, love for oneself has a different form from love for another, just as love for one's friend and love for one's father have different forms. Perhaps the most important difference is that one's relationship with oneself involves a kind of authority that one's relationship with one's friend or parent or even child does not have: I can require sacrifices of myself that I have no right to require of a friend or parent or even child. Another is that correlative with this authority over oneself there is a special responsibility for one's moral development, going beyond that which one has for a friend or parents, and more akin to, though perhaps going further than, one's responsibility for one's children's moral development.

10. CONCLUSIONS

We ought to have an unconditionally committed love for everyone. At the same time, one and the same love can pass through a number of different forms. This innate dynamism must be present if love is to be responsive to reality—if it is to have the connection with knowledge that it ought to have. If we accept the Christian claim that all duties are rooted in love, then a love that lacks this ability to adjust itself in order to take on the appropriate form is insufficient. It falls short of what love ought to be like. This observation shows, too, that when love has a form which does not match the reality of the beloved, the distortion should be remedied as soon as we become aware of it. Any such distortion is objectively bad, even if we are unaware of it, and as lovers we can recognize this by our own lights (though obviously only not in the case at hand if we are unaware of the distortion), since it seems plausible that in loving someone, we recognize that person's value and recognize that we should be responsive to the value that the person has.

We have seen, on philosophical grounds, that we should love everyone. But it is plain that we should not love everyone in the same way. The rest of this book will be an examination of one particular way of loving—the erotic (or romantic or sexual, though I think in the end these are roughly equivalent)—and what is appropriate to it.

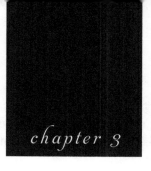

chapter 3

Desire

1. OBJECTIVITY

That I desire something normally helps explain why I pursue it. This much is uncontroversial. But as soon as we try to say anything more, controversies abound. I am going to argue that it is possible not to understand one's own desires—not to know what it is that one desires. Once we have reached this conclusion, we will be able to make some progress in analyzing the concept of a desire. At the same time, it is not my purpose to provide any thorough analysis of desire. I will say just the amount required for my analysis of the morality of sexuality.

It is tempting to say desire is something *felt*. Yet the concept of a subconscious desire seems useful and coherent. Upon looking back at a period in my life I may observe that all my actions were organized around the pursuit of some value, and I may conclude that I did indeed desire to further that value. There seems to have been something in me that explains the multifarious pursuits, and it seems to have played the same explanatory role that a desire would have. Moreover, if one accepts the popular, though I think questionable, thesis that we always act out of a desire, then one must agree that desire surely cannot always be something felt. For, clearly, we often act without any consciously preceding desire for something. And if some desires are unconscious, then it is no surprise that we can be wrong about the content of some of our desires.

But even if all desires did involve something felt, we could still argue that misunderstanding is possible. We fully understand a sentiment like: "I thought I wanted to be a scientist, but it turns out that I just enjoyed fiddling with equipment, and I was an engineer at heart." The phrase "I thought I wanted to . . ." is very common in English.[1] There would be little point to the phrase if there were no distinction between what one actually wants and what one thinks one wants.

Socrates thought that one of the great challenges for us was to know ourselves. We grow in self-understanding, and it seems clear that a part of what we grow in is our understanding of our desires. Plausibly, for instance, we sometimes confuse what we desire to desire with what we actually desire. Or we simply may not know what the object of our desire is. These possibilities exist even in the case of a felt desire. Quite likely, a baby can feel hunger or thirst without realizing that the desire would be satisfied by nutrition or hydration.

If so, then a desire's *proper object*, the thing or state of affairs that the desire is for, will be an objective feature of the desire, a feature about which we could be right or wrong. We may mistakenly pursue something else, while thinking that we are pursuing the object of our desire; this is the first way in which we might err in respect of a desire. We may even succeed in making ourselves think that we have achieved the object and thus fulfilled the desire; the desire may go away then, though it will likely return. This happens even in prosaic cases. I may erroneously think that I want a drink when in fact I want to eat. Drinking some water will fill my stomach and for a short while make the hunger go away. But my blood sugar will remain low and so the hunger will return increased. Or imagine that I make a more general mistake: I erroneously think that each desire's object is the cessation of that desire. Thus, instead of satisfying my appetite with food, I take a hunger suppressant pill. Imaginably—though most improbably— due to this faulty philosophical view of desire, I could think that I have satisfied my hunger and die of starvation.

Second, we might fully understand the object of our desire, but mistake something else for that object. I may feel hungry, understand that what I want is food, and take a bite of the ceramic bagel that my colleague brought in to make a philosophical point. In the case of the ceramic bagel, I will not think I have satisfied my desire by taking a bite. But in other cases, one might even think the desire has been satisfied. Fred always wanted to see the king. Instead, he ended up seeing the king's double, but since he did not know that this was not the king, he thought his desire was satisfied, and the desire went away.

Third, we might be mistaken about how to pursue the goal of a desire. It is possible in this case to pursue a course that does not lead to the satisfaction of the desire, while thinking that one has pursued the right course, and, further, thinking that one has succeeded in achieving one's desire.

Finally, we may fully understand the desire and how to achieve it, but be wrong in thinking that the object is worth desiring. A desire for something immoral is the most obvious example here. This kind of mistake will be discussed more fully in the next section.

Perhaps the most interesting mistake about desire is the first kind, where one does not correctly conceptualize the content of one's own desire. One kind of objectivity in the concept of desire, then, is that it is an objective matter of fact what a person desires, a matter of fact about which the desiring person can sometimes be mistaken. A second kind of objectivity is with respect to satisfaction. One may falsely believe that some object will satisfy one's desire or that some course of action will lead to the satisfaction of the desire, and one may believe afterwards that one's desire has been *satisfied,* when in fact it has merely been *quelled.* The reverse situation is also possible—one may believe one's desire has not been fulfilled, whereas in fact it has. Thus, whether a given person has satisfied a desire or has simply quelled it is an objective matter of fact.

But if we do not have infallible introspective knowledge of desire, how do we know what we desire? Well, we sometimes know what other people are desiring by examining their behavior, and we can surely do the same in our own case. And we can supplement this examination with fallible information derived from introspection. The fact that I seem to myself to desire something is, after all, fallible evidence that I do desire it. The best approach is probably holistic: That hypothesis about the nature of a desire which allows for the best overall fit both to our behavior and the best ethical view is the one to be preferred.

2. EXTERNAL EVALUATION

We can thus query whether the apparent satisfaction of someone's desires was in fact an actual satisfaction of that person's desires. This is an internal evaluation of the satisfaction, though it may proceed based on external evidence. But we can also ask whether the object of the desire is objectively *desirable*, in the sense of being worth desiring, an external evaluation.

In the *Gorgias*, Socrates seems to hold that the two kinds of evaluation come to the same thing. If something is not worth desiring, then it is not what is actually desired, and if something is worth desiring, then it is what is desired. Consider a man with cancer who walks into a store to buy caviar, because a friend falsely advised him that caviar, which he is indifferent to, would cure his cancer. Were he to know all the facts, he would not want caviar. Caviar is expensive and only worthwhile if one enjoys it (and maybe not even then, due to social justice concerns). Socrates would say that the man does not really want caviar. What he wants is health, and he mistakenly thinks that he will be restored to it by the caviar.

The alternative would be to insist that the man behaves in ways that are best explained by a desire for caviar. Socrates will counter that the man's behavior is better explained by his desire for health, together with his belief in caviar's efficacy to cure cancer. Socrates' account seems to make for richer predictions of behavior. It follows from Socrates' account that should the man cease to believe in caviar's efficacy to cure cancer, he would cease to pursue caviar. Nonetheless, such predictions can also be accounted for on a non-Socratic model. The man desires caviar *because* he believes in its efficacy to cure cancer, and were he to lose the belief, he would lose the desire, unless he developed an independent desire for caviar—say, out of a habit of pursuing the eating of caviar. Such an independent but still pointless desire would be one that is harder for Socrates' account to explain, since there seems to be no false belief there for Socrates to appeal to, though maybe Socrates would claim that the man has acquired the belief that eating caviar is intrinsically significantly worthwhile.

A third account of the desire for the caviar tries to combine the Socratic insight that there is something intrinsically different about a desire for a means and a desire for an end, together with the realization that it is indeed right to say that the man desires caviar, in some sense. This account would say that the man desires the caviar *as a cure for cancer*, rather than desiring the caviar (or its consumption) in itself. This desire of his can only be fulfilled in part: he can consume the caviar, but cannot consume the caviar in a way that provides a cure for cancer, since the caviar in fact provides no such cure. Positing the qualified desire is just as effective in explaining the search for caviar as positing an unqualified desire for caviar would be, and just like Socrates' account would, this posit explains why the desire is undercut when one learns that caviar does not cure cancer, as long as no habit has developed.

Moreover, not only can we then explain what happens in a case where the desire remains out of habit, but we can also show why this case is rationally aberrant. For either an independent desire for caviar *simpliciter* has arisen, with no good rational reason for such a desire (just as one might mistakenly move from disapproving of someone as a politician to disapproving of her as a person), or else the person desires caviar as a cure for cancer, while believing that caviar is not a cure for cancer.

It does appear that we should reject Socrates' view that desires are only for ends and not for means, since we now have an account that better fits with our intuitions that there can be instrumental desires, and this account is at least as predictive as the Socratic. On this account, when we have a desire for something that does not, in fact, conduce to the end for which we want it, we have a desire for an object that would be desirable but does not exist. Caviar-that-cures-cancer is indeed desirable, but does not exist. One might erroneously think that a desire *can* be satisfied, but it cannot, because its object cannot be had. The case in which we want something *as* a means to an end when it is not, in fact, a means to that end is one kind of example of this, but it is not the only one. I may, similarly, desire to prove a mathematical falsehood, or to jump higher than is humanly possible.

It is possible to have such a mistaken desire even when one knows that the end is unattainable. Learning that caviar does not cure cancer may alleviate a desire for caviar, but finding out that we cannot avoid death does not remove our desire not to die. There does not seem to be anything conceptually problematic about the existence of a desire for a state of affairs that is *causally* impossible for us, such as avoiding death, though a desire for a logically impossible state of affairs seems more problematic. Once I realize that it is impossible to prove that 2+2=5, to desire to prove it would perhaps be perverse.

Finally, we come back to the initial question. Are there non-instrumental desires that are simply inappropriate to have, not as in the instrumental case because the objects are not an effective means to the end, but simply because the objects are not desirable *simpliciter*? A positive answer also seems correct here. It is not hard to imagine being brainwashed to desire to eat dirt for its own sake, and this noninstrumental desire would be inappropriate (though not something the person can be blamed for given the brainwashing).

3. WAYS OF EVALUATING DESIRE

We are fallible in many different ways in respect of our own desires, and this caution needs to be kept in mind as we look at erotic love and sexual desire specifically. We cannot, for instance, simply assume that people are always right about *what* they desire sexually. The question may require philosophical and maybe even empirical analysis. Bob may think that his sexual desire is only for the pleasures of physical contact,[2] but this does not imply that he is right about himself. Helga may think that she has satisfied her sexual longing by buying an expensive car instead, but surely she has only quelled the desire by distracting herself from it.

Augustine tells us that all our restlessness is a search for God. Sometimes we just want something, have no idea what we want, misidentify the object of our desires quite badly, and end up miserable. All this is very human.

In section 5 of the previous chapter, we saw that sensitivity to the beloved and to one's relationship with the beloved is a crucial part of love. We can now be clearer on one aspect of this sensitivity. Love leads to the desire for good to happen to one's beloved and to the desire for oneself to be united with one's beloved. The sensitivity called for by love requires us to ensure that we correctly understand the objects of these desires, and that their objects be of a sort that can be attained in relationship with this beloved. Having desires that do not fit the relationship with this beloved means that one is loving the beloved as if he or she were someone else. Love for others calls us to the Socratic duty to know ourselves, and hence to understand our own desires.

4. LIBIDO AND DESIRE

Although anybody who is hungry desires food, one can desire food without feeling hungry—for instance, because one recognizes intellectually that one ought to eat at a given time. Hunger is thus a species of *desire for food*. As hunger, its content may be rather more vague than one's desire for food. Thus, while one might desire to eat a particular food or with a particular person, hunger simply calls out for nutrition. It is relatively blind and may be more based in our animal biology than our intellectual faculties.

Likewise, we can try to distinguish libido from the desire for sex. Libido would be a biologically-based appetite for sex, and this would be a species of the desire for sex. A person can desire sex for a variety of reasons, and libido need not enter in at all. No valuation is implied here. Nonlibidinous desires for sex may sometimes be better and sometimes worse than libidinous ones: one might libidinously desire to fulfill the couple's joint emotional need for union, or one might nonlibidinously desire to make a conquest, or one might libidinously desire to humiliate the other, or one might nonlibidinously desire to comfort one's beloved.

Looking forward, we will see that the desire for real union in erotic love includes a desire for sexual intercourse. It does not follow, however, that libido is an essential aspect of erotic love. First of all, it is not clear that the *desire* for union has to be present for love to be there. Love is defined by action and will, and it may be sufficient that one *aims at* or *strives for* union (or maybe aims at or strives for union for its own sake), without one actually *desiring* it. Or it may be that desire is the same thing as one's will being aimed at some goal, in which case all one requires for a desire for union is that one's will be directed at union, and not that one have any libido.

Secondly, kinds of love are distinguished by the kind of union sought and by the aspects of the other person that are appreciated. With or without libido, one can appreciate the same aspects of the other person and seek the same kind of union. Of course, libido can make it easier to appreciate the other's sexual aspects, and can make possible some particular ways of experiencing this appreciation and enhancing the experience of union, and, at least in the male, some libido might be a biologically necessary precondition for the full union (we could likewise imagine an animal that could not swallow when it was not hungry).

Libido can come and go, while a striving, aiming and/or desire for union remains. In fact, when libido is absent, a person might desire sexual union and *therefore* desire to have libido in order to better experience this union. Moreover, it seems that libido is not in and of itself the desire for union that is found in romantic love. For the desire for union that love includes is always a desire to unite with the other as with a person, whereas libido probably lacks this recognition of the personal element. It is, at most, a component of the way that a desire for love's union may exhibit itself on a given occasion, though it never constitutes the whole of that desire, nor is it an essential component.

This shows how sexual love could endure *as sexual love* even if, for physiological reasons, libido became nonexistent. For a couple could still aim and desire to unite sexually so long as they recognized that sexual union would be a good for them. When one recognizes something as good for oneself, one can surely aim at it and desire it. The desire might be one that cannot be fulfilled, but it can still be an appropriate desire, in the sense that sexual union between *this* person and *that* person is logically possible and desirable in itself, though not, under the circumstances, physically possible.

Sexual desire, the desire that seems paradigmatic of the desires associated with sexual love, is a complex that tends to include libido. It is more than libido; nonetheless, libido itself points toward a sexual desire for union. To see this, note that one might propose three plausible candidates for the object that libido directs us to, besides union with another: orgasm, sex, and reproduction. In libido, however, one does more than just desire pleasure. While libido can be quelled for a short while through masturbation (but may come back, in greater strength, later), in typical cases libido pulls one toward another human being of a gender to which one is sexually attracted. Thus, libido is not a desire simply for orgasm. But if it is a desire for sex, then it is a desire for sex with, at least typically, a member of our species, and typically not an entirely unspecified one—the human being is, typically, at least specified in respect of gender, often in respect of age and attractiveness, and quite often in respect of individual identity. And when one reflects on what is relevantly valuable about sex with a human being, sexual *union* may well end up as the most plausible hypothesis for the object of libido.

The final option for libido's goal is reproduction. One might object that libido is too blind for this. However, it is plausible that libido was selected for evolutionarily largely in order to further reproduction, and so it may be that a primary biological purpose of libido is reproduction. This does not imply that reproduction is the *object* of libido. One might have a desire whose object is different from the purpose of having the desire. Think of someone who decides that a hobby would be a good distraction from the troubles of life, and as a result acquires a desire for making paper airplanes, by reflecting on how pleasantly distracting it would be to make paper airplanes. The *object* of the desire is the production of paper airplanes—that is what one desires. The *purpose* of having the desire is distraction from the troubles of life—that is why one has the desire.

Nonetheless, it may be that reproduction *is* actually the object of libido. Whether this is so is a difficult question which I will not answer. However, even if it turns out that this is so, libido implicitly points us toward union with another human being, both because it is reproduction *with another* that is desired—humans reproduce sexually—and because as a matter of fact, for the good of the child, the best context for reproduction is that of interpersonal union between the parents.

5. SEXUAL DESIRE, NEED, AND PLEASURE

There is a temptation to see the desirer's own pleasure as what is central to sexual desire. One way to see that this is mistaken is that sexual desire is not a desire for masturbatory pleasure, but a desire for another[3] or at least for union with another. This seems exactly right phenomenologically. But there is a different argument that one might give as well. Sexual desire can be experienced as a *need,* and while one can certainly want a pleasure, one does not need it in the same sense.

Granted, we do sometimes talk of someone having a need for a certain kind of pleasure. Consider three paradigmatic cases. George needs to enjoy his job to succeed at it. Lydia needs to enjoy a glass of wine to satisfy her curiosity about what the pleasure of tasting wine is like. Patricia needs to derive pleasure from playing with her children in order to fulfill what she takes to be her parental duty to *enjoy* playing with her children. In each of these cases, however, the verb "to need" is used in a sense different from that in which we might say that a person *needs* another sexually—it is simply used to indicate a necessary means (causal or constitutive) to a further end. But sexual need is not like that. At the same time, sexual need is also not like the need for food and water.

If the extent of George's interest in Patricia is that he needs to have sex with her in order to get a raise in his salary or in his self-esteem, he does not need Patricia in the sexually relevant sense of "need." Nor is this a matter of the distinction between needing or desiring a person and needing or desiring sex. George on this story does not even need *sex* with Patricia in the relevant, desirously intense sense in which a lover might say: "I need to make love to you as soon as night falls."

Just as a hungry person says "I need to eat," but not "I need the pleasure of eating," except when speaking facetiously, and just as an alcoholic who says "I need a pleasant drink" is in denial about the object of the desire, which is simply a drink, so too the urgently sexually desirous person does not in the first instance desire the pleasure of sex. Of course, unless the hungry person is at an extremity of hunger, there will be a preference for pleasant food, and an alcoholic who is not too far gone may care that the drink not only be alcoholic but also be pleasant. And likewise, the person who has a sexual desire for a person would prefer to have sex pleasantly. At the same time, a particularly strong concern that the experience be pleasant might put into question whether there really is a felt *need* there. The person who desires another sexually typically takes it for granted that, as a matter of fact, sexual relations with the person would be pleasant, and an undue *concern* for personal pleasure is likely to be a sign of a lack of ardor for the other. What C. S. Lewis says about eros is true of sexual desire:

> No lover in the world sought the embraces of the woman he loved as the result of a calculation, however unconscious, that they would be more pleasurable than those of any other woman. If he raised the question he would, no doubt, expect that this would be so. But to raise it would be to step outside the world of Eros altogether.[4]

At the same time, the fact that sexual desire can be experienced as a need is something we should not take too seriously. The need-aspect of sexual desire may not always be present, and can easily be exaggerated. We know that desires can be distorted. Granted, a human being who never in his or her life unites sexually with another human being is missing out on a basic human good, unless something supernatural takes its place (see chapter 11 on celibacy), but there can often be something misleading about sexual desire's apparent urgency, even when it is present. First, sexual desire is not a need in the strong sense in which we need to eat, drink, know, communicate, love, and be loved, without any of which a human life is very seriously lacking (and in the case of eating and drinking, it is also quickly cut short). Second, the circumstances may be inappropriate for fulfilling the desire. Third, while it is a serious loss for a human being to be unable to eat, drink, know, communicate, love or be loved for even a day, there might be no more loss in abstaining from sex for several years than in abstaining from food for several hours.

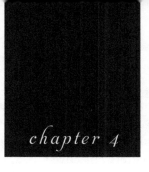

chapter 4

The Meaningfulness of Sexuality

1. MATTERING

They show that what the law requires is written on their hearts,

while their conscience also bears witness and their conflicting

thoughts accuse or perhaps excuse them. (Rom. 2:15)

Some things matter: love, truth, beauty, courage, pain, crime, joy, life, death, and suffering are clear examples. These things do not matter merely because we or our tribe or even the whole human race values or disvalues them. Someone who felt that one of these things did not matter would be blind in a particularly tragic way.

Of course the reader may disagree with me that *all* of these things matter in the final analysis. For instance, some readers may think that beauty is a cultural artifact. Of course, then one could not say that God is objectively beautiful. But let us suppose for the sake of the argument that beauty is a cultural artifact. It does not follow from this that beauty does not matter. For it may be objectively important for a culture to develop a concept of beauty. Even if beauty is not something objective, it may be an essential part of human nature that humans, individually or socially, develop esthetic concepts. The question whether something matters objectively is, thus, different from the question of whether the thing might be socially constituted.

Even if the reader does not accept that beauty matters, the reader should accept that figuring out what really matters is something that matters. If beauty does not really matter, then it matters to know this. It matters because human resources are limited and it is important for us not to spend an excess of resources dealing with things that do not really matter.

Harry Frankfurt has argued that the only things that matter are ones we care about; nothing *objectively* matters, independently of what we care about.[1] But in a revealing footnote he was forced to admit that either we all, deep down, really do care about caring, or else caring is an exception to his theory: something that is worthwhile and matters even when we do not care about it.[2] For, plainly, someone who cares about nothing cannot flourish as much as someone who cares about some things can. The footnote is an implicit admission that there *is* something—namely, caring—that would be worthwhile even if we cared about nothing.

Socrates said that the unexamined life is not worth living. While this is unduly dismissive of the value of the life of, say, a small child, we *do* need to figure out what really matters and to live our lives in reference to this understanding. It may, of course, be that *everything* matters—if all of creation comes from God, and if we are to love God with all of our heart, soul, might, and mind, then this is quite plausible—but even then we need to figure out what matters more and what matters less, in order to apportion our resources appropriately.

Now suppose, though I am pretty sure this will not happen, that I found out that it is not an objective fact that beauty matters, so that beauty only mattered *to me* or *to my tribe* or maybe only *happened* to matter to all of humankind. (Maybe God would reveal it to me that this is so.) I could then abandon my commitment to the pursuit of beauty, and thereby show my concurrence in the judgment that it does not objectively matter.

But could I still rationally allow beauty to matter *to me* if I knew that it did not objectively matter at all? One might think the answer is positive. After all, stamp collecting can matter very much to a person who recognizes that it does not matter very much objectively.[3] And even if some stamp collectors may be said to be "obsessed," surely a rational person can collect stamps to a moderate degree while yet holding that stamps, although of little objective significance, matter *to her*. Consider, however, what such a person is likely to say when the resources she puts into stamp collecting are challenged. It will be quite unsatisfying both to her and her interlocutor if she says, "It matters *to me*." Rather, our stamp collector is apt to say something like this: "It is important to have a hobby," or "Stamps can be quite beautiful," or "Stamps transport me to distant countries," or, least satisfactorily, "Well, it's worth doing something enjoyable with one's spare time."

Each such statement connects stamp collecting with something of less parochial interest, something that can be more plausibly seen as mattering objectively, although it still may be that the stamp collecting does not matter in and of itself, as there are other hobbies and other ways of being mentally transported to distant countries. But suppose the stamp collector said instead: "Most stamps are rectangular and collecting rectangular objects is worthwhile," or "I am collecting the stamps, because I am planning on eating all the stamps in my collection—oh, yes, I know they're not at all tasty or nutritious, nor do they have any hidden power or symbolism." We not only would be unsatisfied with the answer but, unless the speaker were joking, would hold that this was something like a sign of insanity. For these answers connect stamp collecting with something that has even less significance. Thus, not only does the rational justification for engaging in an activity which does not matter in itself have to be in terms of something that has a better claim on mattering, but when the justification fails to do this in a particularly egregious way, we suspect that we are not dealing with a rational person.

It appears that even when something does not matter objectively in itself, if pursuit of it is worthwhile, it will matter for other reasons, reasons that will ultimately make reference to something which matters more objectively. We can thus make a distinction between things that matter in themselves, such as joy, and things that only matter either as means to an end or as fairly arbitrarily chosen examples of a more general type. Thus, to use Aristotle's example,[4] bridles matter as means to horseback riding, while we may think that stamp collecting matters only insofar as it is an example of a hobby and it matters for humans to have hobbies.

When something matters, the obvious question is *why* it matters. Answering this will give us the meaning of the thing that matters and will tell us what is essential to the thing insofar as it matters. Thus, if stamp collecting matters because collecting examples of beauty matters, then the fact that most stamps are rectangular will not be a part of the reason why the activity matters. By contrast, if stamp collecting matters because it is a hobby and it is important to have hobbies, then the pleasure of the collecting will be essential to the activity, assuming it is an important part of a hobby that it be pleasant.

Of course it may be that stamp collecting matters in more than one way. If so, then we can ask which ways, if any, of mattering are more important and salient. Thus, stamp collecting matters to some extent by preventing pieces of paper from going to a landfill. But since the quantities of paper are so small, this cannot justify the importance attached to the activity and the resources invested in it.

Note, too, that the person engaging in the activity may be quite unaware why the activity matters. If we accept the Socratic ideal of explicitly reflective self-knowledge, we will be apt to see such a person as falling short of the human ideal. On the other hand, if St. Paul is right that there is a law written on human hearts (Rom. 2:15), then a person might know *that* the activity matters—that it matters might be written on the heart—without knowing *why* it matters.

One may worry how we can go about figuring out what *really* matters. Harry Frankfurt thinks that the only thing we can do is to see whether a given thing is one that we care about. Consequently, Frankfurt identifies what is important with what we care about.[5] But the consequence does not actually follow. For we might argue in exactly the same way that the only way of figuring out what really exists in physical reality is by examining what we perceive with our senses, and thus mistakenly conclude, with Berkeley, that to exist in physical reality is just to be perceived. We can instead say that the fact that we care about something is *evidence* that the thing is important, just as the fact that we apparently perceive something by our senses is evidence that the object is physically real, while allowing that some unperceived physical objects are real, just as some uncared for things can be quite important.

It is, in fact, quite possible to realize that one used to care about something that was not important and that was not worth caring about. Thus, one might realize that the reason one acted in certain ways was because one cared very much about having a character different from one's father's character, and then later realize that such difference is not worth caring for. The realization is not just a change of preference, as when one replaces an old interest with a new one, not having the time for both and without denying that the old was also worth having. In a mere change of preference, one acknowledges the appropriateness of past cares. But in addition to a change of preference, one can also realize that past cares were cares that one should not have had, that the things one cared about were empty—or worse.[6]

We cannot fully describe the general method for figuring out what is important, what matters, what we should care about. But neither can we fully describe how we can figure out what physical reality contains. We have partial answers in both cases: cares and perceptions provide some evidence, as does fit with a larger, plausible, and integrated ethical, metaphysical, and scientific theory. I cannot fit the claim that it matters to have an even number of hairs into any larger, plausible theory, just as I cannot fit the claim that triangular objects turn square when unobserved into any larger, plausible theory, and, in part for this reason, I dismiss both claims.

2. DOES SEX MATTER?

We have two sets of rules regarding sexuality and its expression: some rules are *moral* in nature, such as the prohibition against rape, and others we see as *customs*, such as the rule that a giving of rings should accompany marital promises, a rule that is parochial though, none-theless, important in its context. We distinguish the two, and then we have a number of disagreements about which rules fall into which category. We will discuss the details of some moral rules in future chapters. But at present both categories will be of interest.

The sheer number of customs and rules suggests that we see sex-uality as something that matters. Even if authors, like Goldman,[7] who think that there are no special moral rules in the area of sexuality ex-cept those that are special cases of general rules of morality—such as the duty to keep promises—are right, the social conventions concern-ing sexuality are a testimony that sexuality matters to just about every society. And the simplest explanation why it matters to so many is that it matters objectively and everyone knows this.

Marcus Aurelius said that "as for sex, it is the rubbing together of pieces of gut, followed by the spasmodic secretion of a little bit of slime."[8] He is right as far as this goes. But the challenge, which this book will seek to answer, is to see how sex is more than that, so that it matters in a way in which the rubbing together of two thumbs thereby producing finger oil is not.

Before we can move on to the portion of the book devoted to answering that challenge, we need to further discuss whether sexuality matters objectively in any way other than the obvious ways relating to the furthering of the human race and avoiding physical and psycho-logical dangers. We will start with considerations of the restrictions on sexuality found in our society and move on to other considerations.

3. CASUAL SEX

A young man once wrote in a paper for me that his fellow students were a little "conservative." It seems that they wished to lose their vir-ginity only with someone they *liked*. While one might giggle at the extent of the "conservatism" implied by this wish, the student was right that the restriction is a significant one. We all prefer to engage in pleasant activities with people we like, but it is not particularly im-portant that the first person with whom we shake hands or go to see a movie should be someone we like. Sex is somehow different from these other activities, and it does not appear that the difference can be accounted for by the physical sequelae in an age of contraception.

Could the attitude here be merely cultural? Even if the attitude were universal among humans, that possibility would remain, since something could happen to matter in every culture without mattering objectively. But let us continue examining the issue. Observe that present-day Western culture is the best subject for the study of male-female sexual behavior in the absence of fear of pregnancy, so limiting our examination to it will be worthwhile if we are trying to find the significance of sex beyond reproduction. Also note that while some of the restrictions on sexuality that I will discuss below might not be found in some other cultures, these cultures are likely to have other restrictions in their place: for instance, they may not object to polygamy, but may have restrictions on what religious differences between partners are permissible.

In general, casual sex is not really so casual when looked at closely. It is still highly selective in the choice of partner. Consider some specifics.

First, casual sex is rare with a partner who is a close relative; given that, as a society, we strongly disapprove of sex with a close relative, it is unlikely that someone will knowingly and *casually* engage in incest.

Second, typically, it is not at all random whether the partner is male or female. This is true even if the person is capable of receiving the pleasurable sensations of sex from persons of either sex. And the majority of people are indeed capable of receiving these sensations from both males and females. After all, if a heterosexual or homosexual person is capable of having sexual pleasure with no partner at all, namely in masturbation, one would presume him or her physically capable of having sexual pleasure with a partner of either sex. Nor is it merely the case that, say, a heterosexual person prefers people of the opposite sex *when possible,* because I assume it is relatively rare for a heterosexual person who goes to a bar to make a pick-up to come back for the night with someone of the same sex when it proved impossible to find one of the opposite sex. (The case of prisons warrants separate examination. There, the point is not just the current nonavailability of opposite-sex partners, but *longer-term* nonavailability, combined with various power issues.)

Third, the partner tends to be of an age attractive to oneself—typically without great age-disparity—and is usually someone with whom one has had at least some prior conversation. The use of alcohol may decrease some of this selectivity, but that only underscores the fact that selectivity is ingrained, absent mind-altering substances.

Moreover, our society simply does not tolerate sexual relations between adults and children. Even though the exact definition of "children" varies, the prohibition almost always includes some postpubescent persons. The standard justification for this restriction is that it is due to a consent requirement: we talk of "statutory rape." However, twelve-year-olds are quite capable of denying consent to eating broccoli and giving consent to eating ice cream, so it is not a complete incapability of giving consent per se that is at issue. Rather, we tend to think of children as incapable of making "important" decisions, and that is why we see a problem with their consent to sex. And this in turn implies that we see sex as important. There is something that matters about the decision whether or not to have sex with someone, something that matters in a way in which it does not matter whether or not to eat ice cream.

Of course, at present, sex, especially with minors, can still lead to physical and psychological harm. But physical harm can be removed technologically (only partially now, but eventually almost completely). The psychological harm is more problematic, but there is little reason to suppose that it would not be at least theoretically possible, through appropriate therapeutic pre-intervention, to ensure that the harm from, say, broken sexual relationships would not exceed that from broken nonsexual friendships—and we do not think it a bad thing for children to enter into the latter. Granted, there is always the danger of exploitation. But if we see sex the way Marcus Aurelius did, it is not quite clear what the "exploitation" would consist in, as long as the minor partner were free to come and go, were not physically or psychologically harmed, and enjoyed the procedure. After all, it is not exploitation to receive nonsexual favors from a child.

These physical and psychological dangers of adult-child relationships could thus, at least theoretically, be removed or limited to a degree that is thought acceptable in other adult-child activities, such as various wilderness activities. And yet sexual relations between an adult and a child would still be wrong, which observation emphasizes the difference we see between sexual relations and other joint activities. Moreover, in other situations where we do not deem children to be capable of giving consent, we accept proxy consent, for example, from parents, and parents can permit children to engage in other potentially physically and/or psychologically injurious activities, such as mountain climbing, playing musical instruments, and participating in competitive sports. But prohibitions on adult-child sex tend to apply even if the parents give consent.[9]

Fourth, in our culture, explicitly sexual activity itself is supposed to be done behind closed doors, and it generally involves only one pair of people at a time and, in fact, typically only one partner per night.

Fifth, where human partners are available, "casual" sex rarely crosses species boundaries, even though "the rubbing together of pieces of gut, followed by the spasmodic secretion of a little bit of slime" that Marcus Aurelius talks about is certainly possible across species. In this way, sexual sharing differs from other forms of sharing which occur, generally with little social opprobrium, between humans and nonhuman animals whenever the nonhumans are capable of reciprocation, and sometimes even when they are not. People talk to their pets, share ice cream with them, stroke them affectionately, seek emotional support from them, exercise physically with them, and so on. Some of us dislike seeing too many resources lavished on a nonhuman, since a nonhuman animal is generally believed to have lesser intrinsic worth than a human, and the resources could be better used on a needy person instead. But we do not object to animal-human sex on the grounds that the sexual favors could have been bestowed on a needy human, for we do not believe there is a duty to bestow sexual favors on others, except perhaps in the context of a preexisting commitment that requires this of one.

Even casual sex, thus, has many restrictions placed on it by most participants. One might think that these restrictions are mistaken leftovers from a culture that was opposed to casual sex due to the danger of pregnancy and disease, or perhaps the restrictions result from genetically implanted instincts tied to the fact that in our evolutionary history the main significance of sex was reproductive. But few really want us to be free from these "leftovers." We cannot, while maintaining our integrity, say that something is a mere cultural artifact and then organize our lives according to it as if it were more than a cultural artifact—and, moreover, legally impose this organization on others (say, in the case of the prohibition against adult-child sex). Thus, if we are to maintain some of these rules, we need to see sex as something that should *not* be a casual matter, even apart from reproductive issues.

My student may have been right: his college was conservative, but only in the way that all of our culture is. If we looked at our culture from the outside, we would see that, perhaps apart from very small pockets of the pornography industry, sexual behavior in just about every segment of our culture is highly restricted, especially as compared to what one who thought sex did not objectively matter would expect it to be, in an age where the physical sequelae are limited.

4. SEXUAL ASSAULT

The difference between our treatment of sexual and nonsexual relations is particularly clear in the criminal code. While any deliberate, harmful, and unauthorized touching of an adult by an adult counts as battery, sexual assault is taken to be much more serious than nonsexual physical assault that causes comparable damage.

Indeed, sexual assault is taken to be a serious crime even when no physical damage is done, though it is sometimes more difficult to prove the fact of rape in such cases. Sexual assault is likewise a serious crime even if there is no psychological damage because the victim *never* finds out about it. Compare the case of an assault where the attacker knocks someone out with the case of an assault where the attacker knocks someone out and then rapes the victim, in such a way that there are no physical sequelae and the victim never finds out about the rape. Clearly the assault plus rape is worse, despite the lack of physical or psychological sequelae of the rape.

We do not think the prohibition on rape a merely parochial rule, and when rape is practiced systematically, we treat the rape as a crime against humanity, the sort of thing for which people could in appropriate circumstances be tried by an international tribunal even if their acts did not contravene the laws of the country in which they were committed.

Now, we might think that the prohibition against rape is grounded in the fact that sexuality happens to matter subjectively to people in all human societies, in such a way that makes it wrong to go against their strong feelings. And we do, in fact, think it is important to respect people's subjective feelings. Even if we think that stamp collecting is objectively unimportant, we would think it wrong for the government to take away a collector's stamps and give her their market value in cash instead, at least without a really strong reason. Likewise, we may think that there is objectively no such thing as "taboo," but consider it badly wrong to force someone who believes something is taboo to do it. Likewise, most atheists would be appalled at someone's secretly serving pork to an Orthodox Jewish guest.

Rape, like breach of promise or theft, is defined in terms of a lack of consent. One has only breached a promise if one has not been released from it, and one has only stolen if the owner has not consented to the removal of the property. One might conclude from this that a sexual activity is a rape only if it goes against the victim's desires, and hence what makes it wrong is the victim's subjective perception of the act.

But actually the issue is more subtle than this argument suggests. First of all, it is not the state of the victim's desires but the lack of *consent* that defines rape, breach of promise, and theft. Suppose your friend really wants you to have a small painting that has been in her family for generations. However, she promised her late father that she would strive to ensure the painting would remain in the family. She herself feels no desire to keep the painting in the family. In fact, she associates unpleasant memories with it and she knows you would enjoy it. Thus, she would much rather that you had it. But she cannot give it away. She tells you all of this. She even tells you that she would not mind if it were stolen, but that given her promise she will guard it legally and physically. You are now suspecting that the reason she is telling you all this is because she consents to your taking it. But she explicitly tells you that she does not consent to it, since she is faithful to her promise. It would then still be theft for you to sneak the painting out of your friend's house, even though in doing so you would be doing something that you know your friend wants done. Conversely, one may desire to hold on to property but reluctantly have to sell it, and to buy it from the reluctant seller is not theft. It is not the desire to hold on to property but the lack of consent that defines theft.

One might think that in some cases there can be implied consent, and so the desire is definitive. Thus, if someone is your best friend, you are very, very hungry and her house happens to be right there, unlocked, while she is away for the holidays, you might reasonably presume that she would consent to your going into her house and eating food from the fridge. I think this is correct. But in the example of the painting, there is no implied consent. Typically, there is only implied consent if it is appropriate to say that consent would be given, were it possible to inquire whether the person consents. But in the case of the painting, consent was expressly withheld. Desire is not definitive, but normally it is defeasible evidence of what the person would say.

Consent, then, is something very different from desire. One can refuse to consent to something that one strongly wants, and one can consent to something one does not want. As a result, the need for sexual consent cannot be grounded in the strength of people's desires.

Futhermore, there is a disanalogy between cases of theft and breach of promise on the one hand, and rape on the other. For there are times when nonconsensual expropriation is not theft, for instance when it is done by the state as a penalty for a crime or as taxation. Likewise, there seem to be times when not keeping a promise is the right thing to do, as when one does not give back a weapon that one promised to give back because the lender has turned homicidal in the meanwhile (to adapt an example from Plato).[10] On the other hand, state-enforced sexual activity between people who do not agree to it is state-enforced rape, pure and simple. This is true whether sexual privileges are extracted as a form of taxation—one thinks of alleged feudal "privileges"—or in punitive cases. One notices that at times people think of prison rape as part of the punishment of the criminal (this may be a part of the reason why the practice has not been reduced as much as it surely could be). The California attorney general apparently said about Enron chairman Kenneth Lay: "I would love to personally escort Lay to an 8-by-10 cell that he could share with a tattooed dude who says, 'Hi, my name is Spike, honey.'"[11] But this is clearly deeply wrong. If prison rape were really to be a just punishment, there would have to be an official of the state whose duty would be to rape criminals in the statutorily required manner and judicially required quantity, clearly a repugnant idea.

State-enforced sexual activity is rape, even if the victim would prefer the activity to a less controversial punishment such as lifetime imprisonment. One might think that in such a case it would not be rape, since the victim would choose the sexual activity freely as an alternative to jail. However, if the alternative to sexual activity is something particularly harsh, we normally consider the event to be a rape. Even if lifetime imprisonment is subjectively worse for someone than nonconsensual sexual activity, it seems morally acceptable to impose the imprisonment, but not the sexual relations.

Consider, too, the sort of cases mentioned earlier in which one should respect that which matters to a person even when it does not matter objectively, or matter very much. In the case of stamp collecting, we do need to respect the hobby. But we do so only to the extent that we generally have to respect private property and to the additional extent to which the stamp collector desires to retain this particular piece of property. The respect is limited. The state can have a compelling reason to take away the stamps, for instance, because, unbeknownst to the collector, there are secret enemy messages on them in microdots or because the collector has failed to pay her taxes. This compelling reason would justify expropriation. But it is not so in the case of rape. Similarly, if I found out that the stamp collector would be murdered for her collection unless I extracted it and handed it over to a thief, arguably this would be morally acceptable in a way in which raping someone who would otherwise be murdered would not be. And all of this is true, even if stamp collecting happens to be subjectively more important to a particular stamp collector than sexuality is to the particular victim of rape. What matters here is the *objective* importance of sexuality.

The fact that the body is involved is insufficient to explain the strength of our intuitions here. Suppose that the only way I could save my life was by sticking my finger in an unconscious stranger's ear. (Maybe the stranger and I are imprisoned by someone who has read too many analytic philosophy books and who threatens to kill me unless I do this.) It would not be obviously wrong for me to do so, whereas raping the stranger to save my life would be wrong, even if it had no negative sequelae for the victim.

Perhaps raping someone, though, is like forcing someone to do something taboo. But the parallel is unhelpful or imperfect. Consider two cases. First, imagine someone who thought that doing the taboo action was immoral. In that case, forcing the person to do it might be wrong for the reason that we should not force people to violate their consciences. The parallel to this case would be only those cases of rape where the victim believes sex would be immoral. But rape is wrong even in cases where the victim believes or even knows sex would not be immoral (e.g., marital cases). The second kind of case of a taboo action would be one where the person falsely believes that the action would result in significant negative consequences. In this case, forcing is generally unkind, but unlike rape, can be morally justified under exceptional circumstances, as when it is needed to save the lives of many.

The case I mentioned earlier of sneaking pork into an Orthodox Jew's food is perhaps the most interesting as a proposed parallel. One might find this appalling even if one did not believe the rules of kashrut to come from God. In fact, this case seems quite parallel to that of rape. We might well think that sneaking the pork into the food would be wrong even if this were necessary to save the guest's life, as long as it was under circumstances in which Judaism did not permit consumption of pork.[12] It would be wrong even if the Jew told us wistfully of a desire for pork and expressed intellectual doubts about

Judaism, but still cleaved to the religion. However, if we have the intuition that *under no circumstances* is such clandestine pork-feeding permissible—and this is an intuition some will lack—I suspect it is because we think *religion* matters objectively. Otherwise, we are apt to treat this like a case of taboo actions where conscience is not involved. In those cases, it is typically inappropriate to make, by force or subterfuge, the person do the taboo action, but where much is at stake, it becomes permissible. But rape is wrong even if much is at stake.

As already noted, the undeniably severe psychological harm that can result from rape does not suffice to explain our attitudes here. In cases where the victim does not find out, for instance because he or she was unconscious at the time and all evidence has been removed, the rape is still wrong. If the psychological harm were what makes rape as bad as it is, then the cause of the harm of rape would consist not only in the rape but also in the victim's attitudes. Both the fact of rape and the attitudes would be necessary conditions for harm, assuming no physiological harm. The cause of the main harm would then be in the victim and not just in the rapist, with the important exception that the rapist is more likely to be responsible for the deed than the victim is for the attitudes. This is an implausible—and, in fact, abhorrent—view of rape.

Moreover, the view that psychological and physiological harm is what grounds the wrongness of rape would strongly suggest that the attitudes that render rape psychologically harmful are irrational. For if what makes rape bad is that it causes harm, and in cases where there is no physiological harm it mainly causes harm because of these attitudes, then one would be better off without the attitudes. If, of course, sexuality mattered objectively, then these psychological attitudes could be a recognition of something important about sexuality— say, its sacredness or its value—and thus they could be rational. But if sexuality does not matter objectively, then these preexisting psychological attitudes in the victim are irrational. And if we could rid potential victims of these attitudes, we would have done about as much to mitigate the total harm of rape in our society as by preventing many occurrences of rape.[13] But this seems quite absurd.

Before closing this section, we need to consider one particular account of the badness of rape that does not require sex to be important. On this account, what lies at the essence of rape is not the sexuality involved, but the attitudes of the perpetrator, such as the perpetrator's hatred of women. Whether all or most rapists (or at least rapists of women) act primarily out of hatred of women is an empirical question that we do not need to decide here. What we do need to note is that even if this is true, it is not sufficient to account for the badness of rape. Consider two misogynists: one is a rapist and the other keeps his hatred to himself all the time, except that he keeps a diary filled with his hateful sentiments, which diary he never shows to anyone out of fear of chastisement. The two might hate women equally. While both are in the wrong, the rapist has done something far worse. Thus rape is not bad simply because it is an expression of hatred, since the diary is equally an expression of hatred.

And even when rape is an expression of hatred, there must be a reason why rape is a particularly fitting expression of hatred, and to get at this reason we need to once again answer the old question about what justifies our attitudes about rape. Moreover, a rapist who is not motivated by hatred for women, and who desires sexual gratification not otherwise available to him, is at the very least *imaginable*, and on college campuses, in the context of date rape, is likely actual. What this rapist does is still terribly wrong, even though hatred is not the motivator.

It appears, then, that an account of the harm of rape requires our seeing sex as objectively important, and important in such a way that, without consent, sexual activity becomes horribly wrong—so wrong that it is wrong to compel people to engage in it even to save many lives.

5. GAY RIGHTS

A different kind of testimony to the way sexuality matters comes from both sides on the gay rights debate. While some opponents of homosexual activity may be driven primarily by a visceral distaste for this activity or a hatred for those who engage in it, it is charitable to suppose that many sincerely think that homosexual activity is a distortion of something objectively important, something that matters, and that it is wrong because it is such a distortion.

At the same time, defenders of homosexual activity themselves are committed to the importance of sexuality. It is clear that they believe that prohibiting engagement in homosexual activity does not just deprive homosexually oriented persons of a privilege, but that it criminalizes love and stifles human flourishing in an important area of life. A desire not to side with the criminalization of love and the stifling of fulfillment is no doubt a major reason for the societal success of proponents of gay rights.

But of course this kind of a defense of gay rights depends on sexuality mattering very much. Suppose that a law prohibited an opposite-sex couple from sharing strawberry ice cream, while allowing same-sex couples to share strawberry ice cream, and allowing any couple whatsoever to share every other flavor of ice cream. We would think the law absurd, irrational, and hence unacceptable. But it would not be a law that severely impeded human flourishing. It would not be a law that imposed a severe hardship on opposite-sex couples. And the reason for this is that the sharing of strawberry ice cream does not matter very much. Of course a law of this sort would be symbolic of a lower status of opposite-sex couples, and would be rightly opposed for that reason, in the way we oppose even those racist laws that are primarily of symbolic significance. But it does not appear plausible that the prohibition of homosexual activity is *simply* symbolic in this way. Rather, if homosexual activity is morally permissible, the prohibition of it is something that directly and not just symbolically infringes on human rights, because sexuality is a central area of human life.

Not all defenders of homosexual activity speak in ways that imply the importance of sexual activity. But some do, and it is the importance of sexual activity that provides one of the most powerful arguments for the pro-gay-rights position—that by prohibiting same-sex sexual activity, one would be barring gays from something of central importance to human life. It is probably this argument that drives much of the popular support for gay rights. Observe, too, that this argument in favor of gay rights is weakened if we see sexuality's importance as merely subjective. For there is no need for society to respect something that is merely a personal predilection. A law to forbid stamp collecting might be irrational and hence unacceptable, but it would not be a serious infringement of human rights, no matter how subjectively important stamp collecting were to individual collectors.

The debate on homosexuality is highly emotionally charged. For instance, an actively gay or lesbian person who is told that homosexuality is immoral is likely to react strongly to this criticism. The criticism will be treated as somehow touching something *important* about them. Compare this to the reaction of many meat-eaters to being told by a vegetarian that they are murderers. One suspects that while most meat-eaters are unhappy to hear this, many do not find this criticism deeply psychologically troubling, even though, in fact, they have just been accused of something morally worse than what active gays and lesbians are accused of by opponents of homosexual activity. Of course there is a disanalogy between the two cases. A meat-eater can stand secure, being in the majority, unlike gays and lesbians who face significant discrimination, but one suspects that even apart from this, there is an important difference between the cases. The choice of sexual partner appears to be more important than the choice of the foods we eat (though the choice whether to eat at all may well be more important than the choice whether to have sex at all, since it is abstinence from food that leads to death).

We see that significant segments on both sides of the gay rights debate are committed to the idea of sex as something innately important. This is to a large part why so much energy is invested in these debates.

6. SOCIAL CONSTRUCTION AND COMMUNICATION

Of course some readers may be quite willing to reorganize society on the assumption that sex does not objectively matter much, and they can insist that we should keep existing prohibitions—say, the ones against incest or adult-child sex, or the very strong opposition to rape—in force as long as a significant body believes in them because *given the beliefs,* sex is psychologically significant. There is not much that I can say to such a reader. Nor is such a position likely to be plausible, I suspect, to a reader who gives much deference to Christian scripture and/or tradition.

More interestingly, other readers may object that although they themselves find it psychologically impossible or undesirable to transcend the sexual taboos, they still see these taboos as largely arbitrary. After all, most readers in Western countries would find the eating of cats significantly more objectionable than the eating of cows, while yet acknowledging that the difference is merely caused by the fact that for pragmatic reasons we have chosen cats to be pets and have not chosen cows to be pets. We could, in principle, overcome the emotional objections, but there is no reason to do so. As long as enough people in our society have cats as pets, there is a good reason, bracketing reasons for general vegetarianism, not to eat the cats out of respect for the feelings of those who have pet cats. It is also desirable that lonely people should have animals as pets, and even if the choice of species is a product of historical contingencies, once a society has settled on cats as pet-worthy, there is no need to switch from cats to cows and switch dietary habits the other way around—even leaving aside the difficulties facing people keeping several cows in a Manhattan apartment and the challenges of large-scale cat farming.

Expanding on this view, there is reason for society to assign significance to certain activities. Apart from pragmatic considerations, some of this assignment seems purely arbitrary. Thus, we assign a negative significance to spitting on someone, even though we could imagine how this might instead have been seen as a beautiful sharing of oneself with a stranger—a weaker form of a blood-brotherhood, say. But once we have chosen where significance is to be bestowed and in what way, we need to live by this choice, out of respect for the need to assign a value to certain activities, such as sex or spitting, that allows them to be appropriate conduits for the expression of certain attitudes. For these activities to serve the role they do, they must be treated as emotionally important in a way that makes them resistant to change. I would find it hard to convince people in our culture that spitting at them is a sign of my deep respect for them, and my refraining from spitting at people I like is important to maintaining the usefulness of spitting at people as one of the strongest means of communicating dislike or hatred. Of course, we could as a society replace spitting with a different gesture stipulated to carry the same meaning—maybe a pat on the shoulder—but what would be the point of going to the bother of such a replacement?

Now, in the case of spitting, there may not be much social value to society's maintaining this particular form of communication; we perhaps do not really need nonverbal ways to communicate this kind of hatred. But in the case of sex, there is much more value. Perhaps we see sex as expressing some kind of strong affection. It is useful to be able to express such a strong affection, and it is valuable to have a gesture that society considers as sacred or almost sacred in order to express this affection. This could ground a socially relativistic argument against casual sex: Sex has a meaning in our culture; it is desirable to maintain something having this meaning; there is no better candidate than sex available at the moment; and so we should not have casual sex lest we divorce sex from that social meaning.[14] One can, after all, consistently say that an institution or custom is arbitrary, but that it is of great importance to support and maintain it.

Let us now consider what someone adhering to this view can say about rape. First, when the victim believes that sex has deep significance *objectively*, then nonconsensual sexual activity would seem to seriously go against the victim's autonomy to pursue what he or she sees as objectively important. On such a view, some cases of rape can be condemned. But this cannot be the whole story, for surely it is also badly wrong to rape an intellectual who believes that sex has only been assigned its meaning arbitrarily, and who does not personally attach such meaning to sex.

It might be that just as consensual sex has a significance assigned to it, so too nonconsensual sex has an opposite significance assigned to it. Plausibly, nonconsensual sex expresses hatred. Or maybe the significance of rape follows naturally from the kind of significance consensual sex has. If consensual sex signals love, rape is a parody of erotic love, taking the sexual trappings of eros while replacing the agapic component with hatred or objectification, and insofar as love is important, it is also important not to parody it.

On this view, there would seem to be two separate reasons to think rape wrong: (1) rape expresses something negative; and (2) rape parodies the expression of something important that we have reason to protect. However, (1) is surely not sufficient to warrant the strength of disapprobation we heap on rape. Carefully chosen words can express hatred with comparable or greater effectiveness, and while such words are, arguably, deeply morally wrong, it is reasonable to think that they should not be punished by law except when they are libelous, slanderous, or inflammatory of something more than words, while it would be unreasonable to think rape should only be punished when it defames a character or inflames bystanders to something more than rape.

The fact noted in option (2) that rape parodies the expression of something important appears correct, but does not give a correct account of the primary source of wrongfulness in rape, since it misidentifies the primary victim of the harm. According to (2), the primary harm seems to be done to society's custom of using sex to convey affection, and hence the primary victim is society. But while rape has bad social consequences, its primary victim is the person raped. Nor should the penalty in rape be mitigated if the rapist attempted to keep the rape secret from everyone but the person raped, in order to avoid harming society's custom of using sex to convey affection.

In other words, if the social view in question is right, then the penalties for and attitudes toward rape seem disproportionate to the penalties assigned to other crimes that strike at important symbols in Western democracies. The danger is that if one sees the meaning of sex as socially constructed, the sacredness of sex becomes like the sacredness of national symbols. In the United States, it is not a crime to burn the national flag, but even if it were a crime, it should surely not be penalized in the way rape is.

These arguments also show something wrong with Robert Solomon's view that sex is a language.[15] In general, it is not wrong to talk to someone who does not wish to listen. Certain ways of talking to someone who does not wish to listen are penalized, for example, when the volume of the speech violates noise-control laws. But this does not typically rise to the level of a felony in the United States, and it would seem inappropriate to jail someone for years just for using a megaphone. Note the further disanalogy with language. Typically, what propositional content an utterance carries does not depend on whether the listener is consenting to listen, though of course there is a greater danger of misunderstanding with lack of consent. But the meaning of a sexual act changes significantly with the other's consent or lack thereof.

7. ROMANTIC LOVE

It is plausible, given a strong ethics of love, that if something significantly matters morally, this significance must be due to the way the thing is connected with love. Thus, if sexuality matters, it does so through a connection with love. But love for whom? After excluding self-love, which seems an implausible option given the other-directedness of sexuality, only four possibilities are plausible: love for the other party with whom the sexual relationship exists or is contemplated, love for the children that could result from such a relationship, love for society, or love for God.

While love for God is always relevant, in those matters that appear primarily to concern our relationship with our neighbor, we love God *through* loving the neighbor that God has created. The central message of the first letter of John is that saving faith, love of God, and love of neighbor each mutually imply the other two. Thus, we should not consider the possibility that sexuality matters simply because of its connection to love for God separately from love for other people.

There are two plausible accounts of how sexuality could matter because of a connection to love for society. On one account, sexuality could matter because it furthers society reproductively. But sexuality matters even when reproduction is impossible—say, due to sterilization. On the other account, sexuality could matter because it cements together the smallest units of society, i.e., families or couples. We do not need to consider the cementing option separately, because this cementing together surely proceeds in and through love for the sexual partner and for the children.

This leaves us with two options for an account of how sexuality is connected with love: it could be connected with love of children and/ or with love of the sexually desired person. Progeny is, of course, *one* of the reasons why sexuality matters. Children are in the image of God, and the constant message of the Hebrew scriptures is that children are the chief earthly blessing. But, as we said, progeny cannot be the only thing that gives importance to sexuality, since sexuality also matters in the absence of fertility.

Thus, sexuality must also matter because of a connection with love for the sexually desired person. This love is variously described as conjugal (or marital), sexual, erotic, or romantic, depending on context and emphasis. Examination of the conjugal case will have to be postponed to our discussion of marriage. In any case, it is not *just* conjugal love with which sexuality is connected, since sexual attraction can (and, in cultures where marriages tend to be love matches, typically does) precede marriage. Sexuality includes more than just sex, and even if we think that sex should be confined to marriage, surely we should still agree that sexuality in its desiring or yearning aspect is appropriately involved in relationships that precede marriage.

While romantic love need neither imply nor be implied by any sexual *behavior*, romantic love has an essential connection with sexuality. Otherwise, we would not be able to distinguish romantic love from other forms of love. Deep, mutual, and emotionally intense interpersonal relationships need not be romantic in nature: they could simply be a deep form of friendship. We cannot define romantic love in terms of depth, mutuality, or emotional intensity. Indeed, we can see an ideal of a nonromantic relationship with all of these features in Aristotle's description of character friendship in *Nicomachean Ethics* VIII and IX, a relationship involving a deep, nonsexually appreciative sharing and intertwining of lives.

Romantic love involves loving the other as embodied, and not just as an intellectual being. The other matters not just as a person but as an embodied person. But while this is true of romantic love, it is still not what defines romantic love as such. Admiration of a sports star need not be romantic in nature, and yet one typically admires the sports star as an embodied person and not just as a mind. Likewise, while our culture tends to stereotype men who appreciate other men's beauty as being gay, all men *ought* to appreciate the beauty of other men. For, beauty is a good thing, and all goodness flows from God. We should appreciate all good things that God has created. Everyone ought to appreciate the beauty in other people, including physical beauty, but not always in a romantic manner (though prudence is required in choosing the kind or degree of appreciation). When we appreciate a piece of modern architecture, our appreciation is not of the romantic sort. One imagines that if there are nonembodied angels[16] who are somehow capable of perceiving physical beauty, they would appreciate the beauty of buildings and bodies in some nonromantic way.

Nor is it implausible that someone might combine this nonromantic appreciation of physical beauty with a deep, mutual, and emotionally intense friendship. This would not by itself be sufficient for the relationship to count as romantic, unless the combination ended up—as could easily happen—leading to further changes in the relationship.

It is, thus, not just the focus on the embodiment of the beloved that makes a love romantic. It appears that it is specifically *sexual* embodiment, with the beloved seen as a sexual being, that is needed for a romantic love. But it is not enough just to see and benefit the other as a sexual being for the love to be romantic. A gynecologist who works pro bono among the poor certainly sees her patients as sexual beings and benefits them as such. For instance, she benefits them precisely as sexual beings when she delivers a baby or treats diseases of the reproductive system, and this benefiting is an essential expression of the kind of love that she has for them. She loves her patients as sexual beings, but it does not follow from this that she has romantic love for her patients. One might think that the gynecologist's relationship to her patients lacks mutuality, and hence if we simply add mutuality to the requirements, we can exclude this case. But we can imagine that the patient reciprocates in some other equally important way, or we can just imagine a perfectly mutual nonromantic relationship between two gynecologists, each of whom is a patient of the other.

Romantic love essentially involves embodiment on both the side of the lover and that of the beloved. It would not be appropriate for a nonembodied angel to have romantic love for a human being. But again, the case of the gynecologist shows that embodiment is not enough, since the gynecologist's love for the patients is tied to the gynecologist's embodiment, as it is with her body that she helps the patients—with her hands, eyes, vocal cords, and so on (an angel who effects miraculous cures of women is not a gynecologist).

Thus, in romantic love, the embodiment needs to be sexual in nature on both the side of the lover and that of the beloved. But, again, even this is not quite enough for the love to be romantic. Consider the case of a marriage counselor working pro bono and helping the client insofar as the client is a sexual being. We may suppose that the marriage counselor's sexuality enters into his work, not in any ethically dubious way, but simply by providing him with a wealth of experiences from his own life that he can draw upon to empathetically help the patient. Moreover, the marriage counselor's sexual life may have motivated him to engage in pro bono work, having sympathy for others who are going through what he has gone through. Thus, the sexual aspects of the lover's identity can be motivating a love and yet the love can remain nonromantic.

What is missing in the cases of admiring a sports star or doing pro bono work for sexual beings insofar as they are sexual is that the *relationship* between the lover and the beloved is in no way sexual. There may be sexual embodiment on both sides, and the relationship may occur in part through this sexual embodiment, but the relationship itself is not sexually embodied.

At the same time the sexual embodiment of a romantic relationship need not be overt. As noted before, it need not involve any sexual activity. But some vague connection with sexuality will not do for the relationship to count as romantic. There can be sexual attraction without romantic love. It is even possible to have sexual attraction *and* deep friendship, yet without romantic love. The attraction and friendly love could simply be compartmentalized, with the attraction not being among the reasons for friendship and the friendship not among the reasons for the attraction; or two people might be friends, and then a flash of sexual attraction might occur for reasons completely unrelated to the ways in which they appreciate each other as friends. These kinds of cases are not cases of romantic love.[17]

Love has aspects of willing the good for the other, appreciating the other, and seeking union with the other, and we have seen that merely having sexuality be involved in the willing of the good is insufficient to make the love romantic.

Nor is adding to the story an appreciation of the other as a sexual being going to be sufficient to make the love sexual. We can imagine the gynecologist who is suddenly struck with admiration for the plumbing arrangement of the sexual systems in the patient, and who thus appreciates the patient as a sexual being, but does so completely nonsexually and nonromantically.

We can do better if we add that the appreciation is itself sexual in nature, so that sexualization is found on the side of the appreciator and not just on the side of the appreciated. Phenomenologically, this is an attractive proposition, since people in love *erotically* appreciate their beloved, including even the beloved's nonsexual aspects, such as intellectual abilities or verbal expression.

But what does it mean to say that the appreciation is sexual in nature? A plausible answer is that the appreciation occurs in and through sexual attraction (to say that it occurs in and through libido would surely constrict the appreciation too much—the appreciation is cognitively too rich for that). Sexual attraction is a pull to the other person as a sexual being, and specifically a pull toward a union that is sexual in nature.

All this reasoning brings us to the unitive aspect of love, the aspect of being pulled sexually to the other as a sexual being. The relevant unity is not just what Aquinas called formal union, but also *real* union. A real sexual union is called for by romantic love. The consummation of romantic love, a fulfillment distinctive of it, will be a unitive sexual activity.

All our previous attempts at characterizing romantic love were successful at describing *aspects* of romantic love. In romantic love, the other's good as a sexual being is willed in a way that involves the lover's sexuality, the other is appreciated as a sexual being in and through the lover's sexual desire, and the lover strives for, or at least is drawn to, a sexual union with the beloved, a union that consummates the love.

And it is this last element, sexual union, on which other elements depend. For the other's good as a sexual being is willed in a way that involves the lover's sexuality, precisely because mutually good sexual union is sought, and the other is appreciated in and through the desire for that union.

Now, if romantic love is distinguished from other loves by a tendency to a form of sexual activity, then we can see that a central way that sexuality matters is precisely through its connection with romantic love. And if we accept an ethic of love, then we will see that a romantic love *does* matter, since it is a love, and every love matters.

Even though romantic love matters because it is love, it does not immediately follow that it matters insofar as it is romantic. Yet a form of love is not to be understood as love plus something other than love, but rather is an integral unity, where the love itself takes a particular shape, the way that the beauty and the colors of a painting are not two separate aspects of it, but the painting has a beauty of a particular kind precisely in virtue of the colors. The form of love thus also matters crucially. Its romantic character gives the love its shape and concreteness.[18]

This leads to a plausible answer why it is that rape is always wrong, even when the victim is physically and psychologically unharmed: Sexual compulsion is directly opposed to the freedom of romantically loving sexual union. Romantic love involves a freedom not present in all forms of love. While, for example, one has a duty to have a filial love for one's parents, one has no duty to love a particular individual romantically apart from a freely accepted commitment, such as that of marriage.

8. CONCLUSIONS

The above arguments strongly suggest that sexuality matters objectively not merely in virtue of people's subjective desires or the physical or psychological consequences.

The importance of sex will not be surprising to the Christian. A seminal biblical text here is that "in the image of God he created him [the human being, *ha-adam*]; male and female he created them" (Gen. 1:27). Maleness and femaleness are the very first individual features of human beings mentioned in Genesis. The fact that humans are distinguished in this way seems to have some textual connection with the human being's being created in the image of God—interestingly, Genesis 1 does not emphasize sexual distinction in any other species. And, in turn, the distinction between male and female is closely connected with sex, with union as "one flesh," in the second chapter of Genesis. If the distinction between male and female matters, so does sex, and vice versa.

We have already got a hint about why sexuality matters: It matters because of a connection with romantic love. But this observation makes us ask why there is any such a form of love as romantic love at all. That romantic interest does give rise to love is clear, but *why* it does so is not. Why does romantic interest produce a unique and deep form of love, in a way in which another kind of interest, say pecuniary, might not? In saying that sexuality matters because sex consummates romantic love we have not resolved the mystery. For it is unclear why the sort of thing consummated by sexual activity would be a distinct form of love. Presumably, sticking a finger in someone's ear does not consummate a distinct form of love, except perhaps in odd circumstances.[19] What makes sex different from sticking a finger in someone's ear? Hopefully the account of sexual union in the next chapter, which forms the center of this book's analysis, will help to answer this question.

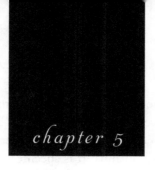

chapter 5

One Flesh, One Body

1. SCRIPTURE ON UNION AS ONE BODY

In Genesis, we read: "Therefore a man leaves his father and his mother and cleaves to his wife, and they become one flesh" (2:24). Christ based a prohibition of divorce precisely on this text:

> Have you not read that he who made them from the beginning made them male and female, and said, "For this reason a man shall leave his father and mother and be joined to his wife, and the two shall become one flesh [*sarx*]"? So they are no longer two but one flesh. What therefore God has joined together, let not man put asunder. (Matt. 19:4–6)

This is the only explicit description of the nature of marriage that is given by Christ in the New Testament, and so we need to take the Gospel and Genesis texts very seriously.

In Genesis, the one-flesh text sets the stage for a history of many different kinds of marital and quasi-marital relationships.[1] In the New Testament, the idea is central to the account of marriage and sexual ethics. It is, for instance, the basis of the command that husbands should "love their wives as their own bodies" (Eph. 5:28). A crucial New Testament theme is the analogy between the Christ-Church and husband-wife relationships. It is specifically essential to Pauline thought that the Church, including Christ as head, is the body of Christ and has the unity of a body that preserves a diversity of functions. The idea of marriage as joining two in one body provides the crucial link between the theological conception of the Church as the bride of Christ and the Church as an organic unity with Christ as head.

St. Paul also applies the one-flesh idea to nonmarital relationships: "Do you not know that he who joins himself to a prostitute becomes one body [sôma] with her? For, as it is written, 'The two shall become one flesh [sarx]'" (1 Cor. 6:16). According to Paul, union as one body should exist only within marriage, and the fact that sex involves a union as one body provides an argument against sex with prostitutes. The notion of sexual activity as constituting a union as one body is thus biblically productive, being connected with theological issues about Christ and the Church, and giving rise to new moral conclusions, such as the wrongness of divorce or of sex with prostitutes.

Observe two further things about Paul's text on patronizing a prostitute. The text presupposes that union as one body is truly bodily and not constituted by emotions, for there need not be any kind of emotional union between a man and a prostitute. Furthermore, Paul does not simply take over the text from Genesis but develops it further, replacing "flesh" (sarx in Greek, basar in Hebrew) with "body" (sôma). Part of the reason for the change may be the specifically negative connotation of "flesh" in Pauline language, whereas "body" is used in a positive sense for the body of Christ. This change suggests that Paul sees sexual union as something that can be valuable, and it is this value that makes it inappropriate with a prostitute. However, "body" is not only a positive term, but a highly significant concept in Pauline thought. A body is neither a simple unity nor a mere collection of parts. It is an articulated entity with parts that work together cooperatively, each performing some function needed by the whole:

For by one Spirit we were all baptized into one body—Jews or Greeks, slaves or free—and all were made to drink of one Spirit. For the body does not consist of one member but of many. If the foot should say, "Because I am not a hand, I do not belong to the body," that would not make it any less a part of the body. And if the ear should say, "Because I am not an eye, I do not belong to the body," that would not make it any less a part of the body. If the whole body were an eye, where would be the hearing? If the whole body were an ear, where would be the sense of smell? But as it is, God arranged the organs in the body, each one of them, as he chose. If all were a single organ, where would the body be? As it is, there are many parts, yet one body. The eye cannot say to the hand, "I have no need of you," nor again the head to the feet, "I have no need of you." . . . Now you are the body of Christ and individually members of it. And God has appointed in the church first apostles, second prophets, third teachers, then workers of miracles, then healers, helpers, administrators, speakers in various kinds of tongues. (1 Cor: 12:13–21, 27–28)

All of this leaves us with a difficult analytical task. After all, in what sense can two people, even united sexually, be said to be "one body"? It seems that even in the middle of intercourse there still are two people, each of whom has his or her own body. We will thus need a sense of "one body" which may not be metaphysically or biologically literal, but which captures the intended significance of the phrase.

2. UNION AS ONE BODY AS THE REASON WHY SEXUALITY MATTERS

If we see sexual activity, or at least sexual activity of some central kind, as an objective one-body union, then we may be able both to see why it matters and why it is naturally connected with a form of love. All love is directed toward some kind of real union. If there were such a thing as a sexual union as one body, and if this union were a good and significant thing, then we would expect this union to be connected with a particular form of love, and sexual love seems the best candidate for that form of love.

Romantic love is embodied in a sexual way. Seeing this embodiment as coming from a tendency toward a one-body union explains much. For instance, it explains how romantic love can get its peculiar shape from the bodily aspect, without downplaying the emotional and intellectual aspect of union. For we are creatures of body *and* soul. Biblically, our souls are not just ghosts moving the machinery of our body, but our souls are that in virtue of which our bodies are alive. According to the Revised Standard Version, God made Adam a "living being" (Gen. 2:7), but the "being" translates the Hebrew *nefesh* while the Greek Septuagint has *psuchê,* and both have often traditionally been translated "soul"—the *psuchê* here seems to be something that lives in and through the body.[2] Occasionally, where older Bible translations of *psuchê* had "soul," as in Matthew 16:26, many contemporary translations have "life,"[3] which correctly picks up on the life-giving nature of the soul. In Catholic dogma, this notion of the soul as the life of the body has become formalized in the teaching of the Council of Vienne (1311–12) that the soul is "the form of the body"— that in virtue of which the body is the kind of living body it is.

Now, if our souls and bodies are intimately related, then it is natural that a union of bodies should be tied to a union of souls. There can be no living human body apart from a human soul, and to unite bodies without uniting souls would be to neglect the body as a living thing, to treat it as something that it is not. Only when a body has changed into a corpse would it be appropriate to treat it in a way that sees it as separate from the soul. A corpse is not a body in the Pauline sense of "body" as an articulated whole of cooperating parts. By using the term *sôma* rather than *sarx,* Paul emphasizes the liveliness, the dynamism of the body. The corpse is flesh but not body. The living person is both flesh and body, and is such in virtue of having a soul. And we may add that even the dead body is associated with the soul that had animated it, as is expressed in our funerary practices.

Thus, a union as one body should naturally come along with a personal or psychological (in a broad sense including the affective and the cognitive) union. If the union as one body is separated from a personal union, the body would be treated as a mere appendage or corpse. Nonetheless, personal union can be found in loves other than the erotic. What defines the specific form of romantic love is the bodily union that it seeks. However, the personal aspects of the love are not mere accidents. They should both precede and succeed the bodily union. In order for the bodily union to be more than two corpses thrown together or even two animals working together, personal union needs to temporally precede bodily union. We can reasonably expect the bodily union to nourish psychological union in the way that our bodies provide for our souls' need to be informed and to have something through which to express their will.

If we see sexuality as concerned with a union as one body, we will avoid spiritualizing sexuality away, in a way that would treat us as nonembodied angels, parallel to an unsatisfactory Christology that considers the fleshly aspects of the Incarnation unimportant. We will also understand why it is that the *physical* aspects of the beloved matter particularly to romantic love.

Futhermore, what is bodily is physical, and the physical provides our paradigm of objectivity. When we hear someone say that a deceased person is *physically* present at a party, what we hear is a strange objective claim, one distinguished from more subjective claims that would be expressed by just saying that the person is "present in spirit" or simply "present." We may wonder whether there are spirits, whether society, law, morality, and higher mathematics might not be mere illusions, but the physical is there, impinging on us, impossible to ignore. A physical body is what it is, just as a dog is what it is. It has an independence from us: we do not get to define what it is. No amount of thinking that my body has three arms will make a third arm sprout. While there are those who claim that physical objects are mere social constructions, few really believe it, and any such view would be profoundly anti-incarnational.

We would expect romantic love to have a fulfillment that is more than merely socially constructed. Here is an argument for this: If the object of romantic love were merely socially constructed, it would be possible for gays and lesbians to consummate romantic love without any sexual activity, simply by society's deeming, say, a Masonic handshake to be a consummation of romantic love. Thus, one could give the defenders of gay and lesbian rights the romantic union they seek without repealing any sodomy laws, a most implausible proposition no matter where one stands on the question of gay and lesbian rights.

In general, lovers want to be *really* united; they do not want others merely to deem them united or themselves merely to think themselves united. For instance, if I wished to work together with a friend on a project, my desire for this expression of friendship would not be satisfied if it only *seemed* that we worked together, whereas I was manipulated into unconsciously doing all the work. Of course I would still *think* that my desire was satisfied in that case, but that is not the same as the desire's actually being satisfied. Robert Nozick offers the thought experiment of a machine capable of producing all experiences we might wish for, with the point that we want more out of life than what the machine can provide.[4] If we desire to be the fastest runner in the world, we do not desire merely the experience of thinking and feeling we are the fastest, but we want the reality. The desire for real union is an important way for reality to enter into love.

If it were possible for a couple to unite as one body in a sexual and important way, then this kind of thing would be what erotic or romantic lovers would desire. For lovers *do* wish to unite in a bodily way as much as possible while remaining within a sexual sphere (thus they might not wish to become Siamese twins, since a union as surgically-produced Siamese twins would take them out of the sexual sphere). Consequently, while scripture presents the union as one body as what sexual activity, or at least some normative kind of sexual activity, produces, looking at romantic love strongly suggests, even apart from Christian teaching, that if a sexual union as one body were possible, then this union would be involved in the sexual activity that fulfills romantic love.

The task for much of the rest of this chapter will be to determine what sexual union as one body could reasonably be taken to be. We will not take the phrase "one body" completely literally in this account,[5] but we will try to take it as seriously as we can, since the text about becoming one flesh is a seminal scriptural text on the nature of human sexuality. This will give us an interpretation of the scriptural text and an argument based on revelation for the resulting account of sexuality. The rest of this chapter will show that there *can* be such a thing as a significant sexual union appropriately described as a "one-body union," and therefore, given the above, this will be what sexuality is primarily about. The central analysis of sexual union will be a philosophical argument, one in principle accessible to everyone, no matter what one's position on the truth of Christian revelation.

3. WHAT WOULD IT TAKE TO PRODUCE A SIGNIFICANT BIOLOGICAL ONE-BODY UNITY?

Suppose we had two cats and wanted to unite them as one body. What would we have to do? Let us first rule out science-fictional scenarios where we somehow mix up their cells and produce a new cat of double the weight. For if that happened, we would not have a union of two cats, but the destruction of two cats and the production of a new cat out of their pieces.

Another unacceptable account would involve a hidden miraculous intervention. Since not everyone thinks cats have souls, I will talk of the human case. Perhaps when a man and a woman engage in sexual intercourse, God joins them together in some empirically undetectable way, for instance by uniting the soul of each to two bodies. But such an account is rather incredible. It posits a hidden miraculous intervention happening in daily life, for believers and nonbelievers alike. The Christian tradition simply never claims that such a miraculous intervention is how the text about God joining two into one flesh should be understood. There may also be serious metaphysical problems with the idea of a body being animated by two souls at once, especially if one takes the soul as the form of the body.

Now, some philosophers believe that the unity of a body is not constituted merely by the way that the parts of the body interact, but by some further metaphysical fact, such as the fact that all of these parts are united with one soul, or the fact that they stand in some irreducible relation of constitution to the whole. It is implausible to suppose that this sort of fact is present in sexual union, unless by a miracle. If these philosophers are right about the nature of the unity of the body, then sexual union does not *literally* produce one body. But we will see that the couple in sexual union can be seen to have at least the crucial *biological* characteristics which a single body has. The couple can be *biologically* or *organically* one body, even if not literally, metaphysically so.

What we are now looking for are the nonmetaphysical aspects of unity as one body. Let us then return to our cats, which we would like to make into one body. Mere physical contact does not make for one body. If we tied their tails together, there would be two squirming bodies, not one. While the flesh matters for sexual union, the kind of union that consists in mere fleshly contact is not what romantic love seeks. Likewise, punching someone in the face produces very forceful fleshly contact. But that is not what lovers seek, and not only because it is not sexual in nature, but because it is not really a union at all.

Would the cats tied together by the tails count biologically as one body if they did not struggle against each other, but each simply happened to walk in the same direction as the other? Surely not. The problem with the case of the two cats tied together by their tails was not that they were struggling against each other, but that they were not acting as one body. The struggle only highlighted this fact. If the cats *happened* to be going in the same direction, this would still not be a union as one body. My heart and lungs are not united as one body merely because they *happen* to be working together. In fact, the parts of a body *can* occasionally struggle against each other in at least some respects, without ceasing to be parts of one body. One can pinch oneself, using one's hands to cause a pain in one's leg. One can breathe too quickly leading to dizziness. And so on.

It would also not suffice for biological union as one body if, instead of the cats being tied together, one held the tail of the other in its mouth. "Overlap," while a more intimate form of contact than mere juxtaposition, is not sufficient for union as one body. A biological union as one body is not achieved by a surgeon putting her hands inside a patient.

Observe now that if the struggle between the parts within one's body becomes too severe, we may wish to say that one or more of the combatants has ceased to be a part *of* the body. For instance, a cancerous tumor growing out of control is probably not a body part. The removal of a tumor is not an amputation; nothing is lost by the person.

The tumor case suggests that one criterion for being biologically a body part is genetic, since a tumor consists of genetically reprogrammed cells. However, genetic sameness is neither necessary nor sufficient for being biologically a single body. Fusion of embryos can produce a chimera that exhibits a unity of organismic function but has different DNA in different cells, such as the famous "geep," produced by fusing sheep and goat embryos, which is biologically a single body.[6] In fact, "cytogenetic mosaics" are not at all outlandish: normally, the cat with tortoiseshell fur results from the X chromosome being deactivated in some but not other cells, and sometimes the tortoiseshell cat is even a chimera of two different cell lines.[7] These cases show that genetic sameness not to be necessary to qualify two things as parts of a single body. The insufficiency of genetic sameness for union as one biological body, on the other hand, follows from the case of identical twins who are genetically identical and yet are not one body.

Neither is having one's material origin in a body either necessary or sufficient for being a biological part of that body. This can be seen in the case of organ transplants: the transplanted organ eventually becomes a biological part of the recipient's body and ceases to be a part of the donor's body, even though in its material origins it comes from the donor's body.

Thus the task of bringing it about that two cats are biologically one body does call on us to genetically modify them or ensure they have a common origin. Let us go back to the case of the cancer. While the DNA of the cancerous cells does differ from that of noncancerous cells, that difference is not our main reason for supposing that the cancerous cells are not a biological part of the patient. What seems to be the source of the supposition is that the unrestricted self-division of the cells neither serves the body's purposes nor is responsive to direction from the rest of the body.

This suggests that we can identify two characteristics of the biological union of the parts of one body. First, there is the parts' responsiveness to the rest of the body. Second, there is a purposefulness in the functioning of the parts that, in some way, either serves or at least should serve the body's purposes. We will consider both characteristics in turn.

In a free-for-all fight between two experienced fighters, each may be responding to all the others by fighting back, but they are not thereby united, because there is no shared goal and each is striving for her own self-preservation at the expense of the other. Here there is responding, but what we need for union as one body is responding *obediently* to direction, and the fighters obviously do not do that. Such obedient responding involves the furthering of the goals of the whole. Thus, even if we focus on responsiveness, we are led to something like a commonality of goals.

It is plausible that responsiveness of the part to the whole, while not sufficient, is a necessary condition for a one-body biological union. And, indeed, there is some likelihood that this would be so in the sexual case. But while this responsiveness may be necessary for a biological one-body union, it is far from biologically sufficient in the absence of obedient response. Not just any responsiveness and control is a characteristic of bodily unity. The sort of control a stronger person exhibits over a weaker person's arm in arm wrestling is not characteristic of bodily unity. The part of the body is not controlled in a way that is foreign to itself. Rather, control in a biological unit involves a harmony.[8]

How can we account for this harmony? It may help to consider the case of an apparently *ruling* part, like the brain in a human being. While the functioning of the brain is *affected* by the functioning of the rest of the body, this is not the same as being directed. When *A* directs *B*, *A*'s direction makes *B* serve *A*'s purposes. But while the brain's function is profoundly affected by oxygen flow, it does not seem quite right to say that the lungs are controlling the brain with the oxygen flow, directing the brain to serve the lungs' purposes. But there is still a sense in which a ruling part is directed by the rest of the body. The ruling part works for the benefit of the whole or, at the least, is a defective instance of the sort of thing that *ought* to work for the benefit of the whole. The brain ought to be sensitive to the body's needs. It is controlled by the parts, but in a subtle way: it receives information about the state and needs of the rest of the body, and strives to direct the parts to fulfill these needs.

Normally, then, the brain is directed in a particularly harmonious way, and directs harmoniously as well. We can think of it as taking on the purposes of the whole body and, unless something has gone wrong, serving them all. The purpose of the whole is, at least to some extent, its purpose. This is true even when, in fact, the brain rebels, as when, due to a malfunction, it impels an animal toward suicide. Here the brain's purpose is to serve the body, but it simply fails to do so. That can happen. In such a case, the control is a normative rather than physical fact. The brain *should* be serving the purposes of the whole.

Something like this normative claim seems to be the way we should account for the intuition that not just any kind of control, but a harmonious control, is a characteristic of the relationship between a biological part and the body. The harmonious direction and responsiveness seem to consist in the fact that it is a part's *purpose* to serve the whole. Thus we come to shared purposes once again.

On the side of purposefulness, it appears to be a necessary condition of something's being a body part that it have service to the body as a purpose. The body's purposes must be its purposes. We should go a step further. Not only must the part have such service as a purpose, but it must actually be striving, if perhaps unsuccessfully and maybe even counterproductively, to promote this purpose. Otherwise the part, as a body part, is dead. One might point to the lungs of a dead person and say that they should be supplying oxygen to the rest of the body. But if they are not *striving* to do that, then they are no longer a part of the body; for there no longer *is* a body in the relevant sense, but simply a corpse, a collection of dead parts. A part that is not striving to fulfill the purpose of the whole is, insofar as it is a biological part, dead.

Sometimes this striving is at a fairly low level. Our hands have as their purpose the manipulation of objects. When we are asleep, our hands are not generally manipulating objects, and when they are, they are not doing so purposefully. However, the hands remain in readiness, full of life. The blood nourishes the cells of the hands, which in turn actively maintain themselves in a state responsive to any nerve signals they may receive. An army in readiness is not an idle army.

Introducing the notion of purpose leads to an understanding of purposeful striving of each part for the promotion of the goals of the whole. At the same time, this striving is controlled by the rest of the body. The control is not alien, because the body controls a striving in a direction that is the actual purpose of the part, insofar as it is a part.

The above was formulated in terms of the biological part-whole relationship. Let us now consider the biological part-part relationship. Two biological parts are united in one body only if they are both striving to fulfill the whole's purposes in a coordinated, mutually regulated way. Suppose now that the two parts constitute the whole body. Then the coordination must be mutual: when we say that the *whole* coordinates or regulates the part, it must be the case that the *other part* exercises some coordination on this part, since the two parts are what make up the whole.

Now consider the striving to fulfill the purposes of the whole. Since this is a harmoniously coordinated striving, and the regulation is exercised by the other part, it follows that the two parts need to have a common purpose. If part A coordinates part B for the sake of purpose X, then X is a purpose of both A and of B. Were the two parts to have nonoverlapping purposes that were somehow to be counted as purposes of the whole, we would wonder in what sense the whole was a single organism. A single organism composed of two parts had better have some purpose that is served by both of them, because otherwise we would simply have two organisms, each fulfilling a different purpose, although perhaps attached together.

Now, prima facie, the following situation is possible. Each of the two parts of the organism could simply serve to benefit the other part and to benefit itself, instead of serving some overarching purpose of the organism as a whole. In that case, the organism as a whole would have two purposes: the benefit of the first part and the benefit of the second part. However, this makes the organism seem to be more like a mutual admiration or, at least, mutual benefit society than like a biological organism. While a biological organism as a whole strives to further the goals of the parts, it furthers the goals of the parts, in particular, *as parts of a whole*. The goal of an organism goes beyond the goals of the parts. In this way, biological unity goes beyond some cases of symbiosis.

In fact, in the case of typical body parts, it does not appear possible to assign a benefit to the part except *as a part*. What could it mean to benefit a heart? If we made the heart stronger, we would be benefiting it as a part by helping it to fulfill the purposes of the whole. It does not seem possible to have a notion of benefiting a heart other than by furthering its function directed at the good of the whole. Thus the relevant kind of well-being of the parts of an organic whole is primarily to be understood in terms of the well-being of the whole.

Let us imagine, however, that the heart does have a purpose distinct from that of fulfilling the purpose of the whole. Maybe we are dealing with a case of symbiosis where the heart is another organism that is a part of a larger organism for which it does the pumping of blood. Indeed, if cells can be counted as individual organisms, something like this happens in us, though in a less striking way. In such a symbiotic case, it might be possible to talk of benefiting the heart in itself. Perhaps the heart would feel pleasure when electrically stimulated in a certain way, and this would be a benefit to it. Let us then suppose the rest of the body only benefited the heart in itself, and not as a part. Could that be enough for union as parts? Surely not. For the whole needs to coordinate the heart's functioning—the functioning of something needs to be coordinated for it to be a biological part—and it needs to coordinate the heart specifically in the fulfilling of its cardiac functions, the functions that it has insofar as it is a part of the whole. But in striving to coordinate the heart's activity, the whole benefits the heart in a cardiac way, benefits the heart as a part, by making it pump blood in a way beneficial to the organism.

It appears, thus, that we can make the further claim that in a union of two parts as one organism, the two parts will be united in a striving not just for the benefit of themselves and each other, but also in a striving for some further goal, a goal of the whole *as a whole*.

Whether biological facts like coordination and purposeful striving are metaphysically sufficient for two parts to *literally* constitute one body depends on difficult philosophical questions about the nature of material constitution. However, we do not need to answer the question here. If there is something further, beyond such biological facts—like the union of parts with a single soul—that is required for a bunch of parts to constitute a *body,* then this something will be metaphysical. But the analogy drawn by the down-to-earth Yahwist author of Genesis 2 and also by Paul between sexuality and a union as one body, is probably an analogy not to an abstruse metaphysical union but to a concrete, biological union, like that between the interdependent parts of one body. We can talk of the parts of our bodies as forming a biological whole without presupposing particular metaphysical theses in the theory of parts and wholes.

The union of actively functioning parts in an organic body involves two crucial features: coordination and striving for a common goal. If the union is to be a good one, then presumably the goal striven for will have to be valuable, and if the union should be an innately significant one, the goal should also have proportionate significance. There may be further biological characteristics needed for union as one body that additional investigation will one day discover. If so, these also may well be present in sexual union, but we shall not need them for the arguments of this book. What we need for this book is the claim that biological union requires coordination and striving for a common goal.

4. PHILOSOPHICAL REFINEMENTS AND DIFFICULTIES

Our bodies have vestigial parts that do not seem to contribute to the functioning of the whole. On the above account of bodily union they do not count as parts of the body at all. That is why in the official summation in the last section I said that this applies to the union of "actively functioning parts." The sense in which a nonfunctional vestigial part, such as *perhaps* the appendix,[9] is a part of the body is a weaker one. Just as is arguably the case for hair, amputation of a non-functional part does not diminish the body. It may be a part of the body, but it does not contribute to the body. When we consider sexual union as one body, we are not interested in the kind of union that keratinized hair cells or useless appendices have to the rest of the human body.

In fact, this is another argument why the metaphysical constitution of parts into a body—say, through some further metaphysical fact or through a metaphysical connection to a soul—is not the sort of union that we are interested in here. For, arguably, even if the appendix is useless, it presumably still has a metaphysical union with a human being, being literally a part of that human being, but a union of this sort is not what we are looking for in the sexual sphere. If the appendix has no function, it has in some ways more in common with arguably dead parts, like keratinized hair cells, than with the heart or arm.

Neither are we, at this point, interested in the union that functional parts have with a whole when they are not actually functioning, assuming there are ever cases when functional parts of a living organism are not functioning (recall that an army in readiness is not an idle army). The notion of such a union would be derivative from the notion of a union where the parts are actually functioning together—maybe the parts are united because they are *supposed* to function together, or because they *tend* to do so. In any case, we do not want to think of sexual union as a passive union: it is a *consummation* and consummation is active (see also sections 4 and 18 of the next chapter).

There remains a serious problem figuring out how to make sense of the notions of function and purpose that are involved. It is commonly thought that one of the main reasons for the successes of science in the modern period has been that the science started to eschew Aristotelian notions like purpose and function. Indeed, the argument goes on, science did not fully abandon these concepts in biology until Darwin—Kant thought that teleological notions were necessary for organizing biological investigations—and it was only then that real progress in biology began.

Two responses can be made. First, one might note that, in practice, biologists do *not* avoid notions of purpose. On the contrary, evolution is held by many to provide a perfectly intelligible sense in which the various parts that make up the body serve a purpose of the whole, the purpose of passing on the genes. Unfortunately, while the teleological language of function and purpose is heuristically helpful in biology, it has been forcefully argued, and I believe the arguments are sound, that evolution does not really give a sufficient grounding for the literal use of words like "function" and "purpose." The function of an organ simply cannot be equated with the way it contributes to the passing on of the organism's genes. One might imagine, for instance, a scenario on which all sheep whose eyes contribute to seeing are slaughtered by an evil scientist. It would then turn out that the eye's seeing does not contribute to the passing on of the genes, even though the eye's function would still be to see, and the sightless sheep would still have a defect, albeit a defect that helped them to survive.[10]

Nonetheless, even if evolutionary purpose and function do not quite match our ordinary notions of purpose and function, these biological notions may be thought to be sufficiently *analogous* to allow us to use the same words "purpose" and "function" in a sense that is analogical rather than purely equivocal.[11]

Secondly, one might argue that even if evolutionary accounts do not *provide* notions of purpose and function, neither do they rule out such notions. There are two ways this argument could be made. The first is based on the notion that evolutionary processes can co-exist with intelligent planning by a divine creator who sets up the initial conditions and arranges the environment in such a way as to get the results he desires. If need be, this can be supplemented by a version of an idea of Del Ratsch.[12] The creator intends to intervene if the evolutionary process is not heading in the desired direction, though perhaps as a matter of fact there is no need for intervention, because everything goes according to plan. Then, one might define purpose and function in the "engineering" sense, in terms of the designer's intentions. Thus, the claim that the immediate function of eyes is to see, with a more remote purpose of providing the mind with information about objects in the environment, could be grounded in the divine creator's plan that eyes should see and thereby provide information about objects in the environment.[13]

A more challenging, but perhaps more philosophically satisfactory, approach would be to allow for an irreducible notion of purpose that reduces neither to selective advantage nor to the purposes a designer might have. This was Aristotle's view. It just is a basic truth that minds are for knowing, eyes are for seeing, and human front teeth are for cutting while the rear ones are for grinding.[14] Teleological properties, the directedness of things toward an objective purpose—a *telos*—are properties just as basic as mass and electric charge are. There are two interrelated difficulties with this account. First, it is difficult to explain the high degree of coordination between selective advantage and objective purposefulness. Eyes have seeing as their objective purpose, *and* the genes coding for eyes have been, presumably, evolutionarily selected for the ability of eyes to see. Is this a coincidence? Second, while it is fairly easy in at least some cases to figure out empirically what provides an evolutionary advantage, to figure out what the objective purposes of things are is difficult. This last criticism applies to the "designer's intention" account of teleological vocabulary as well.

A theist can, however, give a unified answer to both concerns. The question why selective advantage is correlated with objective purpose seems to be rather like the question why our sense perceptions are correlated with reality. The theist can say that divine wisdom caused such a correlation—for instance, in order that we might fallibly know reality via sense perceptions and fallibly know function via selective advantage, or, maybe, more generally, so that the world be more orderly. The same observations can be used to provide us with a fallible method—after all, the correlation between selective advantage and function is probably not 100 percent—for figuring out what the functions of living things are: if a feature evolved because it contributed to fitness through effecting a certain outcome, then it is *probably* the thing's objective purpose to effect that outcome. In fact, this method of figuring out the functions of living things is more or less the one which had been used for centuries before the notion of selective advantage was used by Darwin, because it was believed—this is clear in Thomas Aquinas, for instance[15]—that one purpose of an organism was to live and another was to reproduce, and so as soon as one found a part whose operation tended to contribute to one of these purposes, one could assume that this operation was, in fact, the *function* of the part, that this is what the part was *for*.

God might have given us a faculty of reason capable of directly intuiting at least certain purposes. And maybe he did. Thus, arguably, we simply *know* that an objective purpose of having beliefs is to get reality right. If we did not know this, we would, arguably, not know what a belief is. Likewise, we can see that an objective purpose of us having language is to communicate ideas, intentions, desires, and so on.

In any case, even if we could not give an account of how we know something, the knowledge is not thereby suspect. It is difficult to see that we have any satisfactory account of how we gain mathematical knowledge, for instance, but this fact does not give us reason to question our knowledge that 2+2=4. So even if the above stories of how we know the functions of parts failed, this would not refute the idea that we do know the functions of many parts.

Furthermore, some account of function and purpose is needed to account for a number of ethical and other philosophical phenomena. Probably this must even be an account of the second or third types, i.e., an account in terms of designer's intentions or in terms of basic Aristotelian teleology, given that evolutionary teleology does not seem sufficient for moral significance—evolutionary teleology is merely a matter of ancient prehistory and hence surely irrelevant to medical ethics.

One very particular example of the need for an account of function and purpose is the foundational question of medical ethics: What is a physician's job? It is not the primary job of the physician, as a physician, to make the patient happy or even to benefit the patient. If happiness is understood in a superficial way as a pleasant feeling, then it is not the physician's task to induce that. If happiness is understood as the individual's flourishing, then love for neighbor makes it the task of *all* of us to promote one another's happiness, and indeed to benefit one another, and so this is not the job of the physician *as such*. A much better account of the physician's primary task is that it is to restore the body's function to a *normal* state. Of course, particular doctors might, by virtue of the same training that makes them capable of restoring normalcy, be able to do other things, such as performing cosmetic surgery or executing a criminal. These other things are at best peripheral to the physician's task.

The normalcy account of the physician's task has consequences. For instance, a physician who refuses to act as an executioner or to refer the case of execution to another physician—even if this would make the condemned prisoner die less painfully—is not thereby refusing to help with a medical service, and hence the refusal is not morally problematic in the way that refusing to treat the ulcer of an unlikeable patient would be.

A somewhat more controversial consequence relates to the case of apotemnophilia, a rare psychological condition on which a patient suffers from a desire to have a limb amputated, even though the limb is healthy. It is said that, if patients are carefully screened, their subjective welfare will improve with such amputation. Now let us suppose that one day the best research showed that a class of patients could equally well be helped with psychotherapy to help them accept four limbs, or with surgery to remove the unwanted limb. Both methods would lead to the same long-term patient satisfaction. Both would involve the same amount of complications (amputation can have complications, but so can psychotherapy). In this hypothetical situation, I think it is clear that psychotherapy, not amputation, would be the right solution. And the "normalcy" account explains this: the mind is not functioning properly when it fails to accept the normal complement of limbs, and hence, ideally, the doctor should treat the mind with psychotherapy rather than the limbs with amputation.

But what does it mean for an organ to be normal? One proposal is statistical normalcy, i.e., the mean or median. But it is plainly not the job of the physician to prescribe defocusing glasses for the patient with 20/10 vision, and if normalcy were identified statistically, one would be unlikely[16] to be told, as one currently is, that the majority of American adults are overweight. The physician's implicit criterion of normalcy is not statistical; rather, the doctor looks at a part of the body and tries to determine the state that the part needs to be in to do its job. The patient should not have a statistically average heart, but a heart capable of pumping the volume of blood needed for oxygenating the patient's body.[17] Having a physician perform surgery that moves a patient's vision from 20/20 to 20/10 does not go *against* the physician's primary role, because in doing so the physician is making the eyes *better* perform their function, while changing the vision from 20/20 to 20/40 is clearly contrary to the task of the physician, even though both kinds of surgery produce a departure from the statistical mean.

Thus, it seems that an answer to the foundational questions of medical ethics requires a notion of the function of a body part, and a notion that is not just a matter of ancient prehistory.

All of this is compatible with the idea that something might acquire a usefulness beyond its objective purposes and functions. We can call the function that the thing innately has its "proper" function. It is arguably not the proper function of a horse to be ridden, but we can certainly ride a horse. Nor is it the proper function of the vocal cords to sing arias, but singing arias is a useful thing which the vocal cords of some people can do. It is the proper functions of a thing that define the notion of a defect. A horse that does not allow itself to be ridden is not thereby a diseased or poorly functioning horse in the way in which a horse that refuses to eat or is unable to reproduce would be, nor is it an objective defect in a human being to be unable to sing arias.

Note that an argument can be given that even if there is an evolutionary understanding of the notions of function and purpose, it is surely not the understanding directly relevant to understanding the "one flesh" analogy. The Yahwist author knew nothing of evolution. When he uses the analogy of the couple as one flesh, it is an analogy to the union of the parts of the body *as understood by him*. Now given the way that functional claims about body parts force themselves on us, it is likely that a functional model of the body was not very far from his implicit understanding of a body as a living whole. The same can be said even more confidently of Paul.

5. THEOLOGICAL CONNECTIONS

The functioning parts of the body are interconnected by their coordinated striving for at least one common purpose. It is worth considering two different theological applications to this notion. The direct connection is Paul's understanding of the body of Christ in 1 Corinthians 12:13–28, excerpted in section 1 above. As he says, "The eye cannot say to the hand, 'I have no need of you,' nor again the head to the feet, 'I have no need of you'" (12:21). Paul sees the body (*sôma*) as consisting of parts, each of which makes its own distinctive contribution. The eye contributes sight and the hand manipulation. It would not do for one part to exist without the others. Each has *need* of the others.

If we examine this need, we can see that it has a twofold nature. First of all, many parts have an intrinsic need of others. Without the hand, the person might starve, and the eye would die—and hence the eye needs the hand. But this kind of intrinsic need of each part for the others does not exhaust the neediness there. To see this, consider first the side of the Church. This is a body, and the head is Christ.

> Rather, speaking the truth in love, we are to grow up in every way into him who is the head, into Christ, from whom the whole body, joined and knit together by every joint with which it is supplied, when each part is working properly, makes bodily growth and upbuilds itself in love. (Eph. 4:15–16)[18]

Note that the metaphor of the Church as the body of Christ is not disjoint from that of Christ as the head of the Church. The Church is the body of its head, just as Sweden is the kingdom of Carl XVI Gustav, even though Carl Gustav is himself a part of this kingdom. One of the interrelated parts of the Church is Christ. Now, Paul insists that every part is dependent on the other parts. He explicitly says that the head cannot say that it would be better for there to be no feet (1 Cor. 12:21). This creates a paradox. Christ is in heaven. How can he have a *need* of us? Surely he *can* say to his feet: "I have no need of you." And the problem becomes even more pressing with a more fully developed Nicene theology that acknowledges Christ as God.

The simplest story on which each part needs the others is one where the survival of each part requires the activity of the others: the eye needs the hand because the eye dies if the hand does not feed the body. But this cannot be the whole story in the theological sense. The resurrected Christ would not die if the rest of the ecclesial body of Christ were, *per impossibile,* destroyed. Nor can this be the whole story biologically, since the lungs can survive the destruction of the sexual organs. However, there is a subtler dependency: each part needs the others *as a part,* i.e., as something which is functionally defined by its striving to fulfill the purposes of the whole. Thus, the eye benefits from the hand, not just because the hand is needed to keep it nourished, but because it is only in coordination with the hand that the eye can do full justice to the role of the eye as a part of the whole. The eye sees an object, but the hand is needed to pick it up. Without a hand or some other way of manipulating objects, the eye would be confined to contributing to the intellectual goals of the body. Likewise, while the lungs would survive without the reproductive parts, one of the lung's purposes is to enable the body to fulfill all its basic holistic animal functions, including the reproductive function (say, by helping the body to survive until reproduction can be effected).

This is the way in which Christ, as head of the Church, has a need of us. He has no intrinsic need of us. Being the immutable God and enjoying the joy of heaven, he nonetheless gives his love as a selfless gift. But he needs us in his capacity as a part, albeit the highest part, of the Church. For we contribute to the purposes of the Church as a whole, and in so doing we fulfill the needs of Christ, not any intrinsic needs but needs he has as a part of the Church, a part that he has freely and humbly become. As part of the Church, we have a role in spreading Christ's Gospel and being the loving hands of Christ. There is a sense in which our cooperation is not absolutely essential, in that God could, in principle, directly bring about these effects, or else use a legion of angels. But if he did that, the interconnection and division of roles in the body of Christ would be severely impoverished, and we would be less united to the body of Christ. We are, ourselves, benefited by fulfilling the needs that Christ has as part of the Church, since doing so deepens our incorporation into the body of Christ.

There is a second theological parallel to this book's account of organic union. St. Augustine considered and rejected the notion that husband and wife and the resulting child could be thought of as modeling the Trinity.[19] Augustine's mind is sufficiently fertile that ideas that he rejects are often worth further exploration. If we see husband and wife as united in one body and as mirroring the Trinity, or at least mirroring the Father and the Son, then we can ask whether the union of the persons in the Trinity has most or all the functional characteristics we have identified in an organic union. I will argue that if we understand the Trinity as Thomas Aquinas (who was of course building on Augustine) did, then the answer is positive.

The orthodox view has it that the persons of the Trinity are distinct individuals: the Father is not the Son, the Son is not the Holy Spirit, and the Holy Spirit is not the Father. On an Aristotelian account of natural purposes—and Aquinas is an Aristotelian—the natural purposes of an individual are defined by the individual's nature. All individuals that share a nature also share the associated purposes. All dogs have a canine purpose to their lives, a purpose to function the way flourishing dogs do. All humans flourish by fulfilling the same human purposes, these being, according to Thomas, the attainment of natural and supernatural knowledge of God, though of course they may fulfill these purposes in different ways.

But there is an important qualification to be made. Each human has *his or her own* individual nature or "substantial form." Admittedly, this individual nature is just like the nature of every other human being—we are all equally human—but these natures are truly individual. My humanness, even if it is just like yours, is distinct from yours. This is correlated with the fact that, while my purpose is just like yours, it is still distinct from yours. My primary purposes, on a Thomistic view, are that *I* should attain natural and supernatural knowledge of God, while your purposes are that *you* should attain it. Granted, it may be a part of my purpose to help you attain this knowledge, and a part of yours to help me attain it as well, but there is a special responsibility each of us bears for his or her own state. Even if we disagree with Thomas's intellectualist account of the human purpose and prefer a more Franciscan one on which our purpose in life is to *love*, it will still be true that the direct primary purpose in my life is for *me* to love everyone. The commandment is in the singular: "*Thou* shalt love thy neighbor as thyself" and is not "You should maximize everybody's love for everybody."

Now, in the case of God, there are three persons, three individuals, but one form, one essence, one nature: *divinity*. The Father, Son, and Holy Spirit are one in essence, one in nature. Therefore, like Peter, Paul, and John they have exactly the same purpose. But while in the case of Peter, Paul, and John, there are really three natures— albeit ones that are just like one another, so that their purposes are individualized although exactly alike—it is not so in the case of the divine persons. Because there is but one nature in God, the purpose of the Father is *identical* with the purpose of the Son and of the Holy Spirit. The three divine persons have a single purpose, not just three purposes that are exactly alike.

Furthermore, God is unchanging not in a passive but in an always active way, as Thomas Aquinas insists (see also John 5:17). The three persons always act to fulfill their single purpose, not in a way that would imply the purpose is unfulfilled and constant work is needed to bring it to fruition, but in the way that someone constantly contemplating a beautiful painting, a contemplation complete at each moment, may be continually consummating the appreciation of beauty without that consummation ever being incomplete.

Just as the body is unified by its cooperative activity for a unified purpose, the Father, Son, and Holy Spirit are one by virtue of their single and active essence, which essence makes up their common purpose. At the same time, the activity is ordered, cooperative, and, as it were, controlled. In the Fourth Gospel, we have Jesus saying: "the Son can do nothing of his own accord, but only what he sees the Father doing; for whatever he does, that the Son does likewise" (John 5:19), and indeed on the orthodox account of the Trinity the Son exists from the Father. The Holy Spirit, in turn, proceeds from the Father on the Eastern view, and from the Father and the Son on the Western view, and is active in virtue of the numerically one divine functioning, *energeia,* that he has from the Father or from the Father and the Son.

Thus, something very much like the kind of functional organic unity that we are trying to find in persons engaging in sexual activity is found in the Trinity, though of course, in the case of the Trinity, the unity is more profound, because not only is there one purpose, but there is a single activity, rather than multiple cooperating activities. The above account is based on Thomas Aquinas's philosophy. However, substantially the same kind of parallel can be drawn on patristic accounts. The crucial point is that there is only one divine activity. For if the persons have the same divine activity, they have the same purpose. The unity of divine *energeia* is a part of patristic orthodoxy. This unity is the presupposed background for the Third Council of Constantinople's definition that in Christ there are *two* principles of functioning, a human *energeia* and a divine one, it being taken for granted that the Trinity has only one divine *energeia*. Each *energeia* corresponds to a nature, and as there is only one divine nature common to the three persons of the Trinity, there is only one *energeia* in the Trinity.[20]

6. THE CENTRAL QUESTION

Theologically, at least one central form of sexual activity is supposed to involve a union as one flesh or one body, since scripture so insists in seminal texts, and we have identified this union as a functional, organic union as one body, in part based on Paul's description of the Church as the body of Christ. Erotic love's seeking of bodily union makes it philosophically plausible that if such an organic union is possible in sexual activity, then this is what erotic love seeks. We now need to try to find out whether and how such a union can, in fact, be constituted by a sexual activity.

Consider, then, an instance of morally upright, mutually pleasurable, cooperative, consensual, heterosexual intercourse that is intended both to be expressive of committed conjugal love and to be reproductive, engaged in under circumstances in which the couple both desires and can prudently welcome children. The reason for all of these conditions is that if we include them all, then we can say that just about everyone[21] agrees this would be *an* instance of the normative and meaningful form of sexual activity, though few think that *all* the conditions are necessary. In any case, if union as one body is to be found in some form of sexual activity, it will surely be found here. I will call this the "central case of intercourse," though "central" is used here merely as a term of convenience rather than as a morally loaded term implying some sort of superiority over cases where some of the above-listed ingredients are missing. In fact, on the account I will defend, some of the features included in the description of the ideal case are *not* necessary for the sexual activity to be deeply meaningful.

The problem can now be stated as follows: What is it about the "central" case of intercourse that makes it yield a union as one body that consummates erotic love? And what is the purpose for which the two are functionally cooperating that is needed to produce the union as one body?

I will proceed by considering three main options, each of which draws attention to different features of the central case, and each of which has implications about which other features of the central case are normatively inessential. The first option is one that our culture finds highly plausible: mutual pleasure is the unified purpose toward which the two bodies are unified by striving. The second option is seen in a family of accounts on which some "higher-level" purpose is being striven for, such as spiritual or psychological unity, a mystic union with the cosmos, or the strengthening of the marital relationship. The final option is that a reproductive striving is responsible for the desired union as one body. Each of these options has apparent strengths and weaknesses. I will argue that the first and second options are ultimately unsatisfactory, but that the third is satisfactory in itself, can be defended against obvious objections, and can, in fact, be expanded in such a way as to include the basic insights of the other two. It is worth noting that the final version of the "reproduction" option will make union as one body compatible with the couple's not personally desiring to reproduce.

7. OPTION ONE: PLEASURE

The central case of intercourse, by our stipulation, produces mutual pleasure. This pleasure includes the physical sensations of orgasm, as well as earlier and later physical sensations, and various associated higher-level emotional pleasures. The latter will be covered by the discussion of the next section, and so the primary focus here will be on "physical pleasure." The term is not intended to deny a significant, perhaps crucial, psychological aspect, however, to the pleasure.

We may, thus, construe the two persons, or their bodies, as striving to produce mutual pleasure. This striving is mutually regulated and cooperative. On the suggested account, this is the striving central to union. Unfortunately, our analysis of bodily unity indicates an immediate problem for this account. A genuine organic whole involves coordinated striving for goals that benefit the *whole* as more than just the sum of its parts. But here we have two goals, the pleasure of one person and the pleasure of the other, neither of which is a benefit to the whole, as a whole.

This claim might be disputed in two ways by a defender of the pleasure account. First of all, the defender might claim that *mutual* pleasure is more than just the pleasure of one person and the pleasure of the other person. It is a *joint* pleasure. But a pleasure account like this seems problematic. The feelings of the two persons are separate. There is no merging of consciousnesses. What, then, makes the pleasure joint?

There are two prima facie plausible suggestions here. The first is that what makes the pleasure joint is just that it is a product of a joint and mutual activity. But that threatens circularity—the jointness of activity in organic union essentially involves a jointness of goal. Perhaps this circularity can be overcome. But also note that the joint striving for pleasure will itself have to be valuable, since among the goals of the joint activity is this very joint striving for pleasure. But then the joint activity is, among other things, a joint striving for a joint striving for pleasure. And it does not appear plausible that *biological* unity is achieved by this rather intellectual pursuit, this meta-striving for a striving.

The second, and in general more plausible, suggestion is that a pleasure is joint when there is a single thing in which two people take pleasure. When they read the same book together at the same time, their pleasure is joint in a way in which it is not if they read different books without sharing the contents. On this suggestion, the central case of sexual union would require that there be some *one* thing that is enjoyed, and the enjoyment of which is the unifying purpose of that activity. Now it may well be that there *is* a single unified object of enjoyment. One suggestion is that this object of pleasure is *the union itself.* But it is implausible to suppose that what at least partially constitutes the union is the striving for the pleasure of that very union. For then the content of the union is defined circularly: The union is defined at least in part by a joint striving toward some goal g. Goal g is in turn defined as the pleasure of what is, in part, striving for g. This is viciously circular.

Of course there might be other unified objects proposed for the pleasure, activities distinct from union itself. Thus, the couple might be enjoying striving for reproduction, and *striving for reproduction* is a unified object distinct from the union brought about by striving for pleasures. But then our focus moves away from pleasure and toward the activity in which the pleasure is taken. It is the unity of *that* activity that is responsible for the unity of the pleasure, and hence for the unity of the couple.

Pleasure, thus, shifts our focus away from itself and toward something else. As a stand-alone account, pleasure does not seem satisfactory.

Maybe, though, we can simply say that the couple is taking pleasure in the sexual activity qua joint physical activity. But while it is possible to take pleasure in a joint physical activity as such, for instance in an acrobatic routine, that pleasure is not what sexual pleasure is. Sexual pleasure is not the pleasure of a *performance* well done. Seeing sex primarily as performance seems deeply mistaken as to the nature of sex: an awkward, physically disabled couple can have just as "good sex" as a pair of trained acrobats. In any case, even though the pleasure of performance might be a part of the pleasure a couple feels in having sex, that is not a distinctively sexual pleasure. A related account, that of Alan Goldman, has defined sexual desire in terms of the desire for bodily contact and its pleasure.[22] But that account is mistaken for the same reason—the pleasure of touch is not specifically sexual pleasure. One can enjoy the feel of a cat's fur against one's hand without it being sexual.

Another defense of the pleasure account would be simply to drop the requirement that the goals of the whole have to be different from the benefits to the parts considered in themselves. Thus, the goals of the whole are, just, the individual pleasures of the two. This would weaken the "one body" analogy, perhaps unacceptably, but let us allow such a weakening for the sake of argument.

There will, still, be three criticisms of the pleasure account. First, recall the orgasmatron from Woody Allen's 1973 film *Sleeper*. This is a device that, when entered by one or more persons, rapidly induces orgasms in them. Fairly early on in the film, we see a fully clothed man and woman entering, and then coming out blissfully a few seconds later. Later in the film, our hero is seen coming out black and blue after a long session alone in the orgasmatron. Sexual pleasure does not require more than one person, if the appropriate technology is used. But two people entering the orgasmatron for a few seconds are not united as one body. Perhaps the fact that the other person is not needed for the pleasure is why they do not count as united—there is no essential cooperation there. But imagine an orgasmatron modified so that two people are needed to activate it, maybe because it is activated by a shape-recognition system that requires the presence of (exactly? at least?) two people. It is still implausible to suppose that such a device would provide the kind of bodily union that romantic love seeks, even though entering the device would be a mutual striving for the production of pleasure, and each party could enter in order that the other might receive pleasure. (The case where both want pleasure for themselves would clearly be less unitive.)

Hence mutual striving for the production of pleasure does not seem to be the center of union. Maybe the defender of the pleasure account would insist that the striving for pleasure has to be biologically based or not technologically mediated for it to count as sexually unitive. But a proponent of such a view would say anal sex is sexually unitive, but any activity that essentially involves "sex toys" is not, and this does not seem a plausible combination of views.

Also note that pleasure is a goal that is not, itself, at an organic level. Pleasure essentially requires a mind to perceive it. While that in which pleasure is taken is extra-mental, the pleasure itself is a mental phenomenon. But, arguably, biological organisms are defined by their *biological* goals, goals at a biological level, such as growth, nutrition, and reproduction. My body is not merely a bunch of otherwise disunited parts that work together to benefit my mind. This is true regardless of whether one considers the mind a part of the body or not. If the mind is a part of the body, then a striving solely for the benefit of the mind benefits a mere part rather than the whole. If the mind is not a part of the body, then a striving for pleasure does not seem to be a primarily biological striving. Here we can bring back the physical emphasis of the term *flesh* (*basar, sarx*) in Genesis 2 and in Jesus' recounting of it, which emphasis suggests a biological level.

The defender of the pleasure account can try to argue that the neurochemistry of pleasure is good for one on a bodily level. However, it seems improbable to suppose the bodies involved in sex are, in fact, striving for these relatively minor health benefits, or that these benefits are responsible for the great significance of sexual union. It is probably even healthier to exercise together than to have sex together, but while exercising together can be unitive, it does not have the level of significance that sex does. It may also be the case that science will one day find that human sexual activity decreases lifespan—some evolutionary theories suggest there would be a longevity-cost to reproduction.[23]

But the most serious reason why striving for mutual pleasure is not what produces the union that romantic love seeks is that the conscious experience of pleasure does not, in itself, have an independent value. Consider the three most plausible views of the value of pleasure:

View A: Pleasure is always valuable in itself.
View B: Pleasure is valuable when and only when one is taking pleasure in something that is not itself bad.

View C: Pleasure is valuable when and only when one is taking pleasure in something that is in itself good.

I will argue that only View C is satisfactory. Against View A, consider the following scenario, which is an extension of one given by J. J. C. Smart.[24] (Smart apparently accepts View A notwithstanding such apparent counterexamples.) You find out that you will be locked up for life in a cell near a pediatric oncology ward. On all the walls of your room, as well as the floor and ceiling, you have live-action video feeds showing the suffering in the ward. You can't avoid seeing this, and one of the six feeds has its audio on all the time, except for when you are to sleep. You will have no contact with the outside world, except that food will be brought in. Your captors do, however, make you one offer that will, allegedly, make your lot easier: they can perform neurosurgery on you to increase your *Schadenfreude*, so that you will greatly enjoy the suffering of the children dying from cancer. If pleasure is always good in itself, this would surely be a good thing.

If View A is true, it is intrinsically good to feel pleasure, even if it is pleasure at the pain of others. Granted, under normal circumstances, even if View A is true, you should refuse to have your *Schadenfreude* increased, as it would be likely to make you less effective at helping your fellow human beings. But under the circumstances in this scenario, there is no possibility of your helping anybody else. The intrinsic value of the pleasure seems to be the only thing at issue.

It seems clear that you should refuse to have your *Schadenfreude* increased. It is simply bad to be the sort of person who takes pleasure in the pain of others, regardless of whether this harms others. A disposition to *Schadenfreude* is intrinsically a vice, and vices are intrinsically bad. But if View A holds, then every disposition to pleasure should be intrinsically good (though perhaps instrumentally bad), including a disposition to *Schadenfreude*. Thus, we should reject View A. Taking pleasure in something bad is itself bad. If anything, we should be *pained* by bad things.

View B escapes the worst excesses of View A. Nonetheless, it is still mistaken. There is a certain "warm glow" of satisfaction that we have when we think that we have acted selflessly to benefit another. Consider, then, a "satisfaction pill." You can take it after any action of yours to make yourself feel the pleasant warm glow that we have naturally upon selfless action. Suppose, then, that you have done something morally unobjectionable that, however, was unquestionably done for your own personal benefit. To give yourself a lift, you take the satisfaction pill and feel the pleasure of having acted selflessly. View A would judge this to be intrinsically good, because all pleasure on View A is good. But likewise View B would judge this to be good, because you are taking pleasure in an action that is not bad. But there appears to be something problematic about taking such a pill. First of all, taking such a pill will decrease the motivating force of the warm glow in the future. But that is not of the essence. We may suppose that it does not decrease the motivating force—say, because you are the sort of person who is not moved by the expectation of the warm glow, but simply by the value of the action. Taking such a pill is still objectionable. It is having the feeling of taking pleasure in an activity without the hard work of doing the activity that is objectionable—it is a form of self-deceit in an important matter (namely, whether what if any virtue one has exercised), even if it does not lead to any actually false belief.

Perhaps the reader does not feel that there is anything wrong with taking such a pill. Let us, however, turn it around: Is there anything wrong with *not* taking it? Someone who misses out on something good with no good reason for missing out on it can potentially be accused of insensitivity to the good. But those who refuse to take the satisfaction pill are surely not to be criticized for any kind of insensitivity to the good. And a good explanation why they are not to be criticized is that they have *not* missed out on an occasion for getting something good—because the pill-induced pleasure would be an empty and deceptive pleasure rather than something good.

That leaves View C. Whenever pleasure is good, it is the taking of pleasure *in* something good. Aristotle writes: "Pleasure completes the activity not as the inherent state does, but as an end which supervenes as the bloom of youth does on those in the flower of their age."[25]

This "bloom of youth" is what completes the beauty of those in the flower of their age. The bloom is hard to imagine absent other aspects of beauty, such as a well-proportioned build or an intelligent face, and were the bloom of youth somehow able to be found without these other forms of beauty, the result would likely be grotesque—think of the bloom of youth on a cruel and stupid face. Moreover, the visual effect of the bloom of youth is modulated by the young man's features, just as the pleasure of an activity cannot be separated from the activity. We cannot, to use an example I heard from a student, distill the pleasure of camping from the camping itself.

Consider two very different pleasures, that of eating a chocolate cake and that of solving a mathematical problem. We do not experience a single "feeling of pleasure" in the two cases. Rather, we take pleasure in eating a cake and we also take pleasure in solving a problem, and the ways the pleasures feel are different. Aristotle believes that pleasure is not some kind of a fluid that is present whenever one is enjoying something. Rather, pleasure is enjoyment of an activity, and is given its form by the activity, perhaps somewhat in the way that love of a person is given shape by what the beloved is believed to be like.

If this is correct, then a pleasure takes on its meaning from the underlying activity. And just as the bloom of youth would be grotesque on a young man ugly in body and mind, so too a pleasure in something shameful is itself grotesque, and a pleasure in something of neutral value is not worth pursuing.

One might, though, object that while pleasure takes on its meaning from the underlying activity, the underlying activity need not be *good* in order that one's taking pleasure in it be good. Certain kinds of pleasures, like the "warm glow," are only properly had in the case of a good activity. But other pleasures can be appropriately had in the case of a neutral activity. Still, "neutral" is a nice way of saying "worthless but not positively bad," and insofar as we are taking pleasure in an activity, we have a positive attitude toward the activity. But on what possible grounds could we have a positive attitude toward something that is literally worthless? It is *good* things that are to be appreciated, and if one appreciates something that is not good, one's affections are distorted, just as when one "sees" something that is not there, there is something wrong with one's perceptual faculties.

And, in any case, even if I am wrong and sometimes it is permissible to take pleasure in a worthless activity, it does not appear right to understand sexual union in terms of a pursuit of pleasure in a worthless activity. Even if such pleasure had some value, it would surely have very little significance, and pursuit of it would not give the kind of significance to sex that, as we have seen in chapter 4, sex has.

This leaves View C. We can now divide View C in two further ways. Either we require that the thing in which pleasure is to be taken is good in itself, *independently* of the pleasure, or we allow that it can be the sort of thing that becomes good upon pleasure being taken in it. I now want to argue against this second version of View C. On this view, it is never good to take pleasure in something bad, and it is always good to take pleasure in a good. But some neutral things are such that it is never good to take, at least, a certain kind of pleasure in them (e.g., it is not good to feel the pleasure of selfless activity in doing something solely for one's own benefit), while others are such that they become worthy of our taking pleasure in them, as soon as we take pleasure in them. One might have this view of hobbies. Perhaps there is no intrinsic value in stamp collecting, but when stamp-collecting pleasure is taken in stamp collecting, it becomes valuable.

I think this view of hobbies is mistaken. Granted, certain hobbies are such that it takes training to come to take pleasure in them. But this training is, in part, a training in the appreciation of certain kinds of items or forms of activity, like the training to recognize the valuable features of a particular stamp (a value that, in this case, in large part depends on various social institutions). To say that there is nothing there to be appreciated except when one takes pleasure in the activity, is to do some violence to the phenomenology of hobbies; hobbyists think they are on to something valuable, something that not everybody needs to pursue given that there are many no less valuable alternative ways of spending one's time, but still something that is worth pursuing. Consider the case of a stamp collector who falls into a deep depression, so that it becomes clear her hobby will never again give her any pleasure. However, she comes to have a unique opportunity to acquire a stamp that would be the crowning glory of her collection, a stamp that completes a series for which only she possesses the other stamps. It seems that even if she does not derive pleasure from the acquisition of the stamp, the acquisition can nonetheless be a worthwhile action.

Furthermore, the best explanation why we should reject Views A and B is that pleasure is appropriate when it is pleasure *in a good*. Now the pleasure cannot be a part of the good in which pleasure is taken, at least in ordinary human cases. For while one might take pleasure, in part, in the fact that one is taking pleasure in x, this meta-pleasure is distinct from the first-order pleasure in x, and so this is not a case where the pleasure has itself as an object. One might, of course, also have a meta-meta-pleasure, but that in turn will be distinct from the meta-pleasure. Perhaps in cases that go beyond this earthly life it will be possible to have an infinite-order pleasure, and there, maybe, the pleasure could be a pleasure in the taking of pleasure, and maybe the heavenly joy in God is such that the joy is God himself, so that the joy is joy in itself. But it does seem that in earthly cases it is one thing to have a pleasure and another to take pleasure in having that pleasure. An illustrative case is a person who is learning to appreciate a genre of music, and who suddenly, with pleasure, observes that he does now enjoy it.

On the remaining version of View C, then, a pleasure is valuable when one is taking pleasure in something that is *independently* valuable. A hedonism that takes pleasure, itself, as independently valuable fails to explain *why* pleasure is valuable, while seeing pleasure as deriving its value from that in which one takes delight can give an explanation of this. We will accept View C if (but not only if) we see pleasure as presenting to us the value of an underlying state or activity. It is good to know the truth. It is particularly good to know experientially that good things are good, to taste and see their goodness, because, for instance, they are good insofar as they reflect the goodness of God. When we take pleasure in the good, we are recognizing its goodness, and that, too, is a good thing. If we see pleasure as an affective perception of a good,[26] we will give pleasure its due while preventing it from becoming a tyrant. This account of pleasure as a recognition and appreciation of a good will be an important part of some of the arguments about controversial questions about sex later on in the book.

It is a commonplace that the pursuit of pleasure for its own sake rarely fails to produce misery or at least ennui. A pleasure divorced from the underlying good has a tendency to decrease over time, suggesting that one is missing out on what the activity is really aimed at when one aims only at the pleasure. If one not only accepts the dependence of pleasure's value on an underlying independent good but also agrees that pleasure is an affective perception of that good, then one can provide a further explanation why seeking pleasure for its own sake tends not to lead to fulfillment. For if one continues to have a perception that one knows is false, the perception starts to fade away after a while. One may be frightened the first time by the full-sized and realistically colored tiger sculpture at the corner of Main and 4th Street, but as one walks by it every day, the fear shrinks away, and eventually one hardly notices it. On the other hand, brave people do fear *real* danger, and can continue fearing it as time goes on, though they become better able to cope with it. Our minds are adept at weeding out illusions. Probably by adulthood we no longer consciously perceive the famous stick in the water as broken, even though the first time that we saw it as children we might have been taken in by the illusion. A pleasure without an underlying good is an illusion, and when one realizes that it is an illusion—and repeated exposure is apt to make one do that—then the illusion itself palls. The life of a person centered on the pursuit of excitement for its own sake, without a care for the exciting things in and of themselves, is empty. Such hopeless and ultimately ennui-producing pursuit may well be common among affluent Westerners these days.

The problem with the pursuit of pleasure as separated from any underlying good is particularly clear in the case of pleasures that are more morally significant. Suppose you are not scientifically gifted enough to be a great scientist, but your rich parents create an illusion for you, with the help of an army of actors, a multitude of bribes and occasional chemical help—the illusion that you are the greatest scientist ever, frequently tasting the thrill of discovery, receiving the Nobel prize, and so on. But this will all be a sham. The discoveries by which you will be thrilled are ones that scientists have already made a hundred years ago, though your army of helpers has arranged to maneuver you into "discovering them." Surely this is not worth having. The thrill of scientific discovery is a pitiful thing in the absence of discovery, when one has simply been fed ideas and led on by one's lab "assistants." Such a "scientist" should be pitied. I was once at a conference presentation by a mathematician from an institution too impecunious to have access to the relevant research literature and who was thus presenting discoveries that, unbeknownst to the speaker, had already been made by others. No one pointed this out to the speaker—no one seemed to know what to say. It was a sad occasion, somewhat embarrassing to the audience, and while the audience's silence perhaps spared the speaker's feelings, none of us would have wanted to be that speaker.

Now, if pleasure is only a secondary good, then sexual pleasure is either an empty and meaningless pleasure, or it receives its value from some other, deeper good. If sexual pleasure is empty, but a striving for it lies at the center of union as one body, then, contrary to our experience, this union would not be very significant. On the other hand, if sexual pleasure is an affective reflection of a deeper good, then surely it is the deeper good that is more appropriately seen as the goal of the unitive striving, at least if the union to be produced is a deeper one—and romantic love seeks deep sexual union. Thus, even if pleasure *is* involved, we still need to look for another goal on this view.

But perhaps pleasure is the *biological* goal while the deeper, more important goal is one that is sought by the persons as *persons,* and so the biological union is constituted by a striving for mutual pleasure. However, this is not plausible. Biologically, it seems that pleasure is present in order to motivate one to reproduction, rather being present as the ultimate biological goal in sexual activity.

Observe that the pleasure account currently under examination, insofar as it attempts to be faithful to the notion of organic union as partially constituted by a mutual coordinated striving for some goal of the whole, will make the bodily attempt to achieve pleasure central. It is not the pleasure itself that constitutes the union. To make pleasure itself constitute union would seriously depart from our account of a one body union, and would, in any case, be quite implausible. For let us suppose that, for some reason, one or both persons are incapable of feeling sexual pleasure, for example, due to a severing of certain nerves. They can, nonetheless, engage in something that is just like the central case of intercourse except that no physical pleasure is experienced. It does not appear that such a couple fails to be united "as one body." It would surely not do for the man who visited a prostitute to excuse himself to Paul by saying: "I was not one body with the prostitute, because as it happened neither I nor she felt any pleasure," or for a person to think that Christ's prohibition of divorce does not apply because there was no pleasure in the consummation of the marriage, so no one body is sundered. Sexual pleasure does not appear to be the most significant thing here. This is perhaps particularly clear when we consider the ultimate distortion of sex in rape: whether the victim or the perpetrator feels any physical pleasure is of little moral relevance in itself, though orgasm can contribute to feelings of guilt in the victim and thus increase the harm.

Certainly, at least, the meaningfulness of consensual sexual intercourse is not proportional to the pleasurableness. On a view of union as constituted by pleasure, joint entry into the orgasmatron would constitute sexual union as one body, and that surely is mistaken. And just as a union constituted by mere pleasure cannot be very significant, the *striving* for pleasure cannot be very significant either. It would be strange indeed if it were a morally significant fact about a person or a body that it strives for something, where the thing striven for was quite unimportant.

Let me end this section by considering a different view of pleasure supportive of my basic conclusions. On this view, what is central to the meaning of pleasure is that it is a biological reward mechanism designed to induce us to engage in some activity. Seen this way, the pursuit of pleasure on its own makes little rational sense. To try to activate a reward mechanism only makes sense if the activity being rewarded is worth rewarding. It is surely unfortunate if one is rewarded for an activity that is bad. And it is probably also harmful to be rewarded for an activity that is neutral in value, since the reward would skew one's pursuits in the direction of the value-neutral activity, when one could, instead, have been pursuing something valuable. Besides, the rewarding of a neutral activity might lead to an addiction.

8. OPTION TWO: HIGHER GOALS

If pleasure is not sufficiently morally significant, in and of itself, to be the goal of the striving that is central to the constitution of sexual union, let us turn our attention to prospective goals that would have indisputably moral significance. Various goals of the kind have been proposed, and they can be divided into a number of overlapping headings: cosmic, spiritual, cognitive, emotional, or psychological. I will now give one or more examples of each.

On the cosmic side, one might have grand notions about the universe being ontologically constituted by a balance of male and female, so that sexual intercourse is a part of what constitutes the universe itself as one. Or, moving more to the spiritual side, one might think that some great mystical task is furthered by sexual union, say, the reunion of all things into the Neoplatonic One.

Or perhaps, in a somewhat more down-to-earth spirituality we could say that a spiritual mingling between the two persons is mystically achieved by sexual union. And on a more specifically Christian spirituality, one might also see sexuality as a participation in or symbol of the union between Christ and Israel/Church (e.g., Isa. 54:5, Eph. 5:31–32), as symbolic of intra-Trinitarian union, or as a way of perceiving one or more of these deep spiritual realities—a way of having that reality brought home to one cognitively and emotionally. After all, the passionate love of God for his people is, perhaps, to be understood in the light of the human experience of sexual union.

Perhaps indeed there is a cognitive benefit derived from sexuality. Some facts about God, the universe, or humanity may be made clearer to the participants, possibly along the lines of the above suggestions, or maybe what is made clearer to them is some aspect of the beloved or of the relationship. Alternatively, perhaps sexual activity is linguistic in nature: it can be used to convey a message.[27]

Perhaps the benefit is emotional: the members of the couple find it easier to accept themselves, or to reach out to others. They feel more loved and make their love better appreciated by the beloved. Psychological benefits may also include changes to behavior. Sexual self-giving might help to make one less self-centered, more giving in general. It is, in any case, plausible that sexual activity produces some kind of a psychological bond between the parties. One thinks of Tess in Thomas Hardy's *Tess of the d'Urbervilles,* who would be more accurately described as a victim of rape than as a woman seduced, though the plot of the novel turns on how closely bound she feels to her violator. It may even be that there is an explanation of bonding in normal cases in terms of oxytocin and other neurochemicals.

Now, just as in the case of pleasure, I will not dispute whether one or more of these goals are, in fact, achieved by sexual intercourse. Moreover—and unlike in the case of sexual pleasure—I will not dispute the independent value of the goals. Instead I will argue that the striving toward any of these goals is not the striving that helps make two persons into one body.

As an opening argument, consider the question *why* it is that the central case of sexual activity achieves those of the above goals that it does. Why, for instance, might sexual activity be seen as symbolic of the union between Christ and the Church? The symbolism alleged here is not an arbitrary one, in the way the sign "DOG" indicates a canine, while it could just as well have indicated a frog. For if the symbolism were an arbitrary one, then sexual union would not have the intrinsic significance, the intrinsic way of mattering, that it has. Of course, perhaps if the symbolism were arbitrarily chosen by God, it would matter independently of culture and circumstance. But it does not appear from a Christian perspective that God chooses his symbolism arbitrarily. On the contrary, the symbol reflects the spiritual reality. The waters of baptism reflect spiritual cleansing: we do not baptize by rolling people in mud.

Now if the symbolism is not arbitrary, one may ask what it is about sexual union that makes it fit to have this kind of symbolic significance. And the natural answer is that what makes it fit is that it is a union as one body, and the unitive nature of sexuality reflects a spiritual union. Something similar to this can be said about a number of the other cosmic and spiritual suggestions. Why should sexual union reunite things with the Neoplatonic One? Well, in fact, it perhaps doesn't (except maybe when it happens on some occasion to bring someone closer to God—assuming that we can identify the Neoplatonic One with God), but if it did, it would surely do so because it actually unites two persons in an earthly sense, and this union is a start toward cosmic reunion, or perhaps a revelation of the unity of all things. In these cases, the spiritual or cosmic significance of the act seems to depend on the union of bodies being intelligible apart from that spiritual or cosmic significance.

This objection will not apply to higher-goal accounts on which sex causes the achievement of a higher goal in a nonsymbolic manner, and where the cause is not the fact of union as one body *as such* but something else bound up with sex, such as secretion of chemicals, psychological sharing in an intimate physical activity, intense pleasure, or a mystical experience.

On the mystical side, while the intense feelings involved in sex may sometimes facilitate a mystical experience, it seems to be an undue spiritualization of bodily union to suppose that a striving for a mystical experience is what constitutes the couple into one *flesh*. Besides, it is not clear that the presence of such a mystical experience is normatively a part of central cases of sexual union.

Let us consider the biochemical and psychological options. Sexual activity indeed tends to produce certain effects that are indisputably significant. However, these effects can be produced by activities other than sex. For instance, one of the chemicals proposed as serving a role in natural bonding is oxytocin, but it also appears to be released or activated in other ways, and appears to be present to a significantly greater degree in more supportive couples even outside of intercourse.[28] Psychological bonding and other emotional effects can have a multitude of natural causes, sexual activity being only one of these. It is not clear why sexual activity is singled out as the consummation of a special kind of love if sexual activity is understood in terms of the production of psychological effects. Granted, there may be a particular "flavor" or "tinge" that these effects have when they are produced by sexual activity, but this sexual tinge is only of significance if sexual activity is independently meaningful. And sexual union as one body is a unique union for us, a consummation of a basic human love.

The biochemical version of this account can be understood in two ways. Either the union as one body is constituted by the striving to produce the chemicals or by the striving to produce the emotional effect to which the chemicals contribute. The more directly chemical account seems more plausible, in that the lower-level effect is the immediate purpose that produces *biological* unification, while the higher-level effect is more closely connected to *psychological* rather than fleshly union. But if the union is merely constituted by a striving to secrete some neurochemicals, can it really have as deep a significance as sexual union does?

Next, note that there is a single, decisive objection that simultaneously applies to all of the higher-goal accounts, except for the one on which the secretion of the chemicals is itself the constitutive unifying goal. The problem is that all of these set up the goal that is achieved by the mutual striving at a higher level than the biophysical. The goal in each case is something cosmic, spiritual, intellectual, volitional, and/or emotional. This does not make the union be a fleshly union as one body, since a single body is constituted by the striving of parts to achieve various goals at a biophysical level, such as the oxygenation of the brain or the repelling of invading bacteria.

But sexual union is a union as one *flesh*, not just one mind or one heart. The fleshiness of sexuality is crucial to the uniqueness of sexual union among all the unions available to us. Sexuality involves a particular focus on the body of the beloved. In sexuality, the two unite in a totality that involves them not just as persons, but also as animals. We are embodied beings, and sexuality seems one of the most evident features of this embodiment.

But is it not possible for various bodily parts to be united into one body by, say, a spiritual goal? Indeed, the various members of the Church are thus united. However, at this point the metaphor is expressly weakened: Ephesians 5:32 talks of the connection between marriage and the Christ-Church relationship as a *mystery*. The body of Christ is a *spiritual* body, and hence it is no surprise that it is constituted in unity by spiritual goals. But romantic love is interested in a physical body. The fleshiness of sexual union may, thus, provide a disanalogy between the one-body aspect of sexual union and the one-body aspect of the Church—in the case of sexual union we not only have one organized whole (one *sôma*) but also one flesh (*basar, sarx*), as in Genesis 2:24. Though it must be noted that the disanalogy will not be seen as so great if one accepts that the Church is joined by a Eucharistic sharing in the physical body and blood of Christ (1 Cor. 10:17).

If the relevant kind of sexual union is constituted by some higher goal, animals are unlikely to have a sexual union as one body. But if it really is a union as one *flesh*, and if our flesh is really like that of the animals, then it is plausible that some other animals are indeed capable of that union. Of course that union will not have the same significance in their case as it does for us. Similarly, while the destruction of the body is death in the case of both humans and fleas, it is a less significant event in the case of fleas, because the life and death of a flea is not connected with the range of spiritual and psychological phenomena with which our lives are supposed to be connected. But, in any case, if sexual union as one *body* is seen as a union of which animals, too, are capable, then we are unlikely to suppose that striving for a higher goal is what unifies two into one body.

If the above considerations are sound, sexual union should be something that is found in both humans and nonhuman animals, but that, nonetheless, has human significance. There are such events: birth and death are examples.

In any case, the following is true. A union is more profoundly a union as one flesh the more the union is like that of the parts in a fleshly body. The parts of the human body do cooperate together to produce effects at a higher level—for instance, the hands, eyes, and mouth work together in the singing of hymns, thereby helping to produce a spiritual effect. But that is not the only thing that constitutes the parts into one biological organism, since the hands, eyes, and mouth are unified as one body in animals for which such spiritual functions are absent, and hence lower-level goals, also found in non-human animals, are sufficient to unify the parts. What we have is a layered system, on which there is a fleshly union and there are higher-level effects. Nor are the "lower levels" to be despised, since the basic effect of intercourse at the lower level is *human life,* and surely that life has deep significance.

Without denying the existence of higher goals, we should thus look for a more biological goal to constitute the direction in which the processes constituting fleshly union as one body strive.

9. OPTION THREE: REPRODUCTION

There is, indeed, a natural candidate for the goal toward which the two bodies strive in sexual activity, a candidate that satisfies the twin desiderata that the goal should be at a biological level, so that animals can have this kind of one-body union, and yet be humanly significant. This goal is reproduction. Furthermore, there are independent arguments why we should think considerations of reproduction are relevant to understanding sexual activity.

Suppose we wanted to explain the nature of sexual activity to an alien coming from a race that reproduces asexually.[29] Now, it appears that any explanation of sexual activity will have to mention some of the primary sexual organs. But how would we explain what these organs are to the alien?

Certainly, reference to the physical shape of the organs would not help the alien very much. Andrea Dworkin thought that intercourse was a form of the domination of women, because through it a part of the man occupied the inside of the woman.[30] This would be a geometrical understanding of intercourse as defined by the configuration and contact of organs of such-and-such shape, and, contrary to Dworkin, such a geometric understanding seems quite unhelpful. Mentioning that the organs are pleasure-producing would help the alien somewhat, but not much, because it would not distinguish sexual activity from the sharing of ice cream. Of course if we could tell the alien that we are talking of *sexual* pleasure, that might be thought to help, but our alien knows nothing about how sexual pleasure differs from other kinds. The alien might come back with the question: "Oh, is that like the pleasure of solving mathematical problems, or is it like the pleasure of receiving a particularly clear low-frequency square wave with one's rear antennae?" Likewise, it would not help the alien to be told by Marcus Aurelius that there is a "spasmodic secretion of a little bit of slime," as that would not distinguish sex from spitting.

Now, if we wanted to tell the alien about the social role of sex, we could do that. We could talk about the relationships between sex and power, sex and tenderness, and so on. This would help the alien to some extent. The alien might even start to be able to follow the plots of popular novels. However, sex is objectively important and its meaning is not just social, as we saw in chapter 4.

I have already argued that pleasure is not what gives the central unitive meaning to sex (see section 7 above). Therefore, even if we could somehow modify the alien's brain so that it could feel the pleasure humans feel when they have sex, that would not tell the alien what is important, either. The alien would realize: "Ah, yes, it's very pleasant in a unique sort of way." And if the alien accepted an Aristotelian account of pleasure, it might think that this pleasure, at least when it occurs in humans, somehow reflects a peculiar kind of good. But the alien would not be able to explain what kind of good this is.

It would appear that the only way we could give the crucial information to the alien would be by saying that the sexual organs are *reproductive* organs. Telling the alien that the organs in question are reproductive should transform its attitude toward human sexual practices; the alien should go from seeing them as a mere collection of quaint customs to seeing that they are ways of reacting to and coping with something of genuine importance. That reproduction matters objectively should be clear to any intelligent animal, whether one that reproduces sexually or asexually. One cannot help but see one's own life as mattering, and it is clear that one's own life is no different in this regard from anyone else's,[31] so that the generation of new lives like one's own, and the enlargement of the community, also matter. After all, the life of a person has a sacredness to it, whether

133

we understand this sacredness as Kantian autonomy, or as being in the image and likeness of God, or as being an unrepeatable individual who has the power of voluntarily contributing to the creation of his, her, or its own character.

That intercourse is treated by humans in a special way even when it does not result in reproduction, and indeed even when it is not intended to do so, will be no great surprise given human attitudes to the sacred. A book of the scriptures is seen as sacred because of what it teaches. But religious people also show respect to a sacred book—sometimes including a sacred book from a different religious tradition—even when the book fails to teach, say because it is in a foreign or sacred language. The place where a sacred event occurred is often venerated, as are items that touched something sacred. Sacredness is seen as communicable. This kind of communicability is not limited to the religious sphere: objects previously owned by people now deceased who were important to us can likewise take on a special meaning. If reproduction is sacred, it is understandable that intercourse would partake of that sacredness. And the sacred is surrounded by a multitude of beliefs, customs, mores, and traditions.

But it is one thing to say that the alien will understand something about why we attach importance to sexuality when it sees that sexual activity is done with reproductive organs, and another to say that this importance will be *justified* to the alien. The alien may well understand the way humans see the sacredness of an object, event, or activity as spreading or communicating itself to other objects, events, or activities associated with it, but consider this an aspect of human religious irrationality. Even so, it is plausible that the alien will see an importance in the *organs* that produce intelligent life. In any case, it should now be clear that without the sexual organs being characterized as "the human reproductive organs," it would be much more mysterious why we humans attach so much importance to sexuality. All this strongly suggests the reproductive function of the central case of sexual intercourse has much to do with explaining the importance that the act has for us. And if we take this importance to be objective, as we should in light of chapters 3 and 4, then somehow the connection of reproduction has to enter in a central way into our account of the objective meaning of human sexuality.

Seeing the sexual organs as *reproductive organs* does not imply that other purposes cannot or even ought not be served by them. But it does tell us what these organs are, and suggests that an account of sexual activity should involve a central focus on the organs' reproductive role. It is this role that seems to be the relevant difference between these organs and others. Without it, all we would have is the bits of gut rubbing together and making slime. This rubbing would have social, emotional, or spiritual consequences, but the fleshly act would not be deeply meaningful in itself. On the other hand, human reproduction is both meaningful and a part of the fleshly nature of the act.

Let us, then, use this insight in conjunction with the notion of functional union as one body. In the central case, sexual union is constituted by a certain joining of the reproductive organs. Moreover, they are not joined in just any which way, but in the reproductive way; the penis is within the vagina. The male organs in the central case produce not just any slime but gamete-bearing semen. The female organs, far from being passive, frictionally produce physical stimulation that can be appropriately thought of as striving to elicit this semen—this is already a genuine form of cooperation. The semen then enters the female reproductive tract. Cervical mucus attempts to filter out poorly formed sperm.[32] It appears that, at least in nonpregnant fertile women, the female reproductive system is, by itself, sufficient to transport gametes, even without any activity on the part of the spermatozoa; radioactively marked immotile particles placed in the vagina begin to show up in the uterus within two minutes.[33] During some parts of the reproductive cycle, the particles are further transported by the female reproductive system into the fallopian tubes by peristaltic contractions in the uterus and the muscular layers of the fallopian tubes,[34] which may or may not be independent of intercourse.[35] When the woman is aroused, the female reproductive system also appears to delay the spermatozoal transport so as to allow sperm "to acquire the power to fertilize called capacitation."[36]

What we see in uncontracepted intercourse, then, is a mutual organic striving for reproduction (whether it is there in contracepted intercourse will be discussed in section 13 of chapter 7). This striving is cooperative and mutually regulated in various ways, though certain aspects of the striving are only present at some times (e.g., outside of pregnancy). And the goal of the striving is best understood as a goal of the whole organisms, because their goal is to produce offspring genetically like the father and the mother. The goal is, in significant part, something at the biological level—it is a part of the very concept of biological life that life should produce new life—but at the same time, in human reproduction, the child produced transcends the merely biological, since he or she is also a person, a being in the image and likeness of God. What we have here fits with the analysis of organic union: the man and woman unite in a biological way, much like the way parts of a body are united together. And, in fact, by uniting together in this way, they become more truly a living organism, since it is only when they are so united that human adults[37] naturally reproduce.

I am not claiming that successful reproduction is needed for sexual union. A couple might have sex on Monday and fertilization might not occur until as late as the next Sunday, and it is implausible to tie the sexual union to Sunday's fertilization—after all, the man might even be dead by then. Rather, it is the bodies' mutual *striving* for reproduction that is involved in union. Whether reproduction results or not, the bodies' mutual striving unites them, just as when a mammal's optical nerve is damaged, its eyes still unsuccessfully strive together with the brain to obtain information about the environment, and hence are functionally united with the brain.

Nor is *conscious or deliberate* striving for reproduction needed for union as one body. That the bodies are striving for reproduction is sufficient here. We are, after all, talking of a union as one *flesh*, and this is a union of a type in which earthworms can engage, though the union has much greater significance in our case. At the same time, when one's body strives for something, even unconsciously, we do attribute this striving to the person. We might say of a woman in a coma that she is struggling for breath, and this would not be a metaphor. Human beings are not ghosts dwelling in bodies. Rather, whatever their bodies do, this *the persons* do, even if unconsciously. It is *I* who breathe in my sleep, not just my lungs. We do not always retain this fact linguistically, as, for instance, we do not say that I beat my heart, but the question is one of truth and not linguistics. Our bodies are not alien to us. We are beings of flesh and blood; we are from dust and to dust we shall return. What our bodies do, this we do, though our activity may well go beyond that of the body. It is also worth noting that, aside from the innate plausibility of seeing the body as a part of us and the fact that only if we see it in this way can we understand the full significance of sexual deeds, Catholic Christians have an additional reason for accepting the claim that we do what our bodies do: this claim follows from the teaching of the Council of Vienne that the soul is the form of the body.

The reproductive account can take onboard both the insight that pleasure is significant as well as the insight that many additional "higher aims" are promoted in intercourse. Ideally, we should have a conscious way of experiencing our significant activities. The objective union arising from reproductive striving, as well as the reproductive striving itself, are goods. Goods are humanly experienced by taking pleasure in them. Moreover, to take pleasure in the good of union with another is a way of taking pleasure in the other. Thus, pleasure makes the sexual activity be experienced more fully by the couple, though the activity can still occur without such an experience.

It is no surprise if an activity that has reproduction as its biological goal results in a number of additional goods. Since it would be good for a child to be cared for by two parents, it is quite appropriate that the sexual act should unite a couple psychologically. And it is no surprise if an act so intimately connected to *human* reproduction—the reproduction of a being in the image and likeness of God—should have a sacredness and be capable of carrying deep spiritual significance.

10. THEOLOGICAL CONNECTIONS, ONCE AGAIN

Parallels between sexuality and ecclesiology can continue at the finer level of detail we have now. The New Testament presents the Church as a whole as fruitful. A particularly interesting case is in Revelation 12, where the "woman clothed with the sun" gives birth. The child is clearly Christ (see verse 5: the child "is to rule all the nations with a rod of iron"). But it does not appear that the woman in the text is just Mary. For instance, verse 6 has her fleeing into the wilderness *after* the child is enthroned in heaven, which fits better with the Church—which needs to flee from the powers of Satan as represented by Rome—than with Mary, who had to flee from Herod when her child was not yet glorified. The woman seems to be both Mary and the Church, and gives birth both to Christ (verse 5) and to believers (verse 17). As both Mary and Church, she is fruitful. As Mary, Christ is her fruit. As Church we might understand her giving birth to believers, as well as giving birth to Christ in the hearts of the believers. Moreover, the notion of good works as *fruit* of our transformation in Christ, is constant in the New Testament. This transformation, however, is not merely individual: we are united as the Church, and as the Church we bear fruit collectively.

In the Western version of the doctrine of the Trinity, the Father and the Son are fruitful. The Father and the Son are united in their production of the Holy Spirit—united to such an extent that the Father and the Son are a single originating principle in producing the Holy Spirit. And we can say a similar thing even on some Eastern accounts. St. John of Damascus is open to the notion of the Holy Spirit proceeding from the Father through the Son,[38] and there does not appear to be anything wrong with talking of this proceeding as arising from the Father's love for the Son.

Both Christ's love for the Church and intra-Trinitarian love are, thus, innately fruitful, though, while Trinitarian love is eternally fruitful in the Holy Spirit, Christ's love for the Church need not bear fruit in the hearts of all due to our free will. When we see sexual union as an image of intra-Trinitarian love and the love between Christ and the Church, the reproductive aspects of sexual union become highlighted as well.

11. PLEASURE, DESIRE, AND VALUE

But something is left out by the above focus on reproduction. We *do* have the intuition that sexual pleasure has something important to do with erotic love. While the central case of sexual intercourse would continue to have meaning if pleasure were removed, it would not be quite what the couple seeks. Anticipation of pleasure may be closer to the conscious motivation of the lovers than a mutual striving for reproduction would be. We could say that the lovers are wrong here, but it would be preferable if we found a way to work this fact into the account.

To that end, let us assume an Aristotelian account of pleasure as an affective perception of an independent good. A biological striving for a good goal is, in and of itself, of value, a part of biological life as it is meant to be, and in the sexual case, is also good as productive of the good of union. It becomes plausible that sexual pleasure might be an affective perception of the good of this striving. After all, given the assumed account of pleasure, sexual pleasure had better be an affective perception of some good or other. The fleshly nature of sexual pleasure strongly suggests that the good reflected by sexual pleasure is a biological one. And a striving for reproduction seems to be the best candidate for the biological good here.

Of course the person having sex may be quite unaware that what distinguishes sexual pleasure from other pleasures is that it is a perception of this mutual striving. But that kind of lack of awareness can be found in other cases of perception. For instance, two hundred years ago it was not known that when we feel heat, we are perceiving the kinetic energy of molecules. Likewise, if pleasure is a perception of a good, pain is a perception of something bad. But we do get pains in internal body parts, indicating damage to those parts, without having much of an idea which parts these are. There is a real sense in which sometimes we do not know what it is that we are conscious of.[39]

Moreover, if pleasure and that which is enjoyed are as tightly interconnected as the Aristotelian account suggests, then in desiring sexual pleasure, one is at least implicitly desiring the pleasure of uniting with someone in a unified reproductive striving. Furthermore, the general structure of our desire is such that not only do we desire the pleasure of x, but we also desire x itself, unless we explicitly qualify our desire as that of the *mere* pleasure of x. Normally we want to eat the cake, and not merely have the pleasure of eating the cake. Thus, except for the exceptional case where the couple *merely* wants the pleasure of sexual union, they want the pleasure of sexual union as reflecting whatever mysterious underlying good is there, whether they can conceptualize this good or not. Similarly, in typical cases, the hungry person wants nourishment, not the mere cessation of physical discomfort. And someone who does not know that the physical discomfort in hunger is due to a lack of nourishment would still be wanting food implicitly, without realizing it. Thus, those who desire sexual pleasure in intercourse, unless the structure of their action shows that they are focused on *mere* sexual pleasure, are likely desiring the union or united striving that the pleasure, perhaps unbeknownst to them, reflects.

This account provides an answer to a problem set by juxtaposing insights of Aristotle and Kant. According to Aristotle, the virtuous person *enjoys* doing good things. However, Kant argues that such enjoyment endangers the moral value of the act, because the virtuous person is in danger of acting for the sake of pleasure rather than for the sake of duty. Now consider Michael Stocker's case of visiting a sick friend.[40] A virtuous person enjoys doing this. Moreover, one will be happiest at being visited by friends who come *because* they enjoy being with one. Yet on Kantian grounds, this enjoyment seems to endanger the moral value of the visits, because, then, duty is not in view. Yet if we see pleasure and that in which pleasure is taken as tightly bound together—with the pleasure receiving its meaning from the pleasant activity—then we can see that in normal cases the person who comes to visit because she enjoys being with her friend is *also* desiring to be with her friend. For in normal cases, friends do not merely desire the pleasure of company—they would not take a pleasure-of-visiting-sick-friend pill instead. Rather they desire the veridical case of that pleasure, the case where the pleasure of company actually comes from that company. We cannot separate one's being moved by pleasure from one's being moved by the value of the company, because the pleasure is a perception of that value, and it is because of pleasure being such a perception that this pleasure matters.

In a case where someone wants sexual pleasure, we may often have the familiar phenomenon of someone wanting something but not knowing what it is that he or she wants. It may even be that someone who really wants veridical sexual pleasure misinterprets the desire as one for *merely* sexual pleasure, and then attempts to have such pleasure in isolation, for instance through pornography, only to be disappointed in the end.

Of course, if a couple explicitly wants their bodies *not* to engage in a mutual striving for reproduction, then it is more difficult to describe their sexual desire as a desire for such a striving. But even then it is possible. People do have conflicting desires, sometimes consciously and sometimes not. One might be thirsty and not want to drink—one sees this with some small children. Nonetheless, we need not say that in *all* cases the couple really "deep down" desires such a mutual striving. Perhaps they do not. Maybe they really do merely want pleasure, without sexual union behind it. Note, though, that if someone really wanted pleasure only and did not want *anything at all* behind it, this desire would also falsify the Augustinian conviction that all our desires are ultimately desires for God.

If we see a mutual striving for reproduction as at the heart of sexual union, and see sexual pleasure as the perception of the value of this striving or the union, then it becomes clear why sexual pleasure is valuable in the central case. For in the central case, the sexual pleasure goes together with that striving or union and is a perception of it. But perception of a good thing is itself good and the striving is a good thing, since it is a biological function naturally directed at a good goal, and since it is unitive by making the two biologically into one flesh. Union, in turn, is intrinsically valuable as a deeper way of being, as a form of being-together.

A critic might respond that the biological striving has no value unless it actually achieves its goal. However, a *natural* biological striving in a human being is always valuable in itself (though it may be contextually inappropriate), since it is the normal functioning of a creature made in the image and likeness of God. Furthermore, it is good to work for a good goal even when the goal is unachieved. This is clear if the goal is consciously sought. To work for some social cause, such as the cause of elimination of poverty, is good, even if no progress is actually made. And to work together with someone else to eliminate poverty is even better, since such cooperation is unitive: it makes the two have the same goal: to work together, much as a single body functions. Working for a good goal is good even when the activity is not conscious, and even if the activity does not succeed. It is a good thing that the immune system strives to fight off invaders, even if, in the end, it sadly fails. The cooperation of many organic subsystems makes immunity an impressive thing, a valuable thing, a reflection, howsoever pale, of God's power and wisdom, and in a faint way, even a reflection of the multiplicity of persons in the Godhead, who have but one common activity.

This good of striving in common with the other person is essential to sexuality. Desiring this good for oneself *might,* in a particular case, be very closely allied with desiring it for the other, so that there is a very natural tie between desiring sexual pleasure, desiring the activity that constitutes sexual union for oneself, and desiring the good of this activity for the other. And it is plausible that there is something wrong, maybe even perverse, when these ties are broken.

12. HIGHER GOALS REVISITED

Working together with others on a sports team can develop various virtues, such as perseverance, an ability to fail gracefully ("good sportsmanship"), and a cooperativeness that involves a humble recognition of the need to work with others. These are "higher goals" and in the larger scheme of things, they are much more important than victory in the game or the physical striving for victory. Nonetheless, it would be a mistake to see the members of a soccer team as united by a common striving to learn to fail gracefully, or even by a common striving to learn to cooperate. One best learns to cooperate by actually cooperating in something other than learning to cooperate. The higher-level goals in sports are achieved by a physical striving for victory. And it may well be that the best way to achieve these higher-level goals is by focusing primarily on the lower-level goal of victory, while maintaining a vigilance that one's pursuit of the lower-level goals not be contrary to the higher-level ones.

The lower-level goals, like victory or getting the ball in the net, may not be one's reason for engaging in the activity. One might sign up for a sports team precisely because one thinks—or is told by one's parents—that one needs to develop cooperativeness. But to be playing a game one needs to do something beyond developing cooperativeness: one needs to be *playing the game*, striving to win. This striving need not even be conscious. One might not consciously desire victory. A standard case is one in which a parent is engaging in a competitive game with a child. The parent may hope the child will win. But if it is really to be a case of both playing the game, as opposed to just practicing, the parent cannot throw the match—the parent must strive to win while hoping the child will win.

Take a chess master who plays a game well against a weaker opponent and is too tired to care about the result. She is skillfully engaging in a practice the goal of which is victory, but victory is not explicitly on her mind. If one were to ask her what she was doing, she would say: "I am playing chess," and if one were to ask her what the object of the game is, she could say: "Checkmating the opponent." To play a game involves seeking victory, and she is *implicitly* seeking victory. If, however, she told us that she had placed a large wager that she would lose and that she was aiming to win the wager and not to win the game, then in an important sense she would not really be playing the game but throwing the match.

Thus, in games there often are higher goals—and these may be what motivates a person—but pursuit of these goals is not what constitutes the game as such. What constitutes the game as such is the pursuit of the goal of victory. And neither the pursuit of the higher-level or the lower-level goals needs to be conscious.

Even if what physically unites the couple as one body is just a biological striving for reproduction, this does not rule out the possibility that many other goals, at spiritual, cognitive, emotional, or psychological levels, are also served precisely by that union. One of our objections against some of the spiritual accounts was that they did not make clear what it was about the physical act that made it have the spiritual effects. Why should intercourse produce a result that some other instance of "rubbing together of pieces" of bodily parts would not? But intercourse, seen as an activity biologically aimed at reproduction, is a genuine physical union. And our bodies are intimately connected with our minds or souls, so that it is natural that what we do meaningfully with our bodies should have meaningful effects on our minds or souls.

Sexual pleasure is a correlate of such union. Union is experienced to a significant degree through the physical pleasure, and an experience of physical union can be unitive psychologically and emotionally. Normally, every cooperative activity with another helps the people involved to get to know each other, so cognitive goals will normally be served by sexual union.

It is natural for us as human beings, creatures of flesh and blood, to attain higher goals through lower-level activities. Consider, for instance, the way that a spirit of generous love can be developed by feeding those too young, too old, or too disabled to feed themselves— the messier the physical process, the more generous the activity here. What we do with our bodies in cooperation with others matters, not just on the physical level, but also for us as *persons*. And often the nonbiological effects happen in and through an activity that would not make sense, and would not have the same effect, if it were biologically different. If putting a spoon in someone's mouth were not a way of trying to nourish that person, spoon-feeding a child might be an ascetical practice to develop patience, but it would not have the same relevance to becoming more generous that it does.

Theologically, this is clearest in the Incarnation, where God's love for us is revealed in his taking on our flesh, living a human life, with all its glories and indignities, culminating in a humiliating death which exhibited the naked and tortured flesh to all, and then manifesting a glorification of that very same flesh. A view of sexuality that focused on the higher-level goals to the exclusion of the underlying biological reality would be akin to what one might call a more moderate Docetism.

Full Docetism was the heresy which denied that God really became a human being. Influenced by a Gnostic or Neoplatonic disdain for the body, the Docetics thought God only *seemed* to have taken on flesh. A more moderate Docetism would be an attitude rather than a heresy, an attitude in which the physical Incarnation is largely discounted in favor of a focus on the divinity of Christ. Such a Docetism is also exhibited in an impulse to take stories of the history of salvation and *reduce* them to an underlying spiritual meaning—for instance, taking accounts of physical healing and reducing their content to some doctrine, such as that Christ as God cared for our well-being. Docetism, however, always runs the danger of undercutting what it thinks is most important. A Christological Docetist holds that the illusory earthly life of Christ reveals to us something about God's love for us. However, the deeper meaning of an *illusory* earthly life of love for us would likely be that God's love for us is a deceptive illusion. Similarly, if the fleshly union in sexuality does not, itself, matter, even though it *feels* deeply significant, then the fleshly union becomes a symbol of a deceptive union that is less than it seems.

Finally, however, we must observe that a reproductive focus by itself goes beyond the merely biological, because human beings are not merely biological. In human reproduction, a being in the image and likeness of God is produced. The sexual faculties of the lovers are thus cooperating in a way that, if successful, will involve the creation by God of a new being capable of love and reason. That a physical union centered on such cooperation should have higher-level concomitants is unsurprising.

13. OBJECTIONS

i. Reproductive striving is not what people in love actually want. An account of sexual union should fit with what people who love each other romantically actually want. But while some may want children, that wanting is, arguably, not constitutive of their romantic love for each other; romantic love can surely exist apart from such a desire, sometimes giving rise to it later and sometimes not.

In response, we might remember that it is one thing to desire a goal and another to desire the striving for that goal. In wanting to play soccer, one at least implicitly wants to strive for victory. But one might not actually want victory—one might simply want to have something to strive for. However, this response, while helpful, is not sufficient. For it is not only that the desire to have children might be absent in romantic love, but it seems that one might also not have any explicit desire to engage in activities that involve physical striving for reproduction. Reproduction may be nowhere on the minds of the people involved. This may be either because they desire a form of sexual activity other than heterosexual intercourse, or because they do not know about the reproductive potential of intercourse,[41] or because they know but do not care about this potential.

However, as we saw in chapter 3, people can fail to understand what it is that they desire. One might not know that A is constituted by B, and hence not know that in desiring A one is implicitly desiring B. Someone who wants a room to become warmer is implicitly, and often unwittingly, desiring to increase the kinetic energy of air molecules. It is highly plausible that romantic love involves a desire for sexual union as one body—for a total sharing, total union, at the bodily level. But this union is constituted, I have argued, by a mutual biological striving for reproduction. In desiring union, the members of the couple are implicitly desiring the biological striving that constitutes it.

One might observe a group of people and say to oneself: "I'd like to be a part of that group, to have the kind of togetherness with them that they have with each other." One might make this observation without knowing that the group of people is a soccer team or a group of monks traveling incognito. In desiring the particular kind of togetherness that these people have, one is implicitly desiring the activity that unites them, even if one does not know what this activity is. One might even be conflicted or confused, desiring the kind of togetherness that the soccer team has without wanting to play sports— though playing sports together is largely constitutive of the togetherness. A togetherness could be had without playing sports, but it would not be *that kind* of togetherness. Likewise, it may well be that the couple in love romantically wants to have the kind of togetherness that paradigmatic couples in consummated romantic love have, without realizing that this togetherness involves a union as one body.

ii. Activity other than intercourse. Consider the members of a couple in romantic love, who desire to engage in some other activity than heterosexual intercourse. It seems harder to argue that they implicitly desire sexual union, as understood along the lines of this book.

We will discuss noncoital orgasmic activity at greater length in chapter 8, but right now note that if there is genuine romantic love, then the couple seeks that which consummates romantic love, and this includes, whether they know it or not, sexual union. If sexual union is constituted by a mutual, biological reproductive striving, then this is what the couple implicitly desires.

We can also say that noncoital sexual activity derives significance from its similarity to, and often the use of at least one of the same organs as in, coital sexual activity, as well as from the typically aimed-at pleasure, which is in fact the pleasure associated with mutual, one-body union. This also helps explain the significance of cases of rape that do not involve heterosexual vaginal penetration, but also points to a special kind of badness in the latter kind of rape since it appears to involve an unconsented-to one-body union.

iii. Heterosexual intercourse need not include mutual striving for reproduction. While heterosexual intercourse can sometimes be seen as involving such a mutual striving, arguably this striving is not always present. Consider cases of infertility, pregnancy, menopause, or hysterectomy. In some, and maybe all, of these cases, the objection continues, there is no mutual striving for reproduction. Now, the objection ends by giving a dilemma. Either sexual acts in these cases do not involve a sexual union, or sexual union has been misrepresented by the account defended in this book. But the first horn of the dilemma cannot be accepted. For Christians have never taken sexual activity by infertile couples to be wrong or even taken it as failing to be unitive. For example, the Catholic canon law tradition has held that uncontracepted,[42] freely chosen sexual intercourse by a couple that has had a valid wedding is a consummation regardless of fertility.[43] It would be highly implausible to say that romantic love by, say, a postmenopausal woman could not be consummated. This leaves the second horn of the dilemma, namely, that this book misunderstands sexual union.

To respond, note first that some cases of infertility are easy to handle. These are simply cases where there is a genuine biological striving for reproduction, but reproduction does not result. The sperm swim, but not far enough. The woman takes in the sperm, but her body does not have an ovum ready at the time. After all, the team that lost a soccer game still strove for victory. Even futile striving is real striving: the man struggling to push a ferocious and hungry lion away with his bare hands really *is* striving for survival. This is true even if the activity is purely automatic. In fact, it is even true if the man actually wants to die, say, because he expects a martyr's reward but believes it is his God-given duty to struggle for life. Thus, in more moderate cases of infertility we can just say there is an unsuccessful biological striving for reproduction.

A similar thing can be said about even the most extreme cases, such as that of a woman whose ovaries, fallopian tubes, and uterus were all removed, in which case conception is not physically possible. Even then, the woman's body is striving to elicit genetic material from the man by striving to provide physical stimulation, or maybe just by providing a passageway to the normal location of further reproductive organs, which in this case are missing. The bodily parts involved "do not know" that the further organs are missing; the nature of the striving by the parts that are present is, thus, basically unaffected, and these parts strive reproductively.

Consider the consequences of claiming that the woman's body is not striving reproductively in such cases. It would mean that either (a) her sexual organs are no longer reproductive organs, or (b) they are not engaging in the reproductive type of activity in which they engage when the woman is fertile. If her organs are no longer reproductive organs, then we, once again, have the problem of how to describe these organs to an alien—or to ourselves—in a way that makes their significance clear. In either of cases (a) and (b), sexual intercourse is an essentially different kind of biological process when engaged in by an infertile couple than when engaged in by a fertile couple, since in case (a) it is done with different kinds of organs while in case (b) the organs are doing something other than they would be were the couple fertile. But surely intercourse is not an essentially different kind of biological process in cases of infertility. We should think of these organs as reproductive ones, and as engaged in the activity characteristic of them, even when conception is physically impossible. And the characteristic activity of reproductive organs is to strive for reproduction.

This does not mean that *all* changes to the reproductive systems are compatible with continued sexual union. Should the woman's vagina close up completely, in such a way that it would no longer count at all as cooperating in reproductive activity, or should the man be impotent, sexual union would cease to be possible. And we generally *do* recognize that cases like this are different from the central case of sexual intercourse. The couple can cuddle and kiss, but their sexual love cannot be consummated.

iv. Coitus interruptus. While objection iii claimed that the present account is too restrictive as to what counts as sexual union, one may also give the opposite objection. It seems that coitus interruptus, where coition is stopped accidentally or deliberately before the man ejaculates, should not count as the same kind of activity as "completed" sexual intercourse. Now, Christian tradition has treated coitus interruptus and intercourse differently, holding the interrupted variety to be immoral when planned intentionally. Indeed, it is intuitively clear that there is something incomplete in coitus interruptus. Yet, the objection continues, even in coitus interruptus the two bodies are striving in a reproductive direction, as can be seen from the response to objection iii, and while the striving is incomplete, the case should be no more problematic than cases of infertility. Thus, the present objection continues, by the account of this book, coitus interruptus counts as a consummation of romantic love, which according to the Christian tradition it is not.

There are two ways to respond. First, one might admit that coitus interruptus does produce full sexual union as one body.[44] If so, then in respect of the union, it is on par with cases of completed intercourse in which conception does not result. If one opted to claim that coitus interruptus was productive of sexual union, one could then take two stances toward the traditional Christian condemnation. One might, on the one hand, say that this condemnation is mistaken. Or, on the other hand, one might say that the condemnation still holds, but not due to a lack of full sexual union. There might be *other* reasons why coitus interruptus is wrong. For instance, Grisez, Boyle, Finnis, and May[45] have argued that contraception is wrong because it is an intentional act against human life, and it can be argued that the interruption in coitus interruptus is a case of this.

However, a better way to respond is that something important is missing in coitus interruptus that is present in the central case. The sexual union is interrupted before its normal denouement. Plainly, there can be degrees of physical union. In some way, two bodies are striving together reproductively as soon as two people are mutually sexually attracted to each other—each attracted also by the other's attraction to him or her, as in Nagel's account of sex[46]—even if no contact ensues. But such striving is incomplete and not just because reproduction has yet to occur (for in that sense "completed" sexual intercourse would often be incomplete even in the central case, since fertilization can occur up to six days from intercourse). Rather, the striving is incomplete in that not everything that the two bodies *do together* in the reproductive process has yet been done. In other words, the *mutual* part of the process has not been completed, either in the coitus interruptus case or in the mutual attraction example.

Consider my being intellectually united with fellow teammates as part of a scholastic competition where we together accomplish some task that is to be judged, and where every team member's role is essential to completing the task. My union with my teammates is incomplete if I quit before completing my part of our common striving toward victory. It is true that we have striven together and have been united, but the union was not complete because I did not complete my part, whether because I quit deliberately or was forcibly detained. However, once the common part of the task is complete, what the judges say later does not affect our union as striving teammates. It is quite possible that I might not stick around while the judges are deliberating, but it will be no less true that I was completely united in respect of the intellectual union with my teammates, just as the man that Paul says has been united with a prostitute might not stick around to find out whether she got pregnant or not, but was nonetheless united with her.

v. The penis. The penis is not just a reproductive organ, however, but also a urinary one. As a result, even on a biological level, the objection goes, it is mistaken to focus on its reproductive role.

That the penis has a reproductive and a urinary role is clear. But two points should be made. The first is that the penis's urinary role is simply typically not relevant to understanding what the male does in intercourse. The second is that while sometimes for simplicity one might talk of the penis as if it were the male reproductive organ, it is not in fact *the* male reproductive organ. It is in itself but a part of the male reproductive system, and other parts of the system are also involved in the ejaculatory process. While the penis by itself is also a part of the urinary system, the male reproductive system as a whole is not the same as the urinary system—for instance, the seminal vesicles, ejaculatory ducts, and the vas deferens are not parts of the urinary system.

vi. This account makes female orgasm inessential. Female orgasm does not significantly contribute to the reproductive potential of the act. Thus, in an account centered on reproduction, female orgasm is not essential to the act in the way that male orgasm is. Hence, the argument continues, this account privileges male pleasure, male orgasm being essential and female not.

This objection equivocates between the word "orgasm" as indicative of a muscular phenomenon and a conscious pleasure. While I have typically used the word for the conscious phenomenon of orgasmic pleasure, in the claim that male orgasm is essential, the objection must take the word to indicate the physiological phenomena of ejaculation or release of muscular tension. For it is only the physiological ejaculation that is essential on the part of the man; whether the man is conscious of pleasure is not essential to union on the present account. Orgasm in the sense of ejaculation does not require any consciousness of pleasure. Orgasm in the pleasure sense, thus, is inessential in the case of *both* the man and the woman. But the complaint was that the account privileges male *pleasure*, which does not follow from the claim that physiological ejaculation is essential. Admittedly, there is a strong correlation between male pleasure and physiological ejaculation, but the two phenomena are distinct.

Nonetheless, the subjective pleasure, while inessential, *is* important on the present account, and equally so on both sides, as was remarked in sections 9 and 11 above. For a deep union to be fully human, it should be experienced on all the levels of a human being. Without the pleasure, the union can be experienced intellectually and certainly takes place biologically. But the pleasure provides a vivid *perception* of the good of union or of the striving for reproduction. A consciously perceived phenomenon is one that is more truly ours. We are unsatisfied with mere intellectual knowledge: we want to *see* things. We often say things like: "He has never experienced this, so he does not really understand it." There is a kind of incompleteness in knowledge when it is not perceptually based, given how important the senses are to our lives.

Moreover, there may be *some* functional connection between the physical phenomena accompanying the consciousness of female orgasm and reproduction.[47]

vii. Integration requires the couple to intend procreation. The present account is meant to be compatible with the couple's not intending procreation, so long as they do not oppose procreation. But, the objection continues, the couple needs to be integrated on both a personal and a biological level, and this integration requires that they voluntarily endorse the goals of their bodies, and in particular the reproductive goal, by intending procreation. One should, then, modify the present account by adding this fact, or so the objection goes. In light of arguments in succeeding chapters, this modification would eventually have significant consequences, making it wrong to engage in sexual intercourse except with the intention of procreation. But this would be absurd, since it is plainly possible for a marriage with a woman who is either already pregnant or is past the age of childbearing to be consummated, and it would be a stretch to suppose the couple to be intending procreation. Hence, the objection concludes, the present account needs to be rejected.

The main response to this is that the plausible idea that integration requires the willing of the body's purposes must be mistaken. If the argument were correct, the integration of a human being as an individual of body and mind would seem to be most thorough when each of the purposes of a bodily function were also willed by the human being. But in fact, many of our bodily functions are ones the importance of which we become aware only when things go awry. One may have a very hazy idea of what one's liver does, until it is damaged and the doctor tells one about the consequences of the damage. And, hypochondriac that I am, as soon as I start thinking too hard about my breathing, my breathing becomes erratic, and when I think about the oxygenation breathing is supposed to provide, I start wondering whether I am breathing enough, and I begin to feel funny feelings in my fingertips. When things are going smoothly, many bodily functions proceed to their respective ends with little accompanying awareness of the functioning, and often even less awareness of the purpose.

I can be integrated in mind and body if I simply have a general intention that the body should "do its job" or "do its job well," without much of an idea of what that job is. And the body's doing its job well or even excellently is not measured by success at fulfilling its purposes. For it is possible for *both* sides in a sports game to do their job excellently, and yet, at most, one side will achieve victory, and so the other side will have done its job excellently but unsuccessfully.

A variant of the objection is that if we are to have mind-body integration, not only should we will that the body do its job well, but we should will that it do it successfully. But the successful functioning of the reproductive systems results in actual reproduction.

At least three responses can be made. One, perhaps unsatisfactory, is that it may be possible to intend a whole without intending a part. Maybe one can intend that everyone get a reward, while hoping that Martha doesn't. Thus, one might intend that all the bodily systems' purposes be fulfilled, without intending that reproduction should occur.

The second response is that integration between mind and body really does not require the mind to will the success of the bodily functions even in general terms. We do not know the myriad of bodily functions that go on in our bodies. It would be irresponsible, and hence contrary to the proper functioning of the mind, for us to intend that all of these functions should be successful, since we do not know enough about them all. Integration of mind and body is threatened when the mind and body fight each other, but is not threatened when the mind simply does not will the success of some of the bodily functions, as long as it does not will the lack of success.

There is a third response, and this is to note that the parts and aspects of a human person, however integrated the individual may be, can have purposes that are, on some level, at variance with one another. My ears bring information to the attention of the brain while the brain is trying to sleep. Organic functioning can involve a balance between functions that, at a lower level, are opposed to one another. The integration involved in willing all one's bodily functions to succeed on their own level would be something available only to a nonhuman whose organism lacked opposed functions at any level. Even if romantic love calls for a maximality of union, it calls for that maximality only so far as it is possible within the confines of normal human life. If my parts can have purposes at variance with one another, it seems problematic that I should intend that they all succeed; for to intend is to be willing to promote, and such willingness would involve a lack of integrity in my mind.

What I can do, however, is *wish* that all the purposes of my body be fulfilled, and perhaps bodily integration involves such a wish. The wish need only be a general one, and we *can* wish for conflicting things. We can watch two excellent boxers and wish for each to win. If this is right, then it could be that integration requires the couple to wish for procreation to take place. This is quite compatible with the couple's wishing more strongly to avoid the serious financial difficulties that would result from procreation in their circumstances.

But I do not endorse the conclusion that full personal integration in sexual union requires any procreative wish. For it seems that mere wishes have little significance in the mental life of a person, and hence may not contribute to integration in any significant way.

viii. All this is theologically a great stretch. The scriptural data on which the present account is based is mainly that there is supposed to be a union as "one flesh" and "one body." But there is nothing in the biblical text to suggest that this union is produced in a mutual striving for reproduction.

We can respond by first admitting the claim that the texts do not say that there is a mutual striving and certainly do not say that it is for reproduction. However, what I have done is to take the "one flesh" and "one body" texts seriously. They are seminal texts, ones that the biblical and postbiblical traditions take very seriously. They are, Christians should believe, true, and true in a deep way. And if so, it is up to us to examine their implications. I have argued that the best way to understand the union as one flesh and one body is as a union constituted by cooperative reproductive striving.

We can use reason to draw out many conclusions, some interesting and some trivial, from scriptural texts, conclusions that the texts do not actually mention and that the authors did not know. Thus, from the report that there were twelve apostles, together with empirical observation, we can conclude that the number of apostles is twice the number of legs on a butterfly. In this case, we get a theologically uninteresting truth. Slightly less trivially, our reason-based knowledge of the effects of lead exposure, in conjunction with the scriptural command to love one's neighbor, implies that it is wrong to feed large quantities of lead to children. It does not matter here that the authors of scripture had no idea how lead intake interacts with brain development.

The arguments we have rehearsed earlier in this chapter suggest how the position I am defending might have been implicit in the biblical authors' views. It would have been unreasonable for the authors to have thought that union as one body consists merely in physical contact as such, since physical contact clearly occurs in many contexts without the profound implications of sexual union. It seems quite plausible that they would see sexual union as constituted in some unique way by the act actually performed. And if asked to describe the act, and pressed as to how the organs involved are different from other organs, they might well respond that they are the organs with which progeny are produced. In fact, writing in a context where effective contraception was unavailable, the link between sexual activity and reproduction would not have been far from their minds. After all, the first time the Yahwist author presents Adam and Eve as engaging in sexual relations, he also presents conception as occurring (Gen. 4:1). And, at least until very recently, Christian tradition has pretty much unanimously held that there is a tight normative linkage between sexuality and reproduction.

It is only very recently that it has become possible to think of sex separately from thinking of procreation. Thus, while the present account is not expressly in the scriptural text, it is compatible with the text, and presents what seems to be the best hypothesis as to how the union talked about in the text in fact happens.

14. MORAL IMPLICATIONS

It is tempting at this point to draw various conservative moral conclusions, such as the conclusion that contraception is wrong. But we must not be hasty in this. All we have so far is a characterization of the central case of sexual activity as a reproductive act, and of sexual union as a union in reproductive striving. It does not *immediately* follow that contraception is wrong. At the most, one might argue at this point in the analysis that contraception changes the nature of the act. But there need be nothing obviously wrong with that. After all, everyone agrees that a married couple is at least sometimes morally free to replace a reproductive act with a nonreproductive one: they may, for instance, go out to dinner rather than have fertile sex. If contraception is seen as changing the nature of the act, then we should see the contracepted act as less productive of union as one body. But, again, it does not immediately follow that the act is wrong. Sharing ice cream is less productive of union as one body than intercourse is, but it is not immoral.

Nor does it immediately follow from the characterization of sexual organs and intercourse as "reproductive" that it is wrong to employ them in nonreproductive ways. First of all, organs and bodily processes can have multiple purposes. And, second, there does not appear to be anything immoral, in general, in using an organ or bodily process for a new purpose. Exhalation does not have the blowing out of candles as its primary purpose, but there is nothing wrong with such use.

In particular, the above account of intercourse and union does not beg the question against the proponents of contraception and homosexual activity. If moral conclusions about various controversial issues can be drawn from the above characterization of sexual intercourse, it will take more work to draw them.

However, this is work that I shall argue *can* be done. For while it is acceptable to use exhalation for a completely new function, there is a higher standard for the way we deal with sexual processes. One reason for this higher standard is that sexuality is closely tied to love, and whatever directly concerns love must abide by the highest of standards. Another reason is the sacredness of that which is tied to the production of life. But before we try to draw out moral conclusions from the biological approach, let us look at things from the other direction, that of interpersonal commitment.

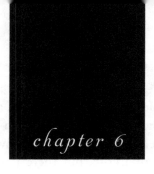

chapter 6

Union, Commitment, and Marriage

1. FORMATION OF A "WE"

I have argued that it is appropriate for higher aspects of the central case of intercourse, such as union of heart and mind, to come about through lower-level ones, like the striving for reproduction. We will not, in fact, analyze the union of heart and mind much further. It is a matter in some ways more suited for exposition in literature than in philosophical argument. But a few remarks might be helpful.

Robert Nozick understands romantic love in terms of the formation of a "common identity," a "we," where the two persons start thinking and acting as if they were parts of a whole, giving up some of their individual autonomy, and taking goods and bads that happen to the other as happening to themselves. That this is, or should be, a feature of romantic love seems quite correct, though Nozick makes the further controversial claim that the full process happens only in the case of *romantic* love. If he is right, then there is a competitor to this book's characterization of romantic love in terms of sexual union—perhaps romantic love can be understood in terms of the mutual surrender of autonomy instead.

It seems that membership in many groups involves some surrender of autonomy and a self-identification as part of the group. Take a stereotypical, traditional English club for men. Membership is by invitation, and it is an honor in terms of which the members identify themselves. There is a concern for the group as a whole and for its unique identity, whether justified or not. This concern is exhibited in upholding of standards of behavior and manners, standards to which one surrenders aspects of one's autonomy, as well as in the exclusion of women, with the conviction that significant changes in the rules for behavior and membership would destroy the club, turning it into a different kind of institution. Social honors or dishonors befalling one member are generally felt as touching all the other members. But we can at least imagine a case, and approximations surely existed, where this is true not just for social goods and bads, but for all goods and bads: in such a club the members will, ideally, treat each other as other selves. Notwithstanding the moral evaluation of this sexist institution, we should say that it could well involve the formation of a "we."

Acquiring a joint identity, surrendering one's autonomy, and having any goods and bads that happen to the other person happen to oneself are features, thus, of other group memberships besides membership in a romantic couple. There may be differences in degree, of course, but it is quite unclear that these features should be definitive of romantic love. The depth of bond between fellow Christians, for instance, that the New Testament presents as an ideal suggests that membership in the Christian Church should involve an even stronger "we" identity than a marriage; the "Pauline privilege," (1 Cor. 7:15) in which a marriage with a non-Christian can be dissolved, is a particularly vivid illustration of this. Nonetheless, even though the formation of a "we" is not an exclusive feature of *romantic* love, a love surely would not be romantic without a tendency toward a "we."

A significant aspect of a union of heart and mind consists of acting together, especially if we understand "acting" broadly enough to include common deliberation and discussion, or maybe just sitting together and feeling the same thing. This sort of union mirrors cooperative sexual activity on a different level. In some cases, the mirroring will be even tighter, in that both the sexual activity and the higher-level activity of the couple will be directed at a closely related goal, the sexual activity being biologically directed at the procreation of offspring while the latter is deliberately directed at care for and education of the offspring, with the education involving physical, emotional, moral, intellectual, and spiritual aspects. In these cases, the union is most integral: all the levels of the two persons are united in at least one set of tightly knit goals.

The higher levels of interpersonal cooperation involved in the union are ultimately more important. Scripturally, this is indicated by the fact that there is no more marriage in heaven (Mark 12:25), but *agapê* remains (1 Cor. 13:13). However, these higher levels are not definitive of romantic love as romantic, because they could exist quite well apart from romantic love—two eunuchs with no sexual interests of any sort could engage in these higher levels of cooperation, including the education of adopted children—even though in our culture couples that raise children are typically in a romantic relationship. Romantic love is defined by a tendency toward the sexual, I have argued. This does not mean that the sexual has to be the most important ingredient, just as soccer is defined by scoring goals and so on, but the associated teamwork is a greater good than victory. Even though romantic love is a unity, we can still think of two aspects of it, the romantic and the agapic. The agapic may be more important, but it is not definitive of romantic love as romantic, since the agapic aspect is common to all other genuine loves.

2. UNCONDITIONALITY, COMMITMENT, AND DEATH

Unconditional love can be seen as a general duty toward all persons, or maybe even all creatures of God (cf. section 8 of chapter 2). At the same time, the unconditionality of love does not imply the unconditionality of the *form* of love. On the contrary, love has an innate responsiveness to the reality of the beloved, and hence may well need to change its form as the lovers change. Thus, while romantic love ought to be unconditional as love, it need not be unconditionally romantic.

Indeed, if romantic love were always unconditionally romantic, then people would be false to their love if they did not marry the first person with whom they were in reciprocated romantic love.

It is plausible that when one talks of, say, the "unconditionality of marital love" or the "unconditionality of paternal love," one means more than just unconditionally having a form of love. The father who assures his children of unconditional love does not simply commit himself to the love that he owes everyone. Rather, he seems to be committed unconditionally to a particular *form* of love. However, this is not entirely correct. For the form of love is conditional on several assumptions here, such as that this person really *is* the same person that has grown up with him. Let us imagine that the father found out that his daughter was kidnapped yesterday and the person in front of him now, to whom he professed unconditional parental love, was not really his daughter, but someone made up to look like her. I think we should not say that he is committed to loving this person *as his daughter*, because this love might be quite inappropriate, especially if his real daughter was returned and the impostor went back to her family. At most there is a commitment to simply *loving* this person in some way or other. And the conditionality of marital love *as marital* follows from there being no marriage in heaven,[1] and hence the love ought to be capable of changing form to a nonmarital form of *agapê*, at least after death.

Nonetheless, marital and parental loves are *relatively* unconditional in form, in the sense that they are grounded in conditions that, at the very least, *should* last for most of a lifetime and, in the case of parental love, even beyond, albeit with adaptations. Marital love carries the condition that the beloved is still alive. This condition, in most cases, is satisfied for a significant length of time. Parental love carries the condition that the beloved either be one's child biologically or have been treated as one's child for a sufficient proportion of the latter's childhood. Again, apart from relatively rare cases, if this condition is once known to be met, it typically will be known to be met for the rest of a natural life.

Scripturally, marriage—and hence presumably also marital and sexual love—stops at death. There is good philosophical reason for this. Sexual love receives its unique identity from the bodies of the two persons. It is plausible that when the body is destroyed at death, the love needs to be transformed. The maximal amount of continuous physical commitment that is possible lasts until the death of one of the parties. Given that romantic love calls for the deepest possible union at all levels of the person, especially including the physical level, it is plausible that romantic love calls for something like this kind of commitment, namely, for a marriage "until death do us part." Granted, after death, there will be a resurrection of the glorified body, Christians believe. However, marriage is a natural state of human beings, while this resurrection is something supernatural. It is no surprise if marriage does not, then, outlast death.

At the same time, the form of love should always take into account the relevant particularities of the persons' relationship. One's love for a deceased spouse, while not a properly marital love, should have a form particular to love for a deceased *spouse,* a love that differs from the love for a deceased *child.* In this life, we might call this "widowed love." We can see that widowed love is not the same as marital love from the fact that widowed love for a deceased spouse can legitimately continue even after one remarries. And it is particularly in the case of remarriage that it is essential that the widow love not be a marital love—it is unfortunate for someone to be married to a person who has a marital love for a deceased spouse.[2] The difficulties involved in this change of form in the love help justify the somewhat grudging nature of the Church's traditional acceptance of remarriage after a spouse's death (e.g., 1 Cor. 7:8–9).

In heaven, the possibility of continuing interaction will presumably transform the widowed love into some other form of love qualified by the shared history of marriage, a form we can only guess at.

3. THE THOROUGHNESS OF SEXUAL UNION

Sexual intercourse is the most thoroughgoing form of biological unity as one body in which two human beings voluntarily, mutually, and equally can engage.[3] To see this, consider the three other deep cases of biological unity: Siamese twins, the union between a pregnant or breastfeeding mother and her child, and a group of people working together at some physical task for a biologically important goal, like killing a bison for food.

Now, the union between Siamese twins is involuntary. Furthermore, while each twin benefits from the parts that they have in common, each would also be better off biologically without the other's noncommon parts. There is, thus, a biological union between the noncommon parts of twin A and the common parts of the twins, but there is no biological union between the noncommon parts of twin A and the noncommon parts of twin B.

The union between a mother and child is short on mutuality: the cooperation of the two is primarily directed at the good of only one of the two. Of course, the mother typically derives psychological and spiritual benefits, but the union is not directed at these benefits.

The case of voluntary cooperation for a biologically important goal requires more analysis. When people work together at a physical task, their cooperation is mentally mediated. What makes it the case that they are *working together* is that they intentionally share the same goal. If one person is chasing a bison toward another, they are only cooperating if they are both intending the same goal, rather than, say, Bob intending to kill the bison that is being chased toward him and Jane intending that the bison should kill Bob. The exact same physical motions can be performed in a case of hunting together and in a case of one party trying to kill another (say, by driving a bison at the victim). What distinguishes the two is a *mental* goal.[4] And this means that the union here is ultimately centered on what happens at the mental level, not the purely biological.

But in sexual union, the common goal is set by the biology. Moreover, though somewhat less significantly since this is merely a matter of degree, the mutual control and cooperation is more thoroughly biological in the sexual case, being less directed by either present deliberation or habits of deliberately arranged activity.

4. DURATION AND COMMITMENT

Sexual union in intercourse is a consummation of romantic love, but it is also an event that lasts for a limited amount of time, and typically only a minuscule proportion of the common life of the lovers is spent in sexual union. Romantic love seeks its consummation, but like any form of love, it also seeks a union extended over time, a union of persons.

Commitment can join momentary actions into a temporally extended whole. If each day my commitments allow me to decide whether I will work that day or not, and each day my boss's commitments allow her to decide whether she will have me work or not, then I am not an employee but a day laborer. The habit of many years may lead me to work and past experience may make me confident that the boss will have me work, but, absent mutual commitment, I am not a member of the staff. Each day involves a separate action. There is something humanly missing from work like this, though we may count as lucky to have it. In uncommitted work like this, my boss and I are not fully joined in a common project.

One of the notable features of a living organism is its tendency to endure over time, a tendency grounded in its ability to preserve itself homeostatically. As a union as "one organism," an act of sexual intercourse by itself falls short in regard to the temporal extension that organisms have. If romantic love's union consisted in a single act of intercourse, that would be disappointing. The couple seeks to be "one flesh" as truly as is possible for them, but biologically the aspect of duration that organisms have is lacking. Consummation is the high point of love's union, but does not exhaust the union that the love seeks.

However, human persons can extend their actions over time through undertaking a commitment. In a *commitment* to a lasting relationship, a couple can extend the biologically momentary nature of the union in intercourse. If they do so, then the union of the couple as one organism involves both of them on the biological level, which yields the common physical striving of the organs of generation, and on the personal level, which commits them to a relationship of the kind of love of which sexual intercourse is the consummation. The temporally extended biological and personal relationship is then a whole, in which the commitment temporally extends the union of intercourse, while intercourse makes the union into a union as one flesh.

Through committed erotic love, then, a couple can be said to be one flesh, in a way unique to persons, not just through biological co-operation but also through commitment. I argued in section 3 of the last chapter that organically united body parts are always cooperating with one another, and this is what largely constitutes the biological union. Now when a human couple is not having sex and is not busy raising children that resulted from their sexual union, they are not biologically united in this active sense. But if we are more careful, we can identify an aspect of biological union present even there, assuming a commitment that only persons are capable of.

Consider my index finger when I am asleep. Its activity consists in its keeping itself in good repair, awaiting orders through the nerves. Now when we consider what the finger's proper function is, what it is there *for*, we find that it is not there to respond to just any old signals that come down the nerve. Rather, it is there to respond to signals originating from the central nervous system—the brain and spinal cord. If the nerves in my finger are electrically stimulated, the finger will respond. However, it is not the finger's proper function to respond to such signals. Indeed, if through evolutionary processes a finger became capable of discriminating the source of nerve signals, and came to respond only to those that originate from the central nervous system, it would thereby be *better* fulfilling its function. Furthermore, the finger's biological function is not just to move in response to signals but to move in ways that promote the biological functioning of the whole organism.

The teleology of my finger—the structure of the purposes of its functioning—thus makes at least two references to things beyond the finger. My finger is there to respond to a particular nervous system, namely my nervous system. It could physically respond to your nervous system if I implanted a radio receiver in your finger and a transmitter in my arm nerves, and, in fact, it could respond to any other electrical source, but that is not what it is there for. And it is there to benefit a particular individual, namely me. It has a connection to the rest of the body, not just in what it actually does but in what it is *supposed to do*. It has a *normative* connection to the other parts.

Full organic union as we know it also includes actual function, which, in the organisms we know, involves constant activity, but also includes this normative aspect of the connection between parts of the body, a normative aspect that is also always present but does not require the united parts to be actually functioning. Rather, it requires each of them to have a directedness at one another. Commitment creates such a normative, teleological connection between individuals. Each individual comes to have the benefit of a particular other as a purpose.

The creation of a new normative connection between individuals in commitment seems to be available only to humans. Nietzsche wrote that the human being became an interesting animal upon acquiring the ability to make promises. Promises are one of our primary ways of creating commitments, and what Nietzsche said about promises surely applies to all ways of undertaking commitments. Through a normative commitment, something that is binding on each of them, two human beings can unite as one flesh in a way mere animals cannot, namely, unite in a union as one flesh that, to some extent, persists outside copulation. Furthermore, if romantic love is directed at as deep a one-flesh union as is possible in a voluntary and mutual context, then it calls for this kind of commitment.

Now while nonhuman animals are, as far as we know, incapable of commitment, they seem to be capable of habit and psychological attachment. Let us then consider whether the enduring kind of one-flesh union can exist simply in virtue of habit and/or psychological attachment, rather than actual commitment. First, it is worth noting that the *first* time a couple engages in sexual activity, they cannot have a habit of engaging in sexual activity with one another. If there were a requirement that for a fully meaningful sexual union, the union must be temporally extended, habit could not do the job the first time. But a first-time sexual union can be fully meaningful.

More importantly, habit lacks the kind of normativity that is present in the union of organic parts. That one has done something many times before does make it more likely that one will do it again. But it does not imply that one *should* do it again. It might be argued, though, that through habit one becomes a certain kind of person, and then one *ought* to act in accordance with the kind of person one is. Given that habits are about as likely to be bad as good, this "ought" does not seem to have much force. But in any case, we can say that if the habit of sexual relations with one person is such as to generate an "ought," so that one *ought* to continue the relationship, then this simply means that the habit has *committed* one to the relationship. Indeed, some habits can do that: by acting in a kind manner to someone, I may well be committing myself to continue acting in a kind manner, as a failure to do so would be a betrayal. But the habit we were considering was one that was supposed to be distinguished from commitment; it was to be the kind of habit an animal can have.

The kind of habit that could produce a temporally enduring union would thus have to be a habit that implies normative commitment, and so we come back to commitment. The same can be said about psychological attachment. Psychological attachment may well induce one to return to the same person. But except insofar as it commits one to loyalty—there may, after all, be a duty to be faithful to certain kinds of attachments—it does not have the normative weight that would direct each person to be there for the sake of the couple in the way in which a finger is there for the benefit of the whole.

Furthermore, the kind of relationship that organic parts bear to the whole is a fairly permanent one. The directedness of parts toward the whole arguably lasts for the lifetime of the part: it is not just the purpose of the part *now* to benefit the whole, but typically it is the purpose of the part to benefit the whole through all of the part's future life. In the case of complex animals, if a severed part survives at all, it might still be said to be directed at the benefit of the whole, and, in any case, severed parts typically perish rapidly.[5] Mere habit and psychological attachment will not make it be the case that one person ought to be united with a particular other person until death.

If the commitment of persons to each other in the union that fulfills romantic love is to mirror, as much as possible, the directedness of body parts to each other and to the whole, it needs to be a "'til death do us part" commitment.

Now is there ambiguity in the word "death"? Whose death? The death of the couple or of the other person or of oneself? A commitment past the death of the body of either person would be problematic in the context of romantic love, which is focused on embodiment. Thus, plausibly, romantic commitment does not go beyond the death of the first member of the couple to die.

But perhaps sometimes the couple dies as a couple before any of the parts do. People do talk of a marriage being dead. A plant might be cut into several pieces, each of which could be planted separately and survive, but the plant as a whole would be destroyed. Could it be that romantic love's commitment is like this, so that each individual is committed to trying to ensure the couple does not fall apart, but if it does, then they are free to go their separate ways?

Here there may be a difference between the biological union and the interpersonal union. The primary commitment in interpersonal love is to a *person*. And while a biological unit is formed in intercourse, that biological unit is not a person: there are two persons there (just as there are three in the unity of the Trinity). The lover's primary commitment is to the beloved, rather than to the couple as such, so that it would not make sense to terminate the commitment should the couplehood be damaged. The disanalogy is not, perhaps, very serious: even a biological part like the finger receives its signals from another part, namely the nervous system, rather than directly from the whole, and hence it has a special connection with another part and not just with the whole, and so in an organism composed of only two parts we would expect each part to be focused on the other. Now, if the commitment is focused on the persons rather than on the couple, the commitment should span the lifetime of the persons.

Thus, one way to extend sexual union temporally is through commitment. Having such a commitment is possible for persons of normal psychological functioning and intelligence (though of course they may end up failing to *keep* the commitment). The second way of extending sexual union is through successful procreation. Sexual union is constituted by a mutual biological striving for reproduction. The procreative striving continues in the couple's mutual contribution to caring for and educating children. And even when the couple has not yet reproduced, a joint commitment to reproducing and raising children when and if that becomes possible, morally licit, and prudent can bind them together, in a way that extends the biological union interpersonally and in time. (In the case of a couple past the natural age of childbearing, that commitment would have to take the form of a conditional: if by some miracle we were able to have a child in a prudent and morally licit way, we would.)

While earlier I have talked of mutual organic striving for procreation as the central aspect of the consummation of romantic love, we can now plausibly add a *second* aspect of consummation: the temporal extension of the union through time, in commitment to one another and to the raising of offspring. If this is right, then a couple that engages in sex without the fullness of commitment—a commitment that I take to require marriage—and that only later takes on this commitment is a couple that has not yet consummated their love. The consummation of their love requires intercourse in the context of the appropriate commitment.

Now one may ask whether the content of the commitment needs to involve sexual exclusivity. Suppose, for instance, that a couple simply commit to have sex with one another for life, but do not commit to not have sex with others. Is this not a sufficient temporal extension of their sexual union?

Granted, such an anemic commitment *is* a temporal extension of their sexual union. But it does not appear sufficient to generate the deep form of union that romantic love seeks. First of all, phenomenologically, while too much exclusivity in friendship can be a deformation of the friendship into cliquishness, a significant exclusivity appears appropriate to romantic love. We are creatures of God, and evil can deform us, but we need to be cautious about ruling basic human attitudes completely wrong. Jealousy seems to be a basic human attitude in romantic relationships; we should thus avoid saying that jealousy is completely wrong. When jealousy goes wrong, it seems to be through a defect of the trust proper to romantic relationship. Part of that trust is a trust in the other's fidelity, and it appears to be a nondefective aspect of romantic relationships that one have an expectation of exclusivity, an expectation that ideally involves trust, but which leads to feelings of jealousy and betrayal when that trust is betrayed. It is very plausible that properly romantic commitment, of the maximal sort that romantic love seeks, would involve exclusivity.

Second, the point of the commitment was to extend organic union temporally into the future of the couple, beyond the short periods of time during which they are having sex. Now, the parts of a body have their function defined by the whole of which they are a part. Cases are rare where something is a proper part of more than one body. The shared organs of Siamese twins are one of the few cases. But one is less closely united with an organ when it is shared. A normative consequence of an organ's being a part of one's body is that others' rights to make use of that organ are limited. To the extent that others are able to make use of a part of one's body, that organ seems less truly one's own.

It seems plausible that the shared organs of Siamese twins are less fully the organs of either to the extent that the other twin is permitted to make use of them. Something that is a part of two different wholes, and is a part of each of them in respect of the same functions, is a part of each whole in a weaker way than something that is a part of only one whole in respect of the same function. A lung that is a part of two bodies is not wholly to be defined as, say, "a lung of Fred." It has an identity as an oxygen extracting organ that goes beyond being a lung of Fred, by also being a lung of Bob. Thus, its union with Fred is less thoroughgoing, less complete, less full.

Likewise, the body of one of the lovers is less fully a part of the united organism constituted by the two bodies if this body is permitted to enter into sexual union with others. The full organic union for which romantic love yearns, with that union having the full personal and normative significance that commitment can give it, requires a commitment not just to future sexual acts but to sexual exclusivity.

The above is an argument against a person being a part of each of two different romantic couples, since in that case that person is less fully a part of each. However, this leaves open the question whether there couldn't be a romantic trio (or quartet, etc.), where all three are united as one body. However, sexual union, which is the consummation of romantic love, is achieved in and through an act where there are precisely two people involved in a primary way. This act is capable of summing up the meaning of the relationship, and that is a binary, not ternary, meaning. It would be different among aliens where three are needed to reproduce; if they have something analogous to our romantic love, it might require a trio.

It is true that other people can be involved in a helping capacity in a sexual act—if the people are disabled, a nurse or other professional might offer some sort of assistance, for instance with undressing or even positioning. But such subsidiary help is a way of helping the two primary agents to have intercourse—the helper is not a part of the act of intercourse. Moreover, an equal relationship would not be signified by such an act, simply because the helper's activity is not on a par with the activity of the two primary agents, as it is only the primary agents' reproductive systems that are fully engaged in the relevant way.

5. IS UNCOMMITTED SEX MORALLY ACCEPTABLE?

Sexual union absent a committed union of persons is, thus, incomplete. Indeed, the couple is uniting as a tragic kind of organism, one with a severely truncated temporal dimension. The act of uniting biologically is a significant act. Through it, two become one. But without the commitment, two become one in a temporary way, soon to be ripped apart. We can see that there is a good found in a married couple's sexual union that is severely curtailed when a couple without a lifetime commitment unites sexually. The question to ask now is whether it is morally licit for a couple to unite sexually absent that lifetime commitment. The mere fact that union is less good for such a couple does not answer the question, since we often need to settle for second best. A partial union, it might be argued, is better than no union at all.

In the case at hand, Vincent Punzo has argued that what we have is not simply second best.[6] A member of a couple that unites physically while lacking the temporal component of the union lacks integrity, not in the sense of being dishonest, but in the sense of not being integrated as a person. The body is not a mere appendage: we are truly embodied beings. But when bodies unite while the persons are not correspondingly united, they are failing to act as united embodied individuals, individuals who have body, mind, and will. (Note that the argument works even if, contrary to the Christian tradition about the existence of the soul, the mind and will are taken to be just neural systems and hence parts of the body—there will still be a disunion between the mind and will, on the one hand, and the rest of the body, on the other hand.)

To unite sexually while choosing not to unite personally is to fail to acknowledge the directedness toward the future that any organism has, including the biologically united organism comprising the man and the woman. There will, of course, be cases where even a married couple knows that their sexual union has no future, for instance, because one of them is going to be executed shortly. However, it is a quite different matter if the lack of a future for the relationship is due to the deliberate choices of the two individuals.

There would arguably be nothing wrong with a couple conceiving a child if they knew that the child would die painlessly at age one due to a genetic defect, assuming that in conceiving the child the couple were not imposing an unfair burden on others. But suppose that it was the couple's own choice not to prevent the genetic abnormality—say, because the treatment was physically painful to them. At this point there *is* a moral problem: the couple is, in an important sense, responsible for their own child's dying at age one. The couple might argue: "It is better for the child to live until age one and then die painlessly than not to have lived at all," but the argument rings hollow when the child dies due to the action or inaction of the parents.

I am not claiming that the noncontinuation of the organic union of husband and wife is a murder, but simply that the argument that it is better to unite partially than not at all is unpersuasive in the same way that the argument of the couple with a genetic defect is unpersuasive, at least in typical cases. For, typically, it is through the unmarried, sexually active couple's own decision that they are uniting absent marriage: they could have married, but they didn't. Granted, they may have had reasons for this decision, just as the couple in the preceding paragraph had reasons not to undergo the genetic treatment. But nonetheless, they are responsible for the nonenduring state of their union, and it is not a good state to be in. And even if one of the members of the couple is to be executed shortly, the couple can still commit for life, rejoicing in the extension of this life if a pardon were to be given.

There is a way to strengthen our above point if we are willing to appeal to a notion of the normal. Marriage is the normal state for human beings—this seems clear from the scriptures, with marriage being the primary remedy for our loneliness and need for others. (This does not imply that everyone should marry, since special circumstances can make it reasonable to refrain from doing something normal, as when one fasts.) Moreover, the combination of romantic desire and romantic love is a normal human state, and it is normal for human beings to live in a state that allows the consummation of this desire and love. In holding back from marriage while having sex, the couple is holding back from something that is normal to human beings. Suppose now that the genetic defect of a procreating couple could have been cured through a *normal* human activity—say, through eating regularly—but the couple has chosen not to engage in that activity. Then the responsibility of the couple for the genetic defect would be particularly clear.

A failure to do what is *normal* is not just an ordinary inaction, but is much more like an action. That while writing the previous paragraph I did not yell "Huzzah!" is a mere inaction of mine. But if it were true that, while writing the previous paragraph, I did not breathe, my nonbreathing would have been an action, a refraining from what is normal. We make this distinction in other cases. To deliberately fail to eat or drink over the period of a week would be tantamount to suicide. To deliberately refuse to be hooked up to a respirator need not be seen as suicide in the same way. Likewise, then, the failure to unite sexual intercourse with commitment when the couple could have done so is more like an action than like a mere refraining, given the normalcy of the commitment.

In any case, even if the above considerations about normalcy are not plausible, the couple that engages in sexual union in the absence of a marriage is typically responsible for the sadly truncated state of their union (one reason for the "typically" qualifier is cases where the two simply are not responsible for their actions, for instance, because of mental illness or immaturity;[7] cases where they are unable to marry will be discussed later in this section). And just as full sexual union of body and person expresses and consummates the conjugal love that is the mature form of romantic love, this sadly truncated union expresses a shortfall of love. By constituting a sexual union, the sexual act places the relationship in the category where conjugal love is salient. But by being responsible for the act's falling short of the consummation of conjugal love, the couple has acted against the salient kind of love. Had the couple abstained from sexual union, but instead held hands and conversed, they might have correctly expressed and lived out a love different from conjugal love: namely, a romantic love that has yet to blossom into conjugality. But the partial consummation—the consummation in body but not in commitment—was worse than nothing at all, since it involved both a giving *and* a holding back.

What, though, of a couple that is incapable of marriage? There the argument that they are *responsible* for their act's falling short in the temporal dimension seems to fail. But here we need to distinguish several different ways in which a couple might be incapable of marriage.

Some couples cannot marry for physical reasons that make the consummation of the marriage impossible. What Jesus said about eunuchs in Matthew 19:12 suggests that he thought eunuchs could not marry. But of course, the question of premarital intercourse does not come up for couples incapable of intercourse.

Some couples are incapable of marrying due to a reasonable legal restriction, either temporary or permanent. In the temporary case, as when the two are below the legal age for marriage, they are still responsible for the fact that they are uniting physically in the absence of marital commitment, since they can unite physically *with* marital commitment, if only they wait. If the restriction is permanent, it is typically grounded in the sorts of reasons that make intercourse morally inadvisable, like reasons of consanguinity.

But now consider a particularly difficult case, that of a couple that is incapable of marrying due to *unreasonable* restrictions or due to mere accident, such as a case where local authorities refuse to celebrate the marriage for racist reasons, or where no one authorized to celebrate the wedding is available. In some such cases, there may be a solution. According to the tradition of the Western Church, a marriage is theologically understood as effected not by the minister (priest or deacon in Catholic tradition), but by the two members of the couple themselves. In order to express the theological significance of marriage, additional regulations were promulgated at different times. Currently, for instance, for a valid marriage of a Catholic to take place, the Latin-rite Catholic Church requires a priest or deacon to bless the marriage, but only if a clergyman is going to be present in their locality at some point over the next month. Essentially, when clergy will be unavailable for a month, the couple can undergo the sacrament of matrimony in the presence of lay witnesses.[8] Moreover, "for a grave and urgent cause" the local bishop can authorize a marriage to be celebrated secretly without civil authorities being informed.[9]

Thus, cases are rare where a marriage would be reasonable but cannot be entered into at all (perhaps without the state's involvement). And in those rare cases, it would still be the choice of the couple not to have privately exchanged vows of commitment for life.

So far, then, we have the ingredients for an argument that premarital sex is wrong, except perhaps in the very exceptional case where a marriage would be reasonable but unreasonable authorities make it impossible, in which case, the couple can only privately exchange vows of commitment for life. In typical cases of premarital intercourse, the couple is doing something that would be a consummation of fully committed romantic love, something that joins the couple as one body, while deliberately leaving out the temporal dimension that commitment would have supplied. In choosing to leave out this temporal dimension, the couple opposes itself to romantic love while acting in a way that partially consummates it. By failing to be committed to each other, the two persons both unite as one body *and* leave it open to themselves to discontinue their union in the future, an option plausibly contrary to the meaning of organic union.

Now there can be forms of loving union in which two people legitimately leave open to themselves the discontinuation of the relationship. After all, it is perfectly fine for two people to date in order to figure out whether they should marry, and when they do this they *ought* to leave open the discontinuation of the relationship. Likewise, there can be forms of loving union where two people, for instance out of prudence, leave the union incomplete—like friendships in which friends withhold certain confidences.

However, the case of sexual union is different. Either the persons who engage in intercourse identify themselves as united as one flesh or they do not. If they do not, then their actions are not grounded in truth, for in truth they *are* united as one flesh, whether they see this or not. Suppose now that they do identify themselves as united in one flesh. By being open to the termination of that one-flesh identity, they are open to the destruction of something closely analogous to a very significant aspect of their own flesh and of the flesh of their sexual partner; they are open to the destruction of the whole united organism as such. And an openness to that destruction is, in itself, contrary to love for self and for the other, especially if one identifies oneself as part of that united organism, both in respect of the benevolence aspect of love and in respect of the unitive aspect of love. To protect oneself psychologically and make it easier to be open to the termination of the one-flesh identity, one might, of course, psychologically dissociate from the fleshly union. But such dissociation is itself wrong. For to dissociate oneself from what one's body does by one's own choice is to deceive oneself into thinking that the body is not really a part of oneself. We could imagine a person who mentally dissociates from certain bodily functions, perhaps thinking them undignified, but such dissociation is a failure of integrity: nothing human should be alien to us.

Furthermore, a nonmarital sexual act is likely to be self-contradictory. For much of what makes sexual activity *exciting* is precisely the way in which we identify with our bodies. It is this identification that makes intercourse more exciting than sex between avatars in a virtual world. In fact, likely, such virtual sex is exciting largely in proportion to the extent to which a person identifies himself or herself, or perhaps the other, with the relevant virtual body, feeling about the virtual body what one normally feels about the real body. Thus, the more satisfying the virtual sex, the more morally problematic it is, since it implies a greater departure from reality through treating what is not a part of one's self as if it were.

Now, a nonmarital sexual act is likely to be engaged in by the couple precisely for the excitement that flows from self-identification with one's body, while at the same time, the couple fails to be committed to acting in ways that are faithful to that self-identification. For insofar as we are identified with the bodies that are united as one organism, permanence is called for.

Can we say anything about the remaining, particularly difficult case of premarital sex, in which the couple is unable to be married solely due to the unreasonableness of others but has united through the private exchange of vows for life? Here I think the best answer is provided by the Catholic tradition, which distinguishes "natural law marriage" from "Christian marriage." Two unbaptized and previously unmarried persons, not too closely related by blood and of sufficient maturity, can always enter into a natural law marriage simply by exchanging private vows. The situation of being blocked from marriage by the unreasonableness of others does not come up for them; an exchange of private vows simply *is* a marriage for them. Hence the argument against premarital sex applies without difficulty to all unbaptized couples of sufficient maturity. And there is good reason why it is inappropriate for two people who lack the maturity to exchange private vows to have sex. Sex is at least a partial way of consummating romantic love, and a couple lacking the maturity to exchange private vows is a couple incapable of freely and responsibly making the decisions surrounding the consummation of romantic love.

Now, when a *baptized* person marries, the act has ecclesial significance, and is not just a natural law marriage. The act signifies the love between Christ and his Church, and must be done in accordance with the authority that Christ has given to the Church. We can reasonably argue that just as, for a Christian, the marriage itself takes on a new theological meaning, so does the act that consummates marriage—intercourse. To engage in that act absent the theological meaning, even if it is not one's fault that one was unable to marry and ensure the act has that theological meaning, is inappropriate. The union of bodies objectively *is* a deeply significant act for an individual, and, as such, it should be permeated with appropriate theological meaning, like every deeply significant human act. In cases where marriage is impossible, one can instead convey theological meaning through abstinence.

6. MODESTY AND MEMORY

That my body is mine is something not merely momentarily true. My body's being mine makes it eminently reasonable for me to care for it in the future—including providing for a respectful funeral. But its being my body also causes my memories to be bound up with it: I remember being in this location, feeling that sensation, and so forth. The claim that my memories are bound up with my body is obvious to the point of silliness: Of course I remember what my body has been up to, there being so little else that I remember. In fact, quite often, I do not even remember my past mental states directly, but infer them from memories about what was going on with me physically at the time—I remember that big, loose dog, and so my mind infers that I must have been scared, without any direct memory of the fear.

The relationship to *my* body clearly differs from the relationship to *my* property, and there are two senses of "my" being used. I bought my car used. Should I care whether it had undergone major repairs in the past? Certainly—but only insofar as the damage and the repairs impact its future performance. If I care about anything more here (and care is different from curiosity), I am treating the car as more than mere property. But I do have reason to care more about what has happened to my body, even if this does not affect its future behavior. To give an extreme case, it would be pathological simply not to care at all after coming out of a coma whether one's physician had committed an outrage against one's body while one was unconscious, even if no traces or damage were left.

Now, in marriage, each spouse has authority over the other's body (1 Cor. 7:4), and "husbands should love their wives as their own bodies" (Eph. 5:28), which is presumably a mutual duty. Moreover, if one is united as one body with a spouse, then one's spouse's body is partly one's own: it is a part of the united body, which united body is partly one's own. There is, thus, an important sense in which it is true to say that the other's body is, partly, one's own. It is not "one's own" in the sense of ownership; rather, the sense in which one's spouse's body is one's own is like the sense in which one's own body is one's own. "One's own" here is a possessive not of ownership but of relation, just as talking of "my father" or "my king" does not imply one owns the father or king.

The history of one's body is significant to one, and if the spouse's body is partly one's own, then its history is also significant. If there were a significant aspect of one's body's history that it would be *inappropriate* for one to know, that would imply an alienation from one's body. Likewise, significant aspects of the history of one's body that it would be inappropriate for one's spouse to know would imply an alienation of one's spouse from one's own body—which is also the spouse's—and therefore from oneself. And since spousal union is sexual in nature, this alienation is particularly unfortunate when the relevant history is sexual. Love calls for knowledge, since love needs to adapt to the beloved (cf. sections 4 and 5 of chapter 2) and since the beloved must be loved as he or she truly is.

On the other hand, there is a presumption of privacy in sexual relationships. On multiple levels, sexual union involves a disclosure of what is hidden. If one would not be embarrassed to have kibitzers in the bedroom, something is wrong with one. There is a loyalty that one should have to those who have disclosed themselves to one sexually. But at the same time, what is done sexually, particularly in the context of a union as one body, is mutual: to be silent about the other is to be silent about oneself.

Past sexual relationships with other persons thus create a conflict of at least prima facie duties within marriage. If the sexual past is kept back, one is alienating one's body and self from one's spouse, and doing so in a spousally relevant context. Yet if the past is disclosed, the privacy of past lovers or partners is infringed on. There is no good solution to this dilemma. And we should avoid *creating* for ourselves moral dilemmas that have no good solution.

I am not claiming here that the dilemma is a conflict between absolute duties. There is no absolute, unconditional duty to reveal every aspect of one's past to one's spouse. Nor is there an absolute, unconditional duty to hide every aspect of a sexual relationship. There can be good reasons for keeping sexual secrets from one's spouse, and there can be good reasons for revealing aspects of sexual history. However, it is always in itself unfortunate to have such secrets or make such revelations.

We must have a good reason to put ourselves into a position where all the options are unfortunate, particularly when they are unfortunate not just for ourselves but in light of what we owe others. The good reason needs to be proportionate to how unfortunate the options are. At times there will be such a good reason in the sexual case. For instance, it is not wrong to engage in sexual relations with one's spouse, even though one might, after all, remarry after that spouse dies, at which time aspects of one's past sexual life will have to be secret from the new spouse. It is not wrong to remarry after one's spouse has died; scripture (1 Tim. 5:14) and the Christian tradition are clear on this point. But there is an indication that there is something unfortunate about such remarriage in the practice of the Eastern Orthodox Church: "Our contemporary rite for blessing second marriages also shows clearly that it is admitted only by condescension. In any case, Christian scripture and tradition agree that faithfulness of the widower or the widow to his or her deceased partner is more than an 'ideal'; it is a Christian norm."[10]

But the typical case of premarital sex does not involve the kind of morally strong reasons that might lead one to remarry, for instance, in order to unite for life with someone one loves or to find a step-parent for one's children. Pleasure certainly is not a good enough reason: pleasure, by itself, lacks the kind of moral significance that would make it appropriate to put oneself at significant risk of the future dilemma whether to reveal what is private or hold back what is relevant.

Suppose, however, that the premarital sex is engaged in for more than just pleasure, as part of a meaningful and loving, albeit nonmarital, relationship. Here the sexual activity does help produce various emotional and other goods. However, notice that in a more meaningful relationship, there is more trust, and hence the presumption of privacy is stronger. Either (a) one is engaging in an intimate and trusting union the privacy of which one will compromise, or (b) one is going to sacrifice an aspect of future union in a more significant (because it would be more committed) relationship for the sake of a union that is only partial (because it is without the temporal aspects that flow from commitment) and that is within a less significant relationship. There is something wrong in either case.

Objection 1. If the disclosure/secrecy argument is correct, then it is wrong for those who are not virgins to marry, since by doing so they put themselves into the dilemma of privacy versus love's union.

There is a kernel of truth in this objection: yes, nonvirginity does create *a* reason not to marry. However, this reason can easily be overridden by the good reasons that one may have to marry. Here one is not talking of sacrificing a more important relationship for a lesser, as when one chooses to have premarital sex, but of gaining the good of marital union. Anyway, in general, rare is the person who has no secrets to keep from a spouse; most of us are the recipients of various confidences from friends and family members.

But to *create* secrets about which one should not talk to one's spouse, one needs to have a proportionate reason. Thus, one needs to have a proportionate reason to receive confidences that one will have to keep from one's spouse, and it would be wrong to accept such confidences without good reason. However, once an unmarried person has received confidences, the need to maintain these confidences generates only a relatively weak reason against marriage. Likewise, the reason against marriage generated by past sexual activity is only weak, but given the typical lack of strong reason for premarital sex, it was likely wrong to have put oneself in the present position.

There is no fully satisfactory solution to the dilemma resulting from the subsequent marriage, and so the person will have to choose the less unsatisfactory one. But since the duties to maintain the privacy of past sexual partners and the duty not to alienate one's spouse from aspects of one's sexual past are not indefeasible, one does not do wrong to choose the less unsatisfactory solution, though one did wrong in putting oneself in the position where marriage would create such a dilemma.

One might here ask: Which is the less unsatisfactory solution? Is it to reveal or withhold the information? Surely there is no general rule here. It is something to discern in the particular situation, with the help of the Holy Spirit.

Objection 2. What if one is having premarital sex to save the life of an innocent person, or for some other really good reason? There seem to be cases where the argument does not apply.

Indeed, the argument only applies to typical cases of premarital sex. It can be permissible to induce a dilemma between the two unsatisfactory outcomes for good reason, and so this argument will fail in cases where there is a sufficiently strong reason for sex, such as to save a life (e.g., because a dictator has told one that unless one has consensual sex with some person, both you and that person will die). It does not follow, however, that sex in those cases is permissible, only that this argument does not prohibit it. Likewise, the argument has no force for someone certain not to marry in the future. But there are few such people.

Moreover, the argument will be harder to apply in cases where the sexual partner has no interest in privacy. But if the intimate sexual bond is, of its nature, such as to call for privacy, one might think that there is something wrong with sexual activity with a partner who does not understand this aspect of sexuality. For if someone does not understand an important aspect of sexuality, then this person's consent is not properly informed, and so the standard consent criteria for the permissibility of sexual activity should rule out the liaison.

Objection 3. What if one is not going to marry? Then the argument seems not to apply at all.

One may wonder how one knows that one is not going to marry. Marriage appears to be the normal state for human beings. Not to enter into the normal state for human beings requires a good reason. But most of the reasons for lifelong avoidance of matrimony are also reasons not to have sex. Thus, if one expects never to have the maturity for marriage, the chances are low that one has the maturity for sex. One might wish to avoid marriage for theological reasons, in order, say, to express a more exclusive union with God, but such a theological reason is also a reason for avoiding sex.

7. PREGNANCY

The oldest and perhaps most practically persuasive argument against nonmarital intercourse has been: "You might get pregnant" or "You might get her pregnant." Easy access to effective contraception, as well as growing acceptance of unmarried parenthood, have made this argument fall on hard times. Nonetheless, I will argue that a version of this simple pragmatic argument *does* give a moral argument against most standard cases of premarital intercourse. The argument is based on an idea of Christopher Kaczor.[11]

Begin with the following moral principle: *It is wrong to risk putting oneself in a position where one will not fulfill one's responsibilities, unless there is sufficiently good reason to put oneself in this position.* There is no general rule for determining which reasons are sufficient. The greater the risk and the graver the potentially unfulfilled responsibilities, the stronger a reason is needed. If I am bringing dessert to a party so that a delay risks only the promised dessert's lateness, it will still be right for me to talk on the phone with a severely distressed friend instead of leaving for the party. Likewise, every time I drive my children to school, I risk my life and theirs, and thereby accept a risk of no longer being able to fulfill my spousal responsibilities to my wife. Nonetheless, the risk is small enough that the educational benefits to my children are sufficient reason to undertake the risk. On the other hand, it would not be appropriate for me to climb Mt. Everest simply for the gratification of a personal desire, since by doing so I would undertake the risk of leaving my children fatherless and my wife widowed without morally sufficient reason. But to climb Mt. Everest to rescue a friend could be justifiable.

The typical case of nonmarital sex involves the risk of pregnancy, and involves a significant risk that if pregnancy results the child will not be raised in a two-parent family. Now each parent bears full responsibility for raising the child—if one of them neglects the responsibility, then the other must shoulder it alone, unfair as that is, an unfairness that the neglectful parent is responsible for. It is difficult enough for two parents living together harmoniously to fulfill their responsibilities with regard to the upbringing of the child, providing the child with love, food, shelter, and clothing, as well as a sufficient religious, moral, and scientific education, and for a parent to fulfill this responsibility alone is near impossible. While this is typically true even in regard to the physical basics, the case of moral education is no less important. Different people have different virtues and vices. With two parents raising the child, the child observes a greater variety of virtues close at hand, all of which the child needs. With only one parent, the child is more likely to regard that parent's vices as normal human features, whereas, while we all have vices, our vices differ. Furthermore, the example of the close and loving interaction of two parents is important for learning interpersonal virtues. There is, thus, intuitive data that it is harmful to a child to be raised by a single parent, and there also appears to be some empirical data.[12]

Moreover, if the child will be raised by only one of the parents, even if that parent can provide the child with all that the child needs, then the other parent will not be fulfilling his or her (typically, his) parental duties toward the child, since the duty is not just to ensure that the child's needs are met, but to *personally* meet the child's needs. We will explore this line of argument in greater detail in section 2 of chapter 10, in connection with gamete donation.

Now, if two unmarried people have a child, the likelihood of the child being raised by two parents who love both each other and the child is significantly lower than in the case of a married couple. Thus, by engaging in sexual activity, the couple risks bringing about a state in which it is unlikely that they will be able to raise their child appropriately. In short, each member of the couple risks putting himself or herself in the position of not fulfilling responsibilities to the child.

It should be noted, however, that the present argument is weaker in the case of couples that are cohabiting with each other, since the likelihood is presumably higher that such couples will stay together. Nonetheless, the argument has some force in those cases, at least in the United States, where the chance that the child will face parental dissolution is significantly higher for cohabiting couples than for married ones (however, it must be observed that in the case of white couples—though not black or Mexican—the difference can be accounted for in terms of other factors than cohabitation versus marriage, such as level of education).[13]

Without contraception, the likelihood of pregnancy resulting from a single act of intercourse by a couple of reproductive age is about 5 percent (that is, for women in their late twenties and early thirties).[14] With contraception, the likelihood decreases. However, contraception does fail. According to a recent U.S. study, "Within 3 months of the initiation of use of a reversible method of contraception, 4.2% of all women experienced a contraceptive failure. . . . At 6 months, 7.3% had experienced a failure, and by 12 months of use, 12.4% had experienced a contraceptive failure."[15] The annual failure rate for the male condom was 17.8 percent, and for the pill it was 8.7 percent. These numbers apply only to the typical case of contraceptive use. If used without mistakes on the part of the couple, the probabilities of failure are much, much smaller, but still nonzero.

It should be noted that the present argument will not apply if both parties know for sure that the members of the couple are, in fact, using a method of contraception that they know for sure will not fail. (This requires that the couple know one another well.) For instance, according to a 2002 report, no studies of the use of the birth control product Implanon have found pregnancies.[16]

But for nonimplantable forms of contraception, even though the probability of conception decreases, it remains significant. Supposing, for instance, using the conservative 1 percent actual annual failure rate of a contraceptive and assuming an average sexual frequency of about twice per week, we can estimate the chance of pregnancy per act of intercourse at about 0.01 percent. This may seem small. But when we consider how serious the responsibilities involved are, the risk is not all that low. In any 10,000 people who engage in the activity, on average one conception will occur. Typically, a person engaging in premarital intercourse does not engage in just one act, but in many. In the case of activities as pleasant and addictive as sex, that the activity will occur "just this once" is unlikely. (Not to mention that, to engage in a sexual act once, knowing that it will be "just this once," is to risk heartbreak in the partner.) The availability of contraception may itself significantly increase the likelihood of sexual activity,[17] and also of repeat sexual activity.

The unfulfilled responsibility that one risks through premarital intercourse is one of the most serious responsibilities a typical human being has. The probability associated with the risk is typically nonnegligible. Thus, in typical cases, a serious reason is needed for sexual relations outside of marriage. Fleeting pleasure, for self and other, does not appear to be a sufficiently serious reason, given the seriousness of the responsibility at issue. Besides, there are unproblematic alternative pleasures available to the loving couple, like sharing low-fat ice cream or discussing a book.

Premarital intercourse, at least as a habitual practice, though probably also as an isolated act, is wrong on account of the risk of pregnancy, at least when the reason for the intercourse is pleasure. Of course, there may be better reasons. Leaving aside rare circumstances, such as the couple having sex because a tyrant will otherwise murder someone, the couple may be pursuing an interpersonal relational goal, such as physical union. But it would have to be but a temporally truncated union, itself morally problematic, as we have seen (see section 5 above), and the risks appear to be out of proportion with the good of such a partial union. Or the good might be some kind of psychological closeness. But it seems not unlikely that a couple could come closer psychologically by a cooperative striving for chastity, and in any case, there are many nonsexual and beneficial activities in which a couple could cooperate—such as working in a soup kitchen or on a political campaign—that could produce psychological closeness.

We could try to move the argument in a social direction instead, at least in the United States. The significant number of children born outside of marriage in this country might arguably be a major contributor to poverty, poorer moral education, and other social ills. By engaging in premarital sex, one takes the risk of being a contributor to this serious social problem. It is true that, more likely than not, procreation will not happen in any given act. However, a significant number of children born outside of marriage are conceived despite the use of contraception. Thus, even engaging in contraceptive intercourse, one is risking being a contributor to the problem. And there one is at least presumptively doing wrong.

We, thus, have two arguments, one in terms of the prima facie impermissibility of undertaking the risk of not fulfilling one's responsibilities, and another in terms of the prima facie wrongness of contributing to major social problems.

Objection 1. The same issues come up within marriage. One *always* risks not fulfilling parental responsibilities. Indeed almost no one fulfills them perfectly. Socrates bewailed the lack of success in Athenian familial moral education, and things seem to be no better now. Besides, any given marriage has a significant chance of divorce and a significant chance of one parent having to raise the children alone.

This is all true, but society requires reproduction to maintain itself over time and assure care for the elderly. It seems plausible that reproduction *within* marriage is, on the whole, a benefit to our society and that the couple reproducing within marriage is, on the whole, contributing to something good. To refrain entirely from reproducing within marriage, barring special reasons not available to most people, might well count as a case of free-riding, since in one's old age one will likely be benefiting from care provided by younger generations who resulted from reproduction by other couples.

Sexual relations within marriage consummate marital love, and this seems a sufficient good to justify taking on various ordinary risks.

At the same time, there may be cases, say, where the couple is destitute, in which a married couple might do well to abstain on account of the risks.

Objection 2. This argument does not apply in all cases. It will not apply, for instance, in the case of a couple absolutely committed to marry should pregnancy result, nor will it apply if the woman is past the age of childbearing or if the couple is firmly engaged to be married. And so on.

This is all correct. The argument only applies to typical cases, but not all cases. It is worth noting, however, that it is not clear how much one can count on a commitment to marry should a child result. Furthermore, such a commitment may be inadvisable, in that a marriage based on such a commitment seems likely to be weaker, given that the couple, for some reason, was not willing to commit to marry unconditionally. And even an ordinary unconditional engagement to marry could legitimately be broken for good reason. In any case, the likelihood of breaking an engagement or having a subsequent divorce, which the unmarried couple risks, is greater than the likelihood of having a divorce, which is what the married couple risks.

Objection 3. Each parent is only responsible for his or her own role, and not for the overall bringing up of the child. Therefore, each *can* fulfill his or her own responsibility, no matter what the other does.

This, however, appears incorrect. Observe that if each parent were only responsible for his or her own role, then each parent would only be obliged to provide half of the food that the child needs to survive. But then if the other parent died, the remaining parent could simply provide half of the needed food, and thus fulfill his or her responsibility. This is surely not right. Each is fully responsible.

Objection 4. Even though contraception can fail, abortion almost never fails. Thus, a couple can ensure that they are not contributing to a serious social problem or to the nonfulfillment of their responsibilities through abortion.

This argument presupposes the moral permissibility of abortion. The early Christian tradition rejected abortion, often as a crime on par with infanticide.[18] For instance, the second-century *Didache* commands: "thou shalt not kill a child by means of abortion, nor slay it after it has been born [*ou phoneuseis teknon en phthora(i), oude gennêthen apokteneis*]."[19] Interestingly, all this was while leading philosophical theories (e.g., those of Aristotle), together with rabbinical Judaism, insisted that the embryo/fetus has no soul either during pregnancy as a whole or at least during the first weeks after conception. The apparent classification of abortion as a sin on par with infanticide, despite the surrounding intellectual and practical culture, makes it likely, given the way the Holy Spirit guides the Christian community in truth (John 16:13; cf. 1 Tim. 3:15), that the Christian prohibition on abortion did not derive from sources other than divine revelation.

There are, of course, philosophical arguments for and against the permissibility of abortion. To examine these in detail would go beyond the scope of this book. But we can say the following without much controversy: It is generally acknowledged that abortion is a tragic choice, one not to be made lightly. It is, indisputably, the destruction of the human organism in an early stage of its development. What is killed is a mammal, a mammal of the species *homo sapiens*. Now even if one could (and I believe one cannot)[20] successfully argue that a distinction is to be made between human persons and members of *homo sapiens*, so that not all members of *homo sapiens* are persons—a distinction that is alien to the Christian tradition—to kill a member of our own species would surely still be an act of great gravity. To risk putting oneself or another in a position where one would have to do such a thing in order not to neglect one's responsibilities is wrong, except perhaps for the gravest of reasons. To risk an abortion for the sake of a couple's pleasure or even for psychological benefits, is plainly wrong, even if abortion were sometimes permissible.

8. "SAVING SEX FOR MARRIAGE"

A table where every seat is at the head of the table would be a table where no seat is at the head of the table. A raise automatically bestowed on every employee would be no compliment, though it would still be nice to get. If I give you my grandmother's ring, the significance of the gift is undercut if my grandmother left me hundreds of rings, and I give one to each person I meet. But if I reserve the gift for someone I care about in a particular way, then even if my grandmother left me hundreds of rings, the ring has a significance due to my reserving it. The more restricted a gift, the more significant it is as a symbol of a particular love. Granted, there are other ways of increasing the significance of a gift, such as by increasing its value; to give one's life for many is significant no matter how many recipients there are, though it is worth noting that in some way there is only one gift there, since we each have only one life to give.

As an initial attempt at another argument for premarital abstinence, consider the apparent fact that having given oneself sexually to multiple people makes one's giving of oneself sexually to one's spouse less significant. It seems that there is a marital good that is lost here, namely, having a physical union with one's spouse that one did not have with anyone else.

Now in some way, it is true that every instance of sexual union is different. In that sense, there is a uniqueness. But *this* kind of uniqueness—the quirks in which acts differ—does not appear sufficient to make an act of marital union into a unique gift. That each of the hundreds of rings one has given has a somewhat different pattern on it will still not ensure the kind of significance in the bestowal of the ring as there would be if one gave just one ring to one person.

Perhaps, though, the uniqueness in marital sexual union is simply that the union is *marital*. It is only marital sexual union that has the temporal dimension commitment gives it. Thus, there is a good of uniqueness there. But there would be a further worthwhile kind of good of uniqueness if the physical act that consummates romantic love had also never been engaged in with anyone else.

As human beings, we exist in time, reaching back into the past with our memories and leaping into the future with our plans.[21] To unite as persons, we should unite, to the extent possible, in all our temporal dimensions. We can dedicate our future to our beloved through commitment, though absent time machines or miracles, we cannot affect the past. But it is quite possible for us to have *prepared* the past in such a way as to deepen union with a person perhaps as yet unknown, making the sexual gift more significant. One can prepare for a temporally extended future union—for a consummation of romantic love that includes the temporal dimension of an exclusivity that embraces the past. One can have a kind of prospective fidelity to one's potential future spouse, even when one does not know who this spouse is.

Such embracing of the past supplies a historical dimension to organic union. Typically, the organic union between parts in a higher animal goes as far back as the parts have existed—sometimes the organism precedes the parts, but apart from cases like those of organ transplants and the embryonic histories of chimeras—the parts do not have a history of independent existence. We cannot have this fully in the case of romantic love—full sexual union clearly can start no earlier than puberty, but also needs to wait for the maturity for a lifetime commitment. But one can produce a historical dimension to union through exclusivity before and after the sexual act, ensuring that one does not unite sexually with anyone else prior to uniting sexually with one's spouse, and one does not unite sexually with anyone else while the spouse is alive.

Through premarital sex, persons make it impossible for either of them to marry someone else while bringing to one's future spouse an exclusivity in the past. But for one to make this exclusivity impossible by having unmarried sex with someone is to impose a significant harm on that other person, limiting his or her freedom to bring this exclusivity to his or her future spouse. Unless one is engaged to one's sexual partner, the probability that one will marry him or her is not overwhelmingly high, so that there is a significant chance one's action of premarital sex will deprive the other of this temporally backwards exclusivity in the other's future marriage. And hence there is very good moral reason not to have sex in the absence of marriage.

Objection 1. While premarital sex does indeed impose a harm on the sexual partner, it is a harm to which the partner consents. But three points can be made to counter this objection. First, even with consent, it is problematic to impose a harm on someone in respect of a deeply significant future relationship for the sake of a partial sexual fulfillment in a present relationship that is of lesser significance: the harm is disproportionate to the benefits. In love, one needs to seek the good of our neighbor, and surely especially that of a neighbor with whom one is having sex. That one's neighbor consents to being deprived of a good does not give one carte blanche to stop pursuing the other's genuine interests. Second, the action of premarital sex goes against the fulfillment of a more mature and complete future romantic love, while giving, at most, a partial fulfillment of a present, immature romantic love. This is a harm it is wrong to impose even on oneself, given that one's vocation as a human being is centered on love, and also wrong to impose on another even with the other's consent. Third, if one's premarital sexual partner marries another, then there is a third party, not presently consenting, who is harmed by the premarital sex—the future spouse of the sexual partner, who is deprived of temporally backwards exclusivity on the part of this spouse. While adultery is a more serious moral offense against the spouse of one's partner in adultery, this kind of premarital sex is also an offense.

Prima facie, this argument works less well in the case of engaged couples very likely to marry. However, three points can be made about such cases. First, engagement is not marriage. The fullness of normative commitment is found in the marriage vows. One way to see this is to note that while it is a serious matter to break off an engagement, almost everyone will agree that it is not as serious as a divorce. Finding out certain unsavory details of one's fiancé(e)'s past—criminal activities, for instance—can be a good reason to break off an engagement instantly, while in the case of a marriage, even if one approves of divorce, it is clear that much more serious thought would need to be put into deciding whether the details are sufficient to divorce. Second, granting that the more likely it is that the couple will marry, the less probability there is of harming a future marriage by robbing it of backwards exclusivity, it is likewise true that the more likely it is that the couple will marry, the easier it should be for the couple to wait for sexual union. Third, such sexual relations limit the other's freedom in marrying, by bringing it about that only with oneself can the other have backwards exclusivity.

Objection 2. This argument presupposes an idealized case of premarital sex between virgins. But only a small percentage of nonmarital sexual acts are between virgins, and in the case of a sexually experienced partner, backwards exclusivity for a future marriage is already impossible, and hence there is no loss.

In response, one might cautiously agree that there is less of a loss in such cases. But one can still talk of degrees of exclusivity or fidelity, in the forwards or backwards directions. It is no excuse for Helga, who has sex with Marcus, a married man, that Marcus has already committed adultery with half a dozen women. In having sex with Marcus, she still imposes an *additional* harm on Marcus, Marcus's spouse, and on the marriage between Marcus and Marcus's spouse. Here we may note in passing that if we take seriously the idea of spouses as one organism, we can talk of "harming the marriage," since there can be harm to the united organism.

At any given time, it is possible for an unmarried nonvirgin to ensure that he or she will be able to give a future spouse exclusivity from that time forward, and sex with someone else at any time afterward removes that possibility.

Objection 3. The present argument points to the ideal of marriage with only one person, and no sexual relations with anyone else before or after marriage. But while the Christian tradition, especially in the East,[22] may agree with this as an ideal, it does not *require* this ideal, allowing remarriage after one's first spouse has died. It seems that one could say that just as not being married to anybody else in the future is ideal but not required, so, too, not having sex prior to marriage is an ideal but not morally required.

But three responses can be given to this argument. First, by engaging in sex before marriage, one is typically sacrificing an aspect of the complete future union of full romantic love for the sake of present pleasure or, at best, a union of incomplete (because not definitively committed) love. And this is wrong. But in remarrying after one's spouse has died, one sacrifices an aspect of the future component of union with the first spouse, but the sacrifice is made for the sake of another union of the same sort, a union of committed conjugal love.

Second, sexual union is tied closely to the body. There is, thus, nothing morally wrong with remarrying after one's spouse has died, because the spouse's body has perished, and the commitment to be a united organism with the spouse makes no sense at this point. If we accept this line of response (and the previous seems preferable), then we might, by parallel, argue that the present argument against premarital sex would not rule out premarital sex prior to the beginning of the life of one's spouse-to-be. That would be a relatively rare case— one would have to know that the person one will marry is not yet in existence. A commitment not to marry anyone yet alive would close one's doors to many otherwise plausible marriage prospects. Moreover, all other things being equal, one should not marry someone significantly younger than oneself, since one is likely to predecease such a person by a significant number of years, thereby depriving the person of love and support in old age.

Third, one might partially concede the point, by allowing that this argument only shows that, just as remaining unmarried after one's spouse dies is something worthwhile, so too abstinence from premarital sex is something to be promoted when there is no sufficient reason to the contrary. (Other arguments may, and I think do, show that there are not, in fact, sufficient reasons to the contrary.) However, there can be circumstances where there is strong reason to remarry after one's spouse has died—for instance, to provide for the financial or emotional needs of children, or simply because of the intrinsic goods of marriage. But in typical cases there is no similarly strong reason to engage in premarital sex. On this response, then, the argument would apply only most of the time.

Objection 4. The argument presupposes a serious possibility for future marriage. What if, instead, both sexual partners are committed never to marry anybody? Then the argument seems to provide no reason to abstain. Granted, the case of people vowed not to marry but not committed to sexual abstinence may be rare (depending on how we understand "committed"), but they are cases we should discuss.

Marriage is one of the basic human goods, since it makes possible the temporally extended and embodied union that fulfills one of the basic forms of human love. To miss out on marriage is indeed to miss out on one of the basic human goods. Nonetheless, one might have good reason not to marry—for instance, in order more effectively to minister to the people of God, or in order to devote more time to cancer research. It would have to be a serious reason, however. One should not completely miss out on a basic human good on account of something minor. It surely would not do to plan to abstain from marriage just to be able to freely engage in nonmarital sex.

Moreover, the reasons for being *committed* not to marry need to be *very* strong. Patricia the cancer researcher cannot know ahead of time how effective she will be at her cancer research. Perhaps, one day, Patricia's work will no longer be advancing her field. She should not, through a commitment to nonmarriage, rule out the possibility of marrying at such a point. In fact, I suspect that the only reason to be *committed* not to marry is a spiritual one, in order to devote oneself to one's neighbor without the intense bond of preferential love for one's spouse, and to unite with God without having to divide one's unitive desires between God and spouse (celibacy will be further discussed in chapter 11).

Furthermore, if one has a commitment not to marry and yet enters into romantic relationships, these relationships are, from the beginning, restrained from developing according to their natural trajectory. One is both loving and holding the very same love back, to prevent it getting too far. And that seems an offense against love, and that is no light thing since love is the center of human life.

Perhaps a pair of people who were not committed to nonmarriage, but who simply had good reason to believe that a good marriage would never be an option for them, might escape the present argument. For instance, such persons might know they have a form of mental illness that would make them dangerous to anyone living with them. Or they might both have good reason to expect to have tasks—such as cancer research—that, while not certain to take up their whole lives, would be nonetheless very likely to do so. By engaging in premarital sex, such persons would only be taking on a small risk of depriving a future marriage of a unitive good, and perhaps that small risk could be justified by only a small benefit derived from premarital sex.

However, a variant of the restraint-of-love argument still applies. While it can be reasonable to enter into a romantic relationship expecting that circumstances beyond one's control will break up the relationship before it can blossom into marriage—say, to engage in a romantic correspondence with a prisoner on death row—it is more problematic to enter into a romantic relationship that one knows one *ought not* to extend into marriage. In the case of mental illness or future cancer research, by entering into the romantic relationship while trying to keep it from leading to marriage—even if one has very good reason to try to keep it from leading to marriage—one is, nonetheless, holding love back, unnaturally, from the deeper form of commitment toward which the love naturally progresses (remember love's openness to change of form from section 5 of chapter 2). One might, of course, hold back emotionally in one's relationship with the death-row prisoner, perhaps for emotional self-protection, but even there, such holding back is problematic. One would probably do better to love and to accept the vulnerability that love implies.

But what about sex outside of any romantic relationship, still in the case of a person who is either committed not to marry or expecting to have good reason not to marry? Here it seems that romantic love is not restrained from progressing to conjugality, because there is no romantic love. But note first that unless there is some further motive for the sex, such as professional advancement or saving oneself from starvation, there is almost no reason at all to have sex outside of a romantic relationship. Pleasure by itself is a very weak reason, if it is an independent reason at all. Second, the same kind of holding back would still be present. In this case, it would not so much be a holding back from romantic love developing into conjugality, as it would be a holding oneself back from falling in love with the person with whom one is having sex. But to engage in sexual relations not only in the absence of romantic love but while actively trying to keep romantic love from arising seems deeply problematic. Through the sexual activity, sexual desire is being fostered—for sexual activity is about *both* the fostering *and* the satisfaction of sexual desire—while the union that the desire seeks is deliberately being kept purely physical, which is unfaithful to a desire that seeks full union. Moreover, by keeping a union purely physical, one is dissociating oneself from one's body; one is treating the body as something independent of the person.

Finally, note that the kind of prospective fidelity called for by the prospect of marriage appears to be a virtuous state preparatory for marriage. But marriage appears to be a part of a normal human life. A virtuous state that is called for by a part of normal human life is one that everyone should have at the appropriate stage in life, even those who expect that their lives will not be normal in the relevant respect. There could be virtuous states geared to specific goals that are not a part of a normal human life. Perhaps the special kind of attention to minute detail that one needs to be a watchmaker or computer programmer is not needed for a normal human life, and if so, then there is no need for a person who does not expect to practice such a profession to develop the virtue. But when a virtuous state is geared to a normal aspect of human life, then it is a normal human virtuous state, and to fail to have that state is to fail to exhibit an aspect of normal human moral excellence—and this is a moral failing. For instance, the need for generosity with property is a part of normal human life. That one expects in the future to be so poor that one will have nothing with which to be generous is no excuse for failing to develop this aspect of generosity. One can be poor and have the habit of generosity, even if one does not expect to exercise it. Likewise, one can have marital virtue without being married, and premarital virtue without expecting to marry. Thus, the virtue of prospective fidelity should be had by all unmarried persons, even ones who do not expect to marry.

9. THE BODY AS THE PICTURE OF THE SOUL

An important insight in the thought of some twentieth-century philosophers such as Wittgenstein and John Paul II is that the body *expresses* the person.[23] Wittgenstein put this very memorably: "The human body is the best picture of the human soul."[24]

There is a trivial sense in which the body expresses the person: yes, of course, we express ourselves with our vocal cords and our gestures, as well as in and through the work of our hands. It is a somewhat less trivial insight to observe that *all* we know about another as a person depends on our observation of their body, barring some kind of supernatural insight. Observe, too, the tight correlation in the Gospels between physical actions such as feeding the hungry or visiting the sick and the state of the soul. We are to be judged on love, and yet this love is paradigmatically expressed in a bodily way.

But there is more to be said here. In the Catholic tradition, for instance, the body is not something wholly separate from the soul, but the life of the body is an activity of the soul. The soul's life and the body's life are not distinct. Indeed, in a real sense, the soul *is* the life of the body, as is emphasized both by the Catholic dogma that the soul is the "form" of the body, and by the New Testament's use of *psuchê* to mean both life (e.g., Matt. 16:26) and soul (e.g., Matt. 26:38). The Book of Genesis describes Adam, made of dust, as a "living soul [*nefesh khaya; psuchên zôsan*]" (Gen. 2:7; RSV has "living being"). When we look at Adam in his clayish body, what we see is a soul embodied.

Our bodies are not mere tools of our persons, nor are they worn like clothes. Christ came to redeem us as persons, for it is precisely as persons that we sin. But it is the Word's *becoming flesh*—and not just the putting on of flesh—that scripture emphasizes. We are in the image and likeness of God; and we are embodied. There is no opposition here: we are in the image and likeness of God as the embodied beings we are.

It seems that every aspect of our bodily existence expresses something about us as persons. Some aspects of our bodily existence express our frailty and our fallenness. Some express our basic dignity as in the image and likeness of God. Some may express both.

Now the task of figuring out just how a given bodily feature expresses the person, or how a given personal attitude is expressed in the body, can be a difficult one. One can ridicule this task by asking what it says about Frank that, right now, the number *n* of living cells in his body is an odd number (is he thus a strange kind of guy?), or about Jennifer that she has a rabbit-shaped birthmark (should she become a rabbit breeder?), or about human beings in general that they have appendixes or that they defecate.

The last of these examples is the easiest to respond to, however: that we expel waste expresses, among other things, that we are not angels, that we live in mutual dependence on a larger ecological system. But what about the more trivial cases: the appendix, the birthmark, and the parity of the number of living cells? A recent theory is that the appendix helps maintain intestinal bacteria.[25] If so, then this expresses mutual dependence within a larger ecosystem. But suppose the appendix has no such function. Then, none of the three features are important to the functioning of the body, and that is precisely why one might think they present a difficulty. But if the body is the picture of the soul, then it is natural to say that those features that are unimportant to the biological functioning of the body, even though they do reflect *something* about the person, may reflect quite trivial facts, such as that the person's soul is the life of an odd number of cells. Furthermore, the appendix, the birthmark, and the oddness of the number of living cells all do make *some* difference to our functioning, but the difference is trivial most of the time, except when the appendix becomes inflamed or the birthmark is made fun of or the total number of cells is very small (think of an embryo with only three cells—that there are three rather than two or four may be important).

In any case, when we deliberately act physically, we express ourselves in and through the body in a deliberate way. This self-expression may be integrated with our bodily functioning, or it may be at variance with it. Perhaps the most extreme case of lack of integrity in the embodied person is suicide; there, the person is opposed to the body's basic striving for survival, and yet lives out this opposition in and through movements of that same body, since suicide is committed not by thinking but by acting physically.[26]

Now, if two people are voluntarily and mutually biologically united as one body, in the most thorough kind of union possible, then, as Punzo has argued,[27] it is appropriate that they also be united, perhaps again as thoroughly as is possible for them, on an interpersonal level. It is plausible that what the most thorough biological union possible expresses is a union of persons. We are integral beings consisting of body and soul, or body and mind. Our bodies are not mere property, and when the bodies of two people are united, it is not as if their cars or even their dogs were united. Rather, the *persons* are united, in respect of the body. There would be something wrong if there were one body with a divided mind: it would be a lack of integrity. Similarly, it would be inappropriate for there to be a voluntarily united body with no commitment to making the union permanent. After all, a genuine biological organism should strive for its own self-preservation.

Without love between two persons engaging in sexual intercourse, there would be a union of body, but one that did not fully encompass them as persons. Yet the body expresses the person.

To allow one's body to be united with another's in the most thorough way possible, without a union of the persons at a higher level, would be to treat the body as something that it is not, as something that is not expressive of oneself. But more seriously, if one is united with the body of another person in such a way that both become one body, then, in an important way, that other body is one's own body. And to fail to love that body is like failing to love oneself in respect of one's own body. But we *should* love ourselves: we *should* pursue the good (nothing else is worth pursuing), and, in particular, we should pursue the good for ourselves. Hence, we should love the body of the other person like our own, as Ephesians 5:28 insists. But one ought not love a body without loving the person, since the body is the expression of the person, and to love it without recognizing this, and hence without loving the person who is expressed, would be to misunderstand what the body is, and thus would be a distortion of love.

Therefore, one can argue that one ought to love the person with whom one unites sexually. This is no surprise: we should love *everyone*. But if our bodies are to be truly expressive of who we are, and if directedness at sexual union is what distinguishes sexual love from other forms of love, then it is very plausible that this should be a sexual love, so that the sexual union would be expressive of a romantic union of two persons *as persons*. Further, it should be not just any romantic union, but a romantic union of the most thoroughgoing kind possible. In particular, the interpersonal union should be of a maximally committed kind, since commitment, in both the objective sense of becoming morally bound, as by making a vow, and in the subjective sense of sincerely acknowledging the bond, is always possible to persons of normal psychological functioning (we would take the absence of the ability to sincerely make a vow a serious defect).[28]

10. POLYGAMY AND PROSTITUTION

I shall argue that the permissibility of sex apart from lifelong commitment would also imply the permissibility of some cases of prostitution and of something functionally equivalent to polygamy. To do this, I will distinguish a more conservative from a more liberal version of the permissive view.

On the more conservative permissive view of sex apart from lifelong commitment, unmarried persons are morally permitted to engage in sexual relations assuming informed consent, prudence with regard to physical, emotional, and other consequences, mutual honesty, and an absence of hatred or disgust, but only if they are within an appropriate relationship. The requirements on an appropriate relationship may include such things as mutual affection, love, and commitment, but will fall short of full "'til death do us part" commitment. On the more liberal permissive view, the requirement of an appropriate relationship is dropped: purely hedonistic sex between people who have just met and who are not planning any continued relationship can be acceptable, assuming the other conditions, especially informed consent, are met.

I shall begin by arguing that the more conservative permissive view is an implausible halfway house between a restrictive view that requires lifelong commitment and the more liberal permissive view.

For consider the question of exactly what requirements are to be put on an appropriate relationship, starting with commitment. Lifelong commitment is not required. But how much commitment *is* required? Where is the line to be drawn? It seems likely that a commitment for the next fifty years would be deemed sufficient, while a commitment for the next fifty seconds would not. But it seems implausible to draw the line in terms of a length of time. It would be strange if sexual activity were always wrong if people were committed to each other for a term of less than twenty-five years, but could be right if people were committed to each other for a term of at least thirty years (the in-between lengths might be a gray area). For where would the numbers, however vague, come from?

Perhaps commitment could be measured not in terms of the length of time for which one is committed—which sounds too much like a prison sentence!—but in terms of the way in which the commitment is conditional. Maybe it is permissible for a couple to have sex if each person is committed to the other, conditionally on the other's behavior not being too nasty. But where is the line of being "too nasty" to be drawn? A tempting answer is to allow the members of every couple to draw it themselves. But to do that would be to count as a sufficient commitment to the other to be faithful as long as the other is perfectly nice, and that is pretty close to not being any commitment at all, since none of us is *perfectly* nice for any length of time.

Similar things can be said about the mutual affection and love required by the defender of the more conservative permissive view. Affection and love come in degrees. Just how much mutual affection and love is required for sex would be an unanswerable question. And if one says that *any* amount of mutual affection and love will suffice, then the restriction to cases where there is affection and love does little work, since mutual sexual attraction is apt to produce *some* affection and a glimmering of romantic love, if, at least, there is no hatred or disgust there.

But perhaps an answer is possible here along something like the following lines. Let's say that, prior to having sex, the members of the couple commit to each other as long as the other person does not commit what Catholic theology calls an objectively "grave sin"—or as long as the other is not physically unfaithful. A fairly bright line could be drawn there (more so for the grave sin suggestion than for the infidelity one, since there is a continuum of physical infidelity ranging from a single instance of standing in too-close physical proximity to a regular habit of sexual intercourse).

However, even if we can draw such a bright line, there is still the question why it is that sex ought always to be limited to couples who have *that* kind of commitment, *that* form of mutual affection, and *that* degree of love. The reason is not merely due to emotional and physical consequences, since both the more conservative and more liberal permissive views require prudence about physical consequences. Rather, it must be that there is something about the nature of sex that limits its appropriateness to couples who exhibit the requisite relationship.

But what would this feature of sex be? Let us restrict the discussion to intercourse. Intercourse is the joining of two bodies through the joint activity of the bodies' reproductive faculties. That which, on the more conservative permissive view, limits intercourse to certain relationships is either based on this fact about intercourse, or on the emotions, pleasures, and other physical reactions concomitant with the joint activity of the bodies' reproductive faculties.

What kind of a limit could be based on the fact that intercourse is a reproductive-type joining? If it is the *joining* that is relevant, then the best proposal on the table is Punzo's idea[29] that a thorough joining of persons needs to accompany a joining of bodies. But this yields more than either defender of the permissive view wants—a *thorough* joining of persons requires much more serious commitment.

Maybe, though, it is the reproductivity of intercourse that yields the restriction. To say this, one has to insist that even when intercourse cannot result in reproduction (e.g., intercourse during a pregnancy or after menopause), the reproductive teleology of intercourse nonetheless has normative implications vis-à-vis the type of relationships in which intercourse is permissible. There, perhaps the best proposal available to us is the idea that intercourse should occur only within the kind of relationship in which childbearing would be appropriate. But again, this threatens to require significantly more than the more conservative defender of the permissive view would like. For it is highly plausible that a loving home, with the family as a whole exhibiting unconditionally committed love, is a moral prerequisite for procreation. Once again, it appears difficult to defend the conservative permissive view against attacks from the more permissive side.

What about the other aspects of intercourse? There, it is very hard, indeed, to see why there would need to be a restriction based on the type of relationship. That sex is very pleasant is surely not a reason for limiting sex to a type of relationship; if anything, it would seem to be a reason for sharing the pleasures widely and unselfishly. That sex tends to create emotional ties will create restrictions, but these will not require the confinement of intercourse to certain kinds of relationships, but rather, *either* to certain kinds of relationships *or* to cases where emotional ties will not be created. And there certainly can be cases where emotional ties will not be created—for instance, if the agents are sufficiently inebriated that they will not remember each other afterwards.

Maybe the more conservative defender of the permissive view will say that although the emotional ties will not, in fact, be created each time the couple has sex, the relationship should be the kind of relationship in which emotional ties would be appropriate, because it is normal for such emotional ties to develop. This would be an emotional-tie variant of the procreation argument above. This is a fine argument, but it appears to show too much for a permissivist to make use of it. For the emotional ties seem to require the security of being able to trust the other unconditionally, and this seems to call for lifetime commitment.

If I am right, then the more conservative version of the permissive view is not tenable, but the more liberal version of the permissive view allows for some cases of prostitution and for something functionally equivalent to polygamy. After all, consent, prudence, honesty, and absence of serious relational problems seem quite possible in cases of paid sex, as well as in familial arrangements in which there are multiple persons committed for life, where, for instance, no person is allowed to have sex with anyone who is not a part of the arrangement. And as a throw-away line, one might ask: If sex that is purely for physical pleasure is permissible between people without a significant relationship, why would it not be permissible to have sex for the sake of the pleasure of having money?

If this is right, then we have to choose between the restrictive view that says sexual intercourse requires lifetime exclusive commitment, and the liberal version of the permissive view that only places restrictions of consent, prudence, honesty, and non-negativity on the liaison.

We can now proceed in one of two ways. We could rely on the implausibility of the liberal version of the permissive view. If sex is so widely permissible, it does not appear likely that it also has the kind of deep meaning we ascribe to it, for instance. And, in any case, a lot of people find prostitution and polygamy to be clearly beyond the pale.

Second, we could continue theologically. If anything is clear, it is clear that the more liberal version of the permissive view is incompatible with the vision of sexuality in the Bible and in Christian tradition. For instance, in the Old Testament prostitution is seen as a paradigm of an impermissible activity, and sex without relational constraints has always been condemned by the Christian tradition.

11. FROM MOST CASES TO ALL CASES

Some of the arguments above establish only that premarital sex is wrong in most cases. There are, however, three tools one can use to try to leverage a prohibition against doing something in most cases into a complete prohibition against that type of action—tools involving natural law, virtue ethics, and divine command ethics.

On the natural law side, Thomas Aquinas argues that fornication is wrong because children are harmed by being conceived in circumstances where they will receive inadequate paternal support (cf. the argument in section 7, above). He also writes: "Nor does it matter if a man having knowledge of a woman by fornication, make sufficient provision for the upbringing of the child: because a matter that comes under the determination of the law is judged according to what happens in general, and not according to what may happen in a particular case."[30]

One way of filling out Aquinas's argument is as follows. Each thing that exists has a nature that specifies and explains its normal functioning. Cats hunt, sheep have four legs, and human beings communicate the truth. Normal functioning tends to be good for the individual and the species. A particular individual can, of course, fall short of normalcy—the cat can be indolent, the sheep can have three legs, and the human can lie. Sometimes this falling short is involuntary—in nonhuman animals, it always is such, since only humans have free will. But it is wrong to voluntarily fall short of normal or natural functioning, i.e., to ensure a deliberate malfunction of one's self.

Now in a sinful world, it can be difficult to figure out what actions are natural. That the majority of cats hunt is good reason to think hunting is natural to cats. But that the majority of humans lie is not good reason to think lying is natural to humans, because humans can sinfully fall short of what is normal. One approach to finding out what is natural for humans, then, is to determine the natural behavior of relevantly similar nonhuman animals. For instance, Aquinas claims birds are monogamous and relevantly similar to us in that their offspring, like ours, requires two parents.[31] Why choose this aspect of similarity rather than, say, the bonobos with their notoriously unconservative sexual habits?[32] Maybe because sexuality for Aquinas is defined by a directedness toward procreation, and hence similarity in respect of the raising of children is more important.

But a better Thomistic approach than to look to animal parallels is to make use of the observation that natural behavior tends to be good for the individual and the species, and unnatural behavior tends to be harmful. Thus, that a form of behavior tends to be bad for the species is strong evidence of its being an unnatural form of behavior, and wrong whenever it is voluntary. Even if the behavior is not harmful on some occasion, it is still an unnatural form of behavior and, thus, still wrong, being contrary to natural law.

This opens the way for arguments of this form: a type of behavior tends to be harmful to the individual or species, and so it is unnatural, and hence it is wrong. Thus, from premarital sex being harmful most of the time, we can conclude that it is an unnatural form of human behavior, and that it is wrong whenever it is engaged in freely. Even if an instance of premarital sex is, in some exceptional case, not harmful, it is still an unnatural form of behavior, and thus wrong. This makes some natural law arguments resemble rule-utilitarian arguments, but we have to note that on this reading, Aquinas is not claiming that what makes premarital sex wrong in exceptional cases is its harmfulness in other cases. That view, congenial as it is to the rule-utilitarian, is implausible—why should the fact that an action is harmful in other circumstances make it be wrong in these? Rather, for Aquinas, the action's harmfulness in more common circumstances is *evidence* for its unnaturalness, and the wrongness results from the unnaturalness.

Nevertheless, there is a serious weakness in arguments of this sort: how well the argument works depends on how one describes the action. (This is also a standard problem for rule-utilitarianism.) Perhaps inserting an object in something tends to be harmless. But let us suppose inserting a knife in someone's heart tends to be harmful. (How one counts the "tends to" is difficult; we might imagine we are living at a time where most cases of cardiac knife insertion are cases of murder.) However, inserting a knife in someone's heart with medical knowledge and for a medical end tends to be beneficial. Yet one and the same action, at the very same time, can be (a) the inserting of an object in something, (b) the inserting of a knife in someone's heart, and (c) the inserting of a knife in someone's heart with medical knowledge and for a medical end. If we say that an action is wrong provided that it tends to be wrong under some description, then we have to say that heart surgery is wrong because cardiac knife-insertion tends to be harmful. And if, on the other hand, we allow an action to escape Aquinas-style harm arguments so long as it is harmless under at least one description, then Aquinas has no argument against pre-marital sex under the description "sex in circumstances where one can ensure the welfare of offspring."

Still, I think Aquinas has two responses available. The nature of an entity explains the characteristic forms of behavior for that entity in something like the way that laws of physics explain the motions of the things falling under those laws.[33] When we infer a law of nature, we seek a balance between simplicity of law and closeness of fit to observations. Thus, if I vary x and measure y, obtaining measurements like $x=7.56$ and $y=15.10$, $x=3.89$ and $y=7.79$, as well as $x=4.01$ and $y=8.00$, I would likely infer that the right law of nature describing the data is $y=2x$, but that my data suffers from slight experimental error in respect of x or y of the order of 0.01 or 0.02. But I could have opted instead for the more complex law $y=25x^2/367+1779x/1468+15011/7340$. This law would, in fact, have fit the data *exactly*. But given that $y=2x$ is so much simpler, we sacrifice closeness of fit to simplicity and infer the simpler law. What I said is not an artifact of there being only three measurements—however many measurements there are, there will be such tradeoffs.[34]

Now, we would expect the nature of an animal to encode the basic parameters for that species' normal sexual behavior, including particular parameters that control who mates with whom. Given the choice between positing a human nature that contains the rule *live monogamously* and one that contains the rule *live monogamously except perhaps when you can take care of the children and when there is a defeater for the "privacy/disclosure" and "saving sex for marriage" arguments,* it is simpler to suppose that it is the former rule our nature contains.

A related simplicity-based tool for moving from a prohibition in most cases to a prohibition in all cases is given by some considerations of virtue. A virtue such as courage or generosity is a habit of thought, affect, and behavior. This habit is beneficial to the individual and to others, but not every beneficial habit is a virtue. Virtues are fairly general habits: generosity in general is a virtue, but there is no specific virtue of being generous to people who weigh 154 pounds, even though that would be a beneficial habit, too. The task of discovering virtues combines empirical discovery of actual patterns of thought, affect, and behavior in people, with moral evaluation of benefits and of the role that the patterns fulfill in life.

Now, virtuous sexual behavior does not seem to be a special case of some more general pattern of virtuous behavior, in the way in which being generous to people who weigh 154 pounds is a special case of being generous. One way to see this is to note that there appear to be generally uncontroversial rules of sexual behavior, such as the prohibition against necrophilia or infertile incest, which do not seem to be special cases of some nonsexual rule. We would thus expect there to be one or more specifically sexual virtues.

The arguments in the preceding sections have shown that nonmarital intercourse, if it were ever justifiable morally, would be morally justifiable only rarely. But there are actually extant human habits of behavior that involve abstaining from all nonmarital intercourse and that are, otherwise, plausible candidates for being virtues. One such habit is a chastity that limits sexual behavior to that which appropriately unitively expresses lifelong mutual commitment. But it does not appear that there are actually extant human habits of sexual behavior that involve almost total abstinence from nonmarital intercourse with exceptions in rare cases that fall through the cracks of all of the preceding arguments. Thus, the exceptionless habit of chastity is a more plausible candidate for a virtue.

In any case, just as we should prefer a simpler candidate for a law of nature, so too, we should prefer a simpler candidate for a virtue, barring a strong argument to the contrary. Habits that limit sex to marriage are simpler candidates for being virtues, and there is no good nonconsequentialist moral argument *against* limiting sex to marriage. Since the ethics of love rejects consequentialism—we must not act unlovingly even if the unloving action has good consequences (think of killing one innocent person to save two, and recall Paul's point in Romans 3:8 that we do not do evil that good may come of it)—we have good reason to adopt the view that a habit that limits sex to marriage is a virtue. But to act in a way contrary to a virtue is to act viciously.

A third approach is through divine commands. Consider, for instance, C. Stephen Evans's view of the relation between God and morality.[35] Evans believes that although God does not make any choices about what is *good or bad,* his commands are relevant to what is morally *right or wrong.* Thus, one might say that knowledge is good independently of divine choices, but it is in part because of God's commands that stealing is wrong. Moreover, Evans thinks there are some basic virtue-based duties that are not dependent on the will of God. One of these is the duty to be grateful for benefits received. We have received all the goods we have from God, and our grateful recognition of this calls us to obedience to God's will. Furthermore, God's will is an innately loving will, and his commands for us are ones that are good for us to have.

Now we can evaluate two hypotheses. Both of these hypotheses note that there are reasons why a typical case of premarital sex is harmful to us and why a loving God would want us to abstain in such a case. On the first hypothesis, God has commanded us to refrain from all premarital sex. On the second, he has commanded us to refrain from almost all premarital sex, with rare exceptions in the cases that fall through the cracks of the arguments.

But now we can argue along rule-utilitarian lines. If we were to strive to follow an almost complete prohibition with some loopholes, we would likely be trying to stretch the loopholes to cover the cases we want. After all, premarital sex is often strongly tempting, and times of sexual temptation are not times of the highest degree of rationality. Rationalization in the sexual sphere is a common phenomenon. And it is easier to rationalize the claim that an act of premarital intercourse falls under one of the exceptions to the rule than it is to rationalize the claim that the act isn't really an act of premarital intercourse. Thus, for every instance of correctly following the exception in the more complex rule, there would likely be multiple instances of wrongly assimilating a present case to an exception. The overall results would be unfortunate. Moreover, it is probably easier to develop the simpler moral habit, one that simply stays away from all premarital sex and that avoids thoughts and occasions leading one toward it.

Therefore, it is likely that a loving God would prohibit us from *all* premarital sex rather than giving us the more complex rule. This plausible argument becomes particularly strong when we observe that scripture, as unanimously interpreted by the Christian tradition, in fact prohibits nonmarital sexual activity: the argument just given gave us prior reason to expect a divine prohibition of premarital sex, and now that we see something that seems to be such a prohibition, Christians have good reason to take it at face value, whether or not they take scripture to be always right.

12. WHAT IS THE MOST THOROUGH KIND OF ROMANTIC COMMITMENT POSSIBLE?

We can now use a method for figuring out the kind of commitment that sexual union should involve similar to that which Anselm of

Canterbury used for figuring out the nature of God. Anselm defined God as that than which nothing greater can be conceived, and from this definition drew conclusions such as that God is all-knowing or all-good, since if he were not these, a greater could be conceived. Likewise, we are going to try to figure out what kind of maximal commitment is practically possible in the sexual case.

We have already seen that the body-focused nature of romantic love quite reasonably sets one limit to that love: death. Is this the only possible limit? Consider first an abstract argument to the contrary. Commitment subjectively construed—a personal cleaving to a rule of behavior—requires, in order to be firm, a moral duty independent of that subjective cleaving. Without a duty, one could simply one day say, "Why should I bother?" In the case of the commitment simply to love a person, this moral duty arguably comes from the general duty to love everyone. But what could be the source of a duty to love someone in a romantic, or at least conjugal, way?

Here, I think of conjugal love as the most mature form of romantic love. Conjugal love, however, may involve inner shifts of form: thus, changing the bedding of a spouse with Alzheimer's is an act of conjugal love, but it is awkward to call it a form of "romantic love." Still, there is a romantic aspect identifiable there. While there may be no sexual desire, there could be a regret as to the other's unromantic state. Sometimes we use the term "romantic love" for the whole love over a lifetime, but often we reserve the term for the more sexually charged aspects. In any case, here I want to talk about the temporally extended love as a whole, including all the conjugal phases, and will use the term "romantic love" for it all.

Now, the duty to love someone romantically does not come from *having had* a romantic love. For it can be a duty to terminate a romantic relationship (this is uncontroversial in the case of uncommitted relationships). Nor does engagement in sexual intercourse imply a duty to love romantically. For while I have argued that sexual intercourse ought to be expressive of a union of persons, it is not plausible that there is an equally strong duty after intercourse to produce a union of persons. Again, sometimes the morally or prudentially right thing to do is to terminate the relationship.

Rather, the most plausible source of this kind of obligation seems to be a *promise,* implicit or explicit. At least, in practice, that *is* how people cement the union on a personal level: they promise fidelity to one another. However, ordinary promises are not absolutely binding, for we can always be released from a promise by the person to whom we made it. This would mean that a commitment grounded in a promise would be conditional on the other person's not declining to have the promise be kept. This is problematic given the maximizing tendency of romantic love, the need to give oneself as wholly and as irrevocably as practically possible, without the possibility of negotiating release. If there is no way of entering into a more absolute commitment, then this may have to do, but we should examine whether something stronger is not practically possible.

But before we do that, let us consider why it might be desirable to have available some stronger form of commitment than a promise from which the other can release one. One of the central messages of the first letter of John is that "[w]e love, because he first loved us" (1 John 4:19; cf. also verse 10). God's love, thus, preceded our love, and by this, the author seems to want to tell us that it was not conditioned on our love. Now, while this only applies directly to *agapê* as such—and does not by itself imply that romantic *agapê* should have a similar unconditionality as *romantic*—we can still arrive at this conclusion about romantic love when we note that a central theme of both the Hebrew and the Christian scriptures is that the love between God and his people is like that which should exist between spouses. If so, then mature romantic love should also, as *romantic* (or at least conjugal, if we insist on a distinction), not be conditioned on the response. And this kind of conditionality *is* threatened by seeing the commitment as contingent on a promise made to the other person from which the other person can release one. A sinner can say to God: "God, I no longer want you to strive to save me," but God will continue to love the sinner, and this is a crucially important feature of God's love for us.

Thus the methodology of looking for the deepest kind of committed interpersonal union in romantic love that we can imagine does allow us, and perhaps even requires us, to consider the possibility of a commitment that is not dependent on the beloved holding one to it. The main objection to this point is twofold, in terms of the cost to oneself and the cost to the beloved that might result from such a commitment. The cost to oneself can be dismissed. For insofar as the deepest kind of romantic love, even as romantic, mirrors the self-sacrificing divine *agapê* that expressed itself in Christ, it is not something that counts the cost.

The cost to one's beloved, however, cannot be dismissed so easily. If what we are dealing with is love, then the love needs to adjust itself to the beloved's needs. But it might be that the beloved no longer has any need of one. Perhaps, on the contrary, one makes the beloved miserable, physically, psychologically, or spiritually. Consider a case where due to mental illness, the lover cannot but abuse the beloved, or a case where the beloved is someone abusive. The former case makes the beloved psychologically and physically miserable. The case where the beloved is abusive is one where one's presence opens an opportunity to the beloved for a life of vice. But if Socrates is right that there is nothing worse than to become a bad person, then in this case not only does the lover suffer, but the beloved is even more miserable spiritually, even if the beloved does not realize this misery. In these cases, it seems, *agapê* calls for one not to be near the beloved. And if romantic love is to be a form of *agapê*, then it seems it cannot require that one impose one's company on the beloved in these circumstances, since it would be unloving to do so.

Thus, the content of the commitment cannot be that one should actually, no matter what, live with the beloved or in any other way impose oneself on the beloved. However, the commitment can require that one exclusively love the beloved romantically—i.e., not engage in romantic relationships with anyone else—and this can be a commitment independent of whether the beloved desires one to continue that commitment, since the burden is imposed on oneself.

There are still, however, two further problems. The first is that by *mutually* undertaking the commitment, one is imposing on the beloved that very same commitment. The burden of exclusivity can be heavy, and it seems as if it may be contrary to love to impose it on one's beloved. This observation does indeed show that it would be contrary to *agapê* to impose the commitment on one's beloved, but it does not show that it would be contrary to *agapê* to allow the beloved to *voluntarily* take on this commitment. It would have been contrary to love if Peter forced Jesus to wash Peter's feet, but *allowing* Jesus to wash Peter's feet was a different matter. The unitive value of the commitment requires that it be mutual. The fact that the union is also on the personal and not just on the biological level requires freedom. When one offers to make the gift of such a commitment to one's beloved, one hopes that one's beloved will want to offer to make the same gift in return. If not, then the mutual union desired will not result, and undertaking such maximal commitment oneself would not be appropriate—instead of undertaking a one-sided commitment incapable of consummation, one would do better to withdraw to a more appropriate form of love. Of course, if mutual commitment has already been undertaken, and one side subjectively falls short of the commitment, the other needs to hold on to his or her side.

The more difficult question is *how* such a maximally committed interpersonal union could be achieved. We seem to have two kinds of commitments to other people. There are the commitments that we have entered voluntarily, and there are ones where our being normatively committed is involuntary, though it may come about as a result of a voluntary action of ours. Two examples of involuntary commitments are when we have an objective normative commitment to our parents, which does not come about as a result of any action of ours, and the case of having to pay for gas when we have pumped it. The latter commitment comes about as a result of our voluntary action, but our consent to the taking on of the commitment is not asked for—pumping the gas results in our acquiring a debt, even if we do not acknowledge the debt. On the other hand, when we make a promise, our voluntary acknowledgment of our commitment is what results in the normative consequence of the commitment, namely, the obligation to do what one has promised.

I will argue that the commitment called for by the deepest kind of romantic love is of the voluntary sort. For let us suppose that it was of the involuntary sort. The duty, then, would either arise from a voluntary action of ours or not. In the latter case, it would not be a truly personal union on the level of the will. Moreover, the Christian tradition does not recognize involuntary marriages, and it is in marriage that Christians have traditionally seen the commitment instantiated. Let us consider, then, the case where the duty is grounded in a voluntary action, but an action that is not relevantly like an action of promising. Which action could that be? Living together with someone, having sex with someone, or even having a child with someone are not plausibly considered to induce an absolute duty to be committed to the person no matter what, until death. The Christian tradition has never seen it that way, and we can imagine cases where all three actions occurred, but where it is uncontroversial that the person should get out of the relationship. If the commitment is not expressly chosen as such, then perhaps it is not the person as a whole that is united—the consent of the will and intellect is not quite there.

Thus, the commitment had better be of the voluntary sort. The commitment is not like a case where one does some action like pumping gas and comes to owe payment, but rather the commitment is something one expressly takes on. But our only real paradigm of such commitments is commitments that come about through promises. And these commitments, it seems, are not absolute until death. They can be undone by the consent of the person to whom they are made. Thus, it appears, there is no way to "engineer" an absolute commitment of the right sort, since it seems we can always be released by the person to whom we make the promise.

Nor will it do to come up with some clever arrangement, like x's having y promise that y won't release x from the promise that x is about to make, for then x can *first* release y from *that* meta-promise, and then y can release x from the first-order promise, and this is not an inescapable commitment. If promises are going to do the job, then they must be made in such a way that the person to whom they are made can in no way release us, and apart from contrived and practically inapplicable cases,[36] this appears to be impossible.

Perhaps the promise could be made to a third party, though. If this third party is any other human being, that will not help, because the human being could release one from the promise. Nor will it help if that person promises not to release one, because one could release that person from this promise. Perhaps one could come up with cases where the person to whom one makes the promise has no moral right to release one from the promise. But it is still possible for people to do things they have no right to do, and so it seems the promisee could still release one, though it would be wrong for him or her to do so. I do not have a knock-down argument that no case involving a promise to another human being could be arranged so that the promise would be relevant to romantic love and release from the promise would be impossible, but the outlook is bleak.

Now, romantic love calls for a commitment for life that is as strong as possible. If it were impossible to have a commitment from which one could not be released, perhaps one would settle for the closest approximation. One such approximation would be a promise to a third party with a continuing interest in one's maintenance of a marital union,[37] and who is unlikely to release one from it. A plausible option here is the community. The community has an interest in the maintenance of marital unions, for unromantic as well as romantic reasons such as ensuring social stability, providing the young with examples of commitment, and making possible an institution that does justice to the deep union that romantic love seeks. If the community is one that is very unlikely to change its laws and customs concerning conjugal commitment, then making a firm promise to both the community and one's beloved will do much to provide the commitment that romantic love seeks.

But a stronger kind of commitment, if it were practically possible, would be desired. Is an absolutely indissoluble union possible?

13. MARRIAGE AND DIVORCE IN THE NEW TESTAMENT

So far the answer to the question of what sort of commitment romantic love calls one to is conditional. It depends on how far it is practically *possible* to be bound to one's beloved until death, a question, in turn, that does not depend entirely on us. Individuals are unable, it seems, to create such a satisfactory bond on their own. We can make promises to one another, but these are not commitments absolutely binding until death, since the other party can release one. An absolute bond seems to require God to accept our voluntary commitment, so that it might have the kind of force that romantic love would ideally seek for it. Romantic love seeks the deepest kind of union that is practically possible and compatible with romantic love. If, in fact, God does not accept such binding from human beings—does not allow us to be bound until death—then romantic love will have to settle for somewhat less on the personal side of the union, like a promise that must be kept unless the other party and/or the community release one, since the kind of union that is sought in romantic love cannot be greater than the kind of union that is possible for human beings.

There is, however, strong evidence that God does make it practically possible for *Christians* to become bound to one another in this strongly indissoluble way. If so, then perhaps a distinction can be made. Perhaps the natural romantic love, which is all that is available absent God's grace, only calls for a union that must be kept until one is released from it by the other, or maybe by an appropriate authority. But the Christian's eros is, plausibly, raised by grace into a supernatural love, a love that is an image of the love between Christ and the Church, and this love calls for the deepest union practically possible for human beings by God's grace. And this union is indissoluble. This idea of a natural love being raised into a supernatural one was already mentioned at the end of section 2 of chapter 2 as perhaps the best way to understand the deep kind of *agapê* that the First Letter of John talks about.

What is the evidence that a union that is indissoluble (except by death) is available to the Christian? One source of evidence is the innate plausibility of the claim that this is the sort of thing we would expect a loving God, when redeeming humankind, to make possible to lovers. If such a union were possible to lovers, the union would be a deep way of fulfilling love, and a way of making our romantic love be more an image both of the Trinitarian love between the Father and the Son and of God's love for his people. The possibility of such a union would be a generous gift of God. Moreover, this is a gift that Christians have traditionally believed God to have given. It is implausible that Christians would have overestimated the generosity of God in respect of allowing our love to blossom more fully.

One may object that such a "gift" is one that would weigh heavily on us, and so God might choose to withhold it. It would weigh heavily on us because, by making it possible for Christians to unite in this deep way, it would mean that the maximal appropriate commitment that Christian lovers seek would *have* to include this commitment, or else they would be unfaithful to the totality of self-giving in romantic love. But of course being committed until death can be a burden. Still, it is central to Christianity that God bears our burdens with us. The hypothesis, then, that God generously makes such a union possible to us, and gives us the grace to live out the union, is a very probable one.

The second source of evidence is revelation. First, note the prohibition on divorce given by Jesus in each of the synoptic Gospels, twice, in fact, in Matthew, and reiterated by Paul (Mark 10:2–12; Matt. 5:31–32, 19:3–9; Luke 16:18; 1 Cor. 7:10). At Matthew 5:31–32, Jesus first acknowledges that the Mosaic Law allowed divorce. But the context is the discourse of Matthew 5:17–48, itself a part of the Sermon on the Mount, on how the listeners' righteousness has to exceed "that of the scribes and Pharisees" (5:20), who are presented as carefully keeping the Mosaic Law. The main part of the discourse consists of six paired claims, the first of which presents an item either accepted by contemporary religious mores or, more strongly, an item from the Law, and the second of which starts with the highly contrastive "But I say to you," with an emphasis on the "I" (*egô* is used as an emphatic pronoun), and gives a more stringent moral requirement. For instance, the prohibition against murder is extended into a prohibition against being "angry" or insulting someone (5:22).

One of these paired claims deals with the Mosaic Law's allowance of divorce: "But I say to you that every one who divorces his wife [*tên gunaika autou*], except on the ground of unchastity [*parektos logou porneias*], makes her an adulteress; and whoever marries a divorced woman commits adultery" (5:32). Now, we could understand the first half of this saying as advice on how to act justly toward women in a society where the prospects for a divorced woman would be bleak because she would be driven to adultery by such a divorce. However, if Jesus' concern here is only to prevent women from falling into the circumstances of divorcées, the second half of the verse would make no sense. For if it were solely concern for the prospects of a divorced woman that were driving the prohibition on divorcing a wife, then someone willing to marry such a woman would be doing something commendable. But on the contrary, such a person is condemned as committing adultery himself.

There does seem to be an exception here: *"parektos logou porneias."* The term *porneia* is a catch-all term for sexual immorality, translated well by "unchastity." Whether a particular sexual practice is an example of *porneia* is unlikely to be something a lexicon can tell us, much as looking up "just war" in a dictionary will not help a politician decide whether a proposed war is just. A sexual practice is *porneia* if and only if it is, in fact, immoral, though it is possible that a reference to some particular kind of immoral activity is contextually implied.

The most significant question to be settled, however, is not the exact sexual immorality implied by *porneia*—though much scholarly ink has been spilled over the question—but the question between which parties the *porneia* is supposed to occur. There are, after all, two prominent possibilities. On the first account, the *porneia* that makes divorce possible takes place between the woman and an unnamed third party. On the second, the *porneia* takes place within the couple whose divorce is in question.

The first account has been important historically, particularly with *porneia* narrowed down to "adultery." On this reading, if a woman committed adultery with a third party, the exception kicked in. In this particular text, the exception meant only that, in those circumstances, the divorcing husband did not *make* her an adulteress, which was obvious since she already was one. The exception is more important in the parallel text later in Matthew: "And I say to you: whoever divorces his wife, except for unchastity [*mê epi porneia(i)*], and marries another, commits adultery" (19:9). Here it seems that the exception is more substantial, in that it appears to allow for remarriage in cases of *porneia*.

But note first that here it is the husband who is said to commit adultery. This idea is, in and of itself, an important egalitarian move. In a patriarchal society, adultery is always an offense committed against a man. Yet here, adultery is said to be committed against a woman.[38] (Mark 10:11 makes the "against" even more explicit.) Exactly the same reasoning would rule out polygamy, for surely the infidelity to his first wife that a man exhibits when he marries another is, if anything, greater if he has not gone to the trouble of divorcing the first wife before marrying the second. Marriage is, thus, seen as mutual, and infidelity can cut both ways. The text was very much a countercultural one.

But back to the exception: we are considering a reading on which the *porneia* in Matthew 5:32 indicates adultery committed by the wife. It is reasonable to take the *porneia* in 19:9 in the same way, though we do not absolutely have to do this. Against having to take it in the same way, we may note that the exceptions in the two texts apply to different things: at 5:32 the man who divorces on account of *porneia* is not making his wife an adulteress, while at 19:9 he is not making himself an adulterer.[39] But let us consider the simpler hypothesis that we should read *porneia* in the same way. Then, at first sight, 19:9 suggests that it is acceptable to divorce one's wife and marry another if one divorced the wife because of her adultery.

However, this has not been the predominant understanding of Christians in the first five centuries, with the notable exceptions of Tertullian, Ambrosiaster, and perhaps Lactantius. Let us consider first these exceptions. Tertullian interprets Jesus' prohibition as a prohibition against remarrying when the first wife was dismissed "unlawfully," i.e., for anything other than adultery.[40] Ambrosiaster argues that while women are prohibited from remarriage, no matter what the cause of the divorce, "a man is not bound by the law as a woman is; for man is head over woman."[41] Lactantius is the least clear case. He does not appear to say that remarriage is permissible after divorce when the divorce is on account of adultery, but neither does he rule it out: "he is an adulterer, who married a woman divorced from her husband, or who divorced a wife on account of any crime except adultery, so that he might marry another; for God did not wish the body

220

to be broken and torn apart."[42] We could read Lactantius in two ways. On one reading, what is forbidden to the man is divorcing with the intention of remarriage, except when the first wife has committed adultery, with the implicature that both divorce and an intention of remarriage are acceptable in the case of the wife's adultery. On the second reading, what is forbidden is divorcing the wife, except in cases of adultery, and "so that he might marry another" is simply an explanatory remark about the most common causes of divorce rather than something permitted.

Based on the sources cited by Jurgens,[43] it appears that—except perhaps for the passage of Tertullian, which does not speak to the issue[44]—it was uncontroversially accepted that at least *women* could not remarry after a divorce, no matter the cause of the divorce. If we accept St. Jerome's principle that, while the laws of Caesar have a double standard about sexual behavior, "[w]ith us, however, what is unlawful for women is equally unlawful for men; and since both are in a like servitude to God, both are reckoned as of equal status,"[45] then we need to generalize the prohibition on remarriage to men as well as women. It would be much more revisionary to generalize the permission of remarriage in cases of adultery to women, since that permission is given to men only by a small minority of patristic writers, and it is all but unanimous that women are not permitted to remarry.

The main line of thought in the first five centuries, as represented by the *Shepherd of Hermas*,[46] Origen,[47] the Council of Elvira,[48] St. Jerome,[49] St. Augustine, and probably St. Basil,[50] was to insist on the indissolubility of marriage between believers in all cases.[51] A distinction was sometimes made between (a) dismissing a wife, i.e., denying her bed and board, and (b) marrying another. The former was taken to be permissible in cases of the wife's adultery. Some even thought it was obligatory. But the marrying of another was still not permitted. Thus, in the *Shepherd of Hermas*, a second-century work occasioned by the controversy over whether a Christian who sinned could still be forgiven, we have the narrator talking with "the Shepherd":

"Sir," said I, "if a man have a wife faithful in the Lord, and he finds her out in some adultery, does the husband sin if he lives with her?" "So long as he is ignorant," said he, "he does not sin, but if the husband knows her sin, and the wife does not repent, but remains in her fornication, and the husband go on living with her, he becomes a partaker of her sin, and shares in her adultery." "What then," said I, "sir, shall the husband do if the wife remain in this disposition?" "Let him put her away," he said, "and let the husband remain by himself. But 'if he put his wife away and marry another he also commits adultery himself.'"[52]

The text goes on to say that if the wife repents, the husband should take her back, though only once. It also gives an argument for not remarrying, namely, to make it possible to forgive the repentant wife (though presumably this argument only applies the first time, since the author does not believe in taking a wife back multiple times).

If the predominant early Christian understanding is taken to give the right interpretation of the Gospels here, then we have a serious difficulty with understanding *porneia* as committed between the wife and a third party and as giving a permission to remarry.

Of course, one could note that, strictly speaking, Matthew 19:9 does not say that it is *not* adultery when a man divorces an adulteress and marries another. The text on the present reading makes the claim that *if* one divorces, not on account of adultery, and remarries, then one is an adulterer, but does not claim that these are the *only* circumstances in which one is an adulterer. In fact, the word "except" in the Revised Standard Version is an overtranslation of what is a mere limiting clause: "not because of *porneia*." Perhaps the case where one divorces not on account of adultery is just the most egregious circumstance, the one most particularly to be condemned. Remember that the very notion of a man committing adultery against a woman is itself a significant innovation in a patriarchal society. To use the term "adultery," as the text does, when the woman is one that had been divorced is an even greater innovation. There is no reason for this text then to make a *third* innovation and use the word "adultery" in the case of the man who divorces his wife because of her adultery and marries another woman. Such a man's motives, at least, might be more honorable than those of a man who simply divorces his wife for no reason at all, at least if not wishing to be a "cuckold" is honorable. The text might wish to confine itself to the case where the man's vice is more evident, and leave open the question of what happens in the case of the more honorable divorcé.

There is good scriptural reason to accept the predominant early Christian view as correct. Outside of Matthew, none of the other relevant New Testament texts prohibiting divorce and remarriage, namely, those in Paul and in Mark and Luke, make any exemption for *porneia*. This strongly suggests that the exemption was, in some sense, not really significant, but perhaps some kind of a minor clarification. An exception for the wife's adultery would not be a minor clarification: on the contrary, adultery has surely always been one of the leading causes of divorce. For more conservative readers of this book, one can now offer the following argument. If scripture is *inerrant*, then it must in particular be true that "[e]very one who divorces his wife and marries another commits adultery, and he who marries a woman divorced from her husband commits adultery" (Luke 16:18). But if the combination of divorce and remarriage is not adultery when the wife is an adulteress, then it is false that *everyone* who divorces and remarries is an adulterer, and the Lucan text is wrong. On an inerrantist view, then, the text in Matthew must be making reference to some case that is, in some essential way, different from the case of divorcing one's own wife. We will shortly see how this could be. But the main body of our argument will ride on this, because the exegetical strategy of this book does not presuppose inerrancy of scripture.

Still, even without inerrancy, one needs to explain why Paul, Mark, and Luke omitted the *porneia* exception, if that exception was indeed generally operative in the Christian community. A plausible explanation is that the exception covered a relatively rare case, which Paul, Mark, and Luke omitted to mention. But that explanation fits poorly with the hypothesis that *porneia* is adultery between a member of the couple and someone outside the couple. For it seems intuitively likely that adultery would have been involved in a significant percentage of the cases of divorce.

If Matthew 19:9 is read as permitting divorce only when the woman commits adultery, then Jesus' position is not very different from that of the School of Shammai, and it is not a position that should have been so shocking to his disciples, who immediately exclaim: "If such is the case of a man with his wife, it is not expedient to marry" (v. 10). There is something shockingly extreme about the position espoused by Jesus. This is even clearer in the context of Matthew 5:32. Recall that there we had a discourse where Jesus gives commandments that are *much* stricter than the Law or contemporary practice. They are not mere adjustments. The Deuteronomic Code allows divorce when the man "has found some indecency" in the woman (Deut. 24:1). There was debate in the Judaism of the time as to what exactly the "indecency ['*ervah*]" indicated, with the School of Shammai holding that it indicated sexual immorality, probably because the term literally meant nakedness or genitals.[53] Eventually, Rabbinical Judaism allowed for a more subjective reading on which it was up to the husband to decide what he found "obnoxious" (the term used in the Jewish Publication Society translation).[54] In any case, if Jesus merely took something like the position of the Shammaiites, then his action could be taken to be no more than tightening up the interpretation of the word '*ervah*, rather than giving a radically stricter command. But the rest of the discourse involves *radical* tightening of commands: from not murdering to not being angry, from not committing adultery to not looking lustfully, from not swearing falsely to absolute truthfulness in all statements or not swearing at all (depending on one's interpretation) and from retributive justice to offering the other cheek. None of these cases involve a simple tightening-up of conditions.[55]

There are, thus, three kinds of difficulties for the reading of Matthew that takes *porneia* to take place between the woman and a third party: (1) it fits less well with early Christian practice, (2) it is incompatible with inerrancy, given parallel texts in Mark, Luke, and Paul, and in any case gives rise to a puzzle as to why Mark, Luke, and Paul did not mention it, and (3) it makes Christ's view on divorce significantly less radical than the other parts of the Matthew 5 discourse.

Consider now the second reading, on which the *porneia* mentioned takes place not between the woman and a third party, but between the woman and the man who is thinking about divorcing her.

This explains why the term *porneia* is used, instead of a term specifically meaning adultery, since this woman and man are not seen as committing adultery with each other, as there is no one in view in the text for this adultery to be committed against. However, they can still commit other sorts of sexual immorality together. One speculative suggestion could be that they might be jointly committing what Christian tradition would come to call "unnatural acts," such as coitus interruptus. But given that Christian tradition, while condemning such acts, did not make them a ground of divorce, this is an unlikely reading. But if it is not a physical type of act that defines *porneia*, then it must be that the sexual activity, though it may be "natural intercourse," is immoral on other grounds. And here one of the most obvious candidates is that the couple is not validly married.

The concept of the validity of marriage was codified in Judaism in the Tannaitic period (AD 70–200), with the conclusion that not only was a marriage between a Jew and a nonconverted Gentile morally impermissible, but it was literally *impossible*.[56] The Jew and Gentile could go through the motions of marriage, both the wedding ritual and the life together, but the motions would be ineffective—they would not come to be *married*. It would be unsurprising if the ideas of validity were already under discussion among first-century Jews in the time of Jesus.

Validity has developed into an important concept in Jewish and Catholic thought. Catholics would say that, except when nothing else is available, it is wrong, or *illicit*, to baptize someone with dirty water, since the symbolism of spiritual cleansing is damaged, but as long as it is still water and not mud, the baptism is *valid*, nonetheless—the person really does become joined to the body of Christ. On the other hand, an attempt to baptize someone with honey would not only be illicit, but would be *invalid*—the person would not actually be baptized. In military law, likewise, we could make a distinction between a valid order that needs to be obeyed and an invalid order that need not be obeyed, like one where the bounds of the officer's authority are overstepped.

Now in a Christian context, the case of a Gentile-Jew marriage would probably not count as invalid, but there would be other cases of invalidity. Thus, a "marriage" between two people so closely related as to make the relationship incest would be invalid. This idea is found among the tannaim of the second century, and Epstein believes the idea came from an earlier principle.[57]

The term "invalid marriage" is somewhat misleading, since an invalid marriage is not a marriage. It must be understood along the lines of "fake money," where fake money is not really money. If nonmarital sex is wrong, and there is every indication that the early Christians saw it as such, then sex within an invalid marriage is sexual immorality, i.e., *porneia,* since this sex is literally nonmarital sex.

It is worth noting that the notion of the validity of a marriage underscores the claim that marriage is a *reality* independent of our thoughts and perceptions. If a couple can go through a ceremony and still not be validly married, this suggests marriage is something independent of our thinking and perceptions, something truly *real.*

The interpretation of *porneia* in the text as sexual relations within either any kind of invalid marriage or some particular kind of invalid marriage of relevance to the community has several considerations in its favor. First, it allows one to understand why the exception for *porneia* can be freely included or left out, just as it is included in Matthew and left out in Mark, Luke, and Paul. For one can say, equally truly, that "An Oxford diploma has traditionally been a sign of a quality education" and that "An Oxford diploma, fakes aside, has traditionally been a sign of a quality education." The "fakes aside" clause does not actually exclude any Oxford diplomas, but merely clarifies the meaning. The exception for *porneia* on this reading is not really an exception, because when there is the relevant kind of *porneia* between the man and woman, they are not husband and wife.

The most exegetically conservative thing to say about the exception clause is to say that when Jesus actually made the speech about divorce, he included the clause for precision. The other synoptic Gospels, then, either abridge the saying or else are reports of the saying as made on another occasion—for, of course, a teacher repeats his lessons. However, at least in the Sermon on the Mount version (Matt. 5:31–32), the exception stands out from the rest of the discourse stylistically by dampening the fiery language, language that includes talk about cutting off the right hand (v. 30) and being liable to hellfire for insulting a person (v. 22). At the same time, in the context of the discussion with the Pharisees in Matthew 19:9, assuming that was the original context for that saying, if the *porneia* exception were included in the historical dialogue, we would expect the obvious question: "But what, Jesus, is *porneia*?" since the point of the Pharisees' question was precisely where Jesus stood on the dispute about what counts as *'ervah* in Deuteronomy.

These observations suggest, but do not come close to proving, that the *porneia* exception was not a part of the historical Jesus' words on these occasions. Thus, unless one insists on a very conservative reading of the text, it is quite reasonable to suppose that Jesus did not himself include the *porneia* exception, which would explain both the stylistic issues and the clause's absence from the other synoptics. Rather, on this interpretation, the *porneia* exception was inserted by the human author of the first Gospel as a gloss on Jesus' statement.[58] On the invalidity reading, this gloss in no way affects the meaning of what is said but only clarifies that *real* marriages are the only marriages involved, and so even a conservative interpreter could allow that it was an authorial insertion, though the conservative interpreter will insist that the insertion was divinely inspired. After all, Greek had no quotation marks or brackets, and to satisfy a particularly conservative exegete, one could punctuate the text as: "[Jesus said,] 'But I say to you that every one who divorces his wife [except on the ground of unchastity] makes her an adulteress; and whoever marries a divorced woman commits adultery'" (5:32). One could read 19:9 similarly. And it would not be difficult to find a reason for the insertion. It might be that cases of invalid marriage were coming up, say, between pagans who converted to Christianity but were married to close relatives, and it was necessary to emphasize that divorce was not wrong in those cases. Indeed, in those cases, divorce would have been a duty.

Of course, even if one does not accept the hypothesis that the exception is an authorial gloss, the other arguments in favor of reading the *porneia* case as a case of invalid marriage remain. Whether the phrase is a gloss by the human author or was included by Jesus, it is clearly parenthetical. And the parenthetical nature of the exception would explain why we do not have an explicit discussion of invalidity. Moreover, in the Sermon on Mount version, such an explicit discussion would destroy the flow of the radical discourse, and in the Matthew 19:9 version, it would damage the more general point that Jesus was *not* engaging in the kind of detailed analysis of precise conditions in which the Pharisees, who initiated the discussion, were interested, but rather Jesus was getting to the heart of the matter, the original root of the union of man and woman in God's joining of the two as one flesh (vv. 5–6).

On the other hand, it could be argued that Jesus' saying: "What therefore God has joined together, let not man put asunder" (Matt. 19:6, Mark 10:9) implies that it is possible, though not morally permissible, to break apart a marriage. This would seem to go against an interpretation on which Jesus is making divorce impossible or invalid, and would force one to read the claim that the sex in a remarriage after a divorce is adultery (presumably against the first spouse) metaphorically. Two responses are available. First, the "let no man put asunder" can be reasonably read as prohibiting the *attempt* to put asunder what God has joined, without implying the possibility of the attempt's success. We might likewise say something like "Don't be wiser than God!" without implying that it is possible to be wiser than God. Second, and more importantly, Jesus may be seen as generally saying that one should not do things contrary to marital unity. Thus, while a literal severing of the objective normative commitment is impossible—the commitment remains binding even if one rejects it—it is quite possible to fail to subjectively acknowledge the commitment.

Overall, there is very good reason to think that Jesus did in fact claim that divorce within a valid marriage, when followed by a remarriage, constituted adultery. But if it constituted adultery, this means that the marriage bond remained standing despite the writ of divorce being served. Using the distinction between the valid and the invalid, we could say that Jesus decreed that, at least for his disciples, henceforth divorce, understood as a dissolution of marriage, would be invalid in the sense that it would not really dissolve a marriage. If so, and if (as Christians believe) what Jesus said reflects the will of God, then a marriage vow from which God would not release two people is the kind of marriage vow Christians make. Hence, that which romantic love ideally wants is indeed available to Christians, given Jesus' view of divorce.

Perhaps even more theologically important than the explicit prohibition on divorce, however, is the biblical centrality of the analogy between the husband-wife relationship and the relationship between God or Christ and his people. It is of the essence of the relationship between God and his people that it not be conditional in any way. Neither can God's people release God from his promises, nor will God release us from our duty to love him, since this duty comes from our very nature as creatures made in his image and likeness. Note that, in particular, allowing divorce in cases of the spouse's adultery would destroy the analogy, because it is crucial that God does not abandon his people when they pursue false gods, which pursuit is taken to be closely analogous to adultery in the Hebrew scriptures (Jer. 13:27, Ezek. 23:43)

The above considerations give scriptural reasons to believe that the kind of commitment romantic love ultimately calls for is possible— that God does indeed allow us to make something like a marriage vow that unites until death. If romantic love is most deeply fulfilled through a union that cannot be dissolved by any power other than death, we would expect the God of love to make such a union possible. The New Testament fulfills this expectation.

14. NON-CHRISTIAN MARRIAGE

The previous section applies to Christian marriage. But what about the marriage of non-Christians? After all, they too enter into relationships of romantic love. Yet the New Testament implies that at least some non-Christian marriages can be dissolved and a new marriage entered into. Thus, the Pauline privilege allows a convert to divorce a recalcitrant non-Christian spouse (1 Cor. 7:15), and the Christian tradition has understood this passage such that remarriage is to be allowed in this case. Moreover, to enter into a commitment voluntarily requires a certain understanding of the commitment. The non-Christian couple may not understand themselves as entering into a commitment before God from which God will not release them.

Still, romantic love calls for a commitment until death, the maximal commitment practically available. To a Christian couple, this is indissoluble Christian marriage. A non-Christian couple will have to settle for less. One option, suggested at the end of section 12 above, is a marriage commitment made to a community unwilling to release one from it. This option is not fully satisfactory in those contemporary societies where civil release from marriage is easy. However, the community is more than the state, and a commitment to the community can go beyond a commitment to the laws of the state.

A second option is to suppose that even non-Christians can at least implicitly recognize God's role in receiving the commitment of marriage. While perhaps in such cases God does not hold the couple bound absolutely, the couple may recognize that their marriage commitment goes beyond them in some mysterious way, without recognizing that it goes beyond them through being a commitment made to God.

Questions of non-Christian marriage, and the even tougher question of the marriage between Christians and non-Christians, would require a detailed study that would go beyond the scope of the present book. But the basic principle of the maximality of commitment may well remain.

15. HOW DOES ONE MARRY?

We do not have any evidence at all that an absolute commitment of the sort we are talking about in the case of Christians is possible except through marriage. In fact, it would be hard to see how it could be, given that a commitment of this magnitude, if accepted by God in a way that makes it indissoluble, would surely constitute marriage definitionally. The New Testament does not explicitly provide us with any set form to which a marriage ceremony must adhere in order for a valid and indissoluble Christian marriage to result. Two different views have developed in the Catholic and Orthodox Churches. On the Orthodox view, what is central is the priest's performing the marriage with respect to the man and woman, though the couple's consent is required.

On the other hand, according to the Catholic view, marriage is undertaken by the man and woman who are marrying each other. A priest may bless the couple and their marriage, but the cause of the marriage is the exchange of consent. In fact, until the Council of Trent, marriages without any ceremony beyond a private exchange of vows and with no third parties present were considered valid, though it was also considered sinful to exclude the larger community in this way. At the same time, the Catholic Church held that it can introduce requirements that a marriage must satisfy to be valid. From Trent on, the Catholic Church has ruled invalid future marriages between Catholics that do not meet certain minimal ceremonial standards, except in cases where there is a danger of death or lack of clergy. These standards include the presence of a priest or deacon, when one is available.

Both the Catholic and Orthodox approaches have considerations in their favor. If we focus on the need for God to accept the promise and the fact that God accepts the promise only within a certain context, we are more likely to say with the Orthodox that it is the priest, acting in the name of God, who confers marriage on the couple. On the other hand, if we focus on the making of the promise, we will find the Catholic approach perhaps more congenial. However, both views acknowledge that it is only in a (perhaps changeable) context set by the Christian community that God accepts these promises.

It is interesting to note that given present Catholic canon law, there appear to be no requirements imposed for the validity of an exchange of marital vows by two non-Catholics, beyond such conditions as their knowing what they are doing and doing it freely, their not being already married, and their not being within a prohibited degree of kinship. Thus, in practice, there is no problem for Catholics with the notion of Protestants marrying without much ceremony.

Whether it is the Catholics or the Orthodox or neither who are right depends in part on difficult ecclesiological and sacramental questions beyond the scope of this book. However, we can say the following without getting into the detailed questions. Without settling the question of what kind of ceremony is required, it is plausible to say that to omit customary ceremonies is a sign of an unwillingness to enter into the kind of commitment before God that these customary ceremonies indicate. Thus, even if Catholics are right that a Protestant couple can marry with no ceremony at all, for the couple to exchange vows without ceremony, except in a setting like that of a desert island, is significant evidence that they do not mean to marry.

16. WHAT IS THE CONTENT OF
THE MARRIAGE VOW?

The traditional marriage ceremony in English in the *Book of Common Prayer* has the exchange of vows worded as follows:

[T]he curate shall say to the Man,

M. Wilt thou have this woman to thy wedded wife, to live together after God's ordinance in the holy estate of Matrimony? Wilt thou love her, comfort her, honour, and keep her in sickness and in health; and, forsaking all other, keep thee only unto her, so long as ye both shall live?

The Man shall answer,

I will.

Then shall the priest say to the Woman,

N. Wilt thou have this man to thy wedded husband, to live together after God's ordinance in the holy estate of Matrimony? Wilt thou obey him, and serve him, love, honour, and keep him in sickness and in health; and, forsaking all other, keep thee only unto him, so long as ye both shall live?

The Woman shall answer,

I will.[59]

Most Christian marriage ceremonies in the English-speaking world continue to include promises of roughly this form, occasionally omitting some items (especially the obedience and service part of the woman's promise) or adding others.

It seems prima facie unlikely that the exact covenant entered into should differ significantly depending on the exact phrasing that the particular couple used. For the covenant needs to be ratified by God, I have argued, and there is no evidence in scripture or Christian tradition that there is more than one kind of Christian marriage covenant that God ratifies. Moreover, even while the words of the vows are stated, it is likely that what the couple is really meaning to promise is: "We will be good Christian spouses." If it should turn out that, say, obedience is not a part of being a Christian wife, then perhaps we need not take it as something that has really been promised, even if the words were said. And if it should turn out that obedience *is* a part of it, we should take it as having been implicitly promised by undertaking to be a Christian wife, even if the words were *not* said. For a central part of the life of a Christian spouse is a process of learning what a Christian conjugal life should be like, and striving to live that way, whatever it might turn out to be (this is related to love's humility, as discussed in section 5 of chapter 2).

The primary part of the question asked by the priest in these vows is whether the couple is willing "to live together after God's ordinance in the holy estate of Matrimony"; the second part, on this reading, is more of a gloss. Thus, Luther thought that all that was needed for marriage was a much simpler exchange:

Hans, do you want to have Greta as your wedded wife? Let him say: "Yes."

Greta, do you want to have Hans as your wedded husband? Let her say: "Yes."[60]

Nonetheless, the wording of the vows that are exchanged is one witness to the likely content of the obligations of marriage, and we shall now consider some of these, without any pretence to exhaustiveness. Here, the arguments will rely more heavily on revelation. After all, if the marriage vows are a covenant that God ratifies, we may need to rely on revelation to figure out what the content of the covenant is.

17. "FORSAKING ALL OTHER"

It seems quite clear that the sexual exclusion of others is essential to a Christian marriage. Even if this is not explicit in the vows, the very notion of "adultery," understood as a sin that either spouse can commit against the other, presupposes this. And we have seen that Jesus' sayings on divorce do understand adultery in this way. Furthermore, in section 4 above, I have argued that the commitment of romantic love calls for exclusivity.

This means that polygyny and polyandry are ruled out. In a polygynous setting, there would, arguably, be no such thing as a man committing adultery against a woman, since his having relations with another woman is surely no more a *betrayal* of her than his marrying another would be. For the same reason, polyandry makes no sense of a prohibition on a woman's committing adultery against a man.

Moreover, it is plausible to think of Christian marriage as involving equal mutual possession: the man's body is not his, but his wife's, and his wife's body is not hers, but his. It is quite unclear how this mutual possession could exist in a polyandrous or polygynous setting. Furthermore, polyandry has never been a biblically permitted practice, and there is no evidence that it began to be permitted in Christian times. Thus, the only real question is about polygyny, but given the mutuality in Christian marriage, it does not appear possible that men would have been allowed several wives while women were not allowed several husbands.[61] But if, on the other hand, one is also sceptical of the prohibition on polyandry, then we need only gesture at the impossible complications of a system where there is both polyandry and polygyny. It seems one could have such bizarre arrangements as one where Bob is married to Jane and Martha, while Jane is married to Bob and Fred, but Martha is only married to Bob.[62]

These arguments do present a strong case that polyandry and polygyny are unacceptable for Christians, but except for the mutual possession argument, the arguments, perhaps, do not quite get to the heart of the reason why these practices are unacceptable. However, given the centrality of the seeking after the deepest kind of union possible in a sexual setting, we can see the inappropriateness of a polyandric or polygynous arrangement.

Polygyny was a socially accepted earlier Hebrew practice and was apparently considered permissible by Jews in the first century. If we see Jesus' insistence on a restoration of the original ideal of a one-flesh union as revisionary in the case of divorce, we should likewise see it as revisionary in the case of polygyny. For the two cases are closely parallel. Indeed, the moral permissibility of polygyny plus a prohibition of divorce would largely impose a burden only on women, since they would be bound to a man who could, with moral impunity, take another and ignore the existence of the previous wife, except maybe for financial support and sexual duties. But the man might have no objection to fulfilling the sexual "duties," and the financial support is something that he might still owe in the case of divorce, given a sufficiently explicit marriage contract.

If polygyny is unacceptable in the case of Christians, we can ask the further question whether it is acceptable in the case of non-Christians. Is it because of the supernatural aspect of Christian marriage that the polygyny is unacceptable, or was it morally unacceptable all along?

One way to focus the question is to ask about the polygyny in the Hebrew scriptures. A basic question is whether polygyny was actually morally permitted to the Hebrews, or whether it was merely divinely tolerated. Exactly the same question can be asked about divorce, and Jesus' explanation that the permission of divorce was given because of people's "hardness of heart" (Matt. 19:8) does not settle the question, since it is possible (a) that out of the hardness of people's hearts God decided not to punish divorce, or (b) that out of the hardness of people's hearts God actually *permitted* people to contract divorces. I suspect that the latter is the right reading but do not have a particularly strong argument.

In the case of polygyny, a powerful scriptural argument that the practice was not always immoral can be based on the levirate duty: "If brothers dwell together, and one of them dies and has no son, the wife of the dead shall not be married outside the family to a stranger; her husband's brother shall go in to her, and take her as his wife, and perform the duty of a husband's brother to her" (Deut. 25:5). No limitation is given in the text to the case where the husband's brother is unmarried. Given the acceptance of polygyny among the original audience for this commandment, if such a limitation were meant, it would have to be expressly stated. Rather, it appears that even if the husband's brother already had a wife, he was still called upon to take another. Granted, the duty is not absolute, as the man could opt to be publicly shamed instead (Deut. 25:9), but the text makes it clear that taking the woman as wife was the resolution preferred by the author.[63]

At the same time, there is a sense that polygyny is not an ideal situation. The case of the levirate duty is no exception to this, since it depends on the clearly nonideal circumstances of a brother dying childless, apart from which circumstances the union would be prohibited as incest (Lev. 18:16). There seems to be a paucity of scriptural examples of happy polygynous marriages entered into under close to ideal circumstances, where more than one wife is truly a well-loved partner.[64] Consider, for instance, Leah, Rachel, and Jacob (Gen. 29–31). Polygyny ensued because of the deception by Laban, but it was Rachel for whom Jacob really cared. On a different note, Epstein suggests that polygyny "was distasteful to the Hebrews," being seen as an "excess" of the "ruling class."[65] He reminds the reader of the biblical warning to rulers not to multiply wives (Deut. 17:17).

If this is correct, then while polygyny was not only divinely tolerated among the Hebrews but actually morally permissible, it was not something that was advisable apart from rare circumstances. This suggests that polygyny is not something intrinsically immoral. However, it is something generally inadvisable, and it is difficult to see how it could realistically obtain, except in truly exceptional circumstances, in a setting where women are fully respected as equal partners. But matters are different for Christians, given that Jesus made the original ideal of a one-flesh union normative, and for Christians polygamy is not an option.

While some prominent theologians, possibly including John Paul II, have held other views, the position that polygyny was permitted to the ancient Hebrews is similar to that held by Thomas Aquinas, who argued that whether monogamy is morally required depends on the circumstances. In circumstances where there was a need for the Chosen People to quickly populate the land, polygyny was morally permissible. But there is no similar imperative for us to quickly populate any land, perhaps because Christianity is not supposed to be an ethnic phenomenon, and the Christian Church is quite capable of significant growth not only through reproduction but also through conversion.

A serious difficulty with this position, however, is that it makes trouble for the contention that romantic love seeks the deepest kind of commitment possible, and apart from that deepest kind of commitment, sex is impermissible. We might argue, however, that at certain times in history, for good reason, God has limited the deepest kind of commitment that is possible, not making it possible for couples to commit to exclusivity when, say, there was a need for rapid population growth. On this response, polygyny would also not be permitted to non-Christians in our time.

18. THE MARRIAGE "DEBT"

The positive side of the sexual exclusion of all others is the sexual relationship with the spouse. This is not particularly explicit in the Anglican vows, but implied by "keep thee only unto her/him" and perhaps in "live together after God's ordinance."

Paul sensibly believed that there was a duty for a married couple to engage in sexual relations. It appears that a sexual duty is even incumbent on the couple when neither spouse has made any sexual request, "lest Satan tempt" the persons, presumably to some kind of illicit sexual behavior:

It is well for a man not to touch a woman. But because of the temptation to immorality, each man should have his own wife and each woman her own husband. The husband should give to his wife her conjugal rights [*tên opheilên*], and likewise the wife to her husband. For the wife does not rule [*exousiazei*] over her own body, but the husband does; likewise the husband does not rule [*exousiazei*] over his own body, but the wife does. Do not refuse one another except perhaps by agreement for a season [*pros kairon*], that you may devote yourselves to prayer; but then come together again, lest Satan tempt you through lack of self-control. (1 Cor. 7:1b–5)

At the same time, the duty is not an absolute one, because it is acceptable for the couple to agree not to engage in sexual relations *pros kairon* for reasons of devotion to prayer. It being somewhat unlikely that Paul was worried about the rather small amount of time that sexual relations take away from prayer, this suggests an ascetical practice of refraining from sexual relations practiced by some couples in the early Church, one that continued until at least the Middle Ages.[66]

One obvious question is what length of time the "season" may be. But the word *kairos* does not indicate a specific length of time. Thus, in Luke 8:13, we are told of those who "believe for a while [*pros kairon*] and in time of temptation fall away." This "while" could, surely, be days, or months, or years.

Thus, Paul is not setting down any requirement of a specific sexual frequency. Rather, it seems, the couple may abstain from sexual relations for as long as both (a) their devotion to prayer requires and (b) they can safely keep away from temptation. What this length of time would be clearly depends on specific circumstances. It is even conceivable that if temptation were not likely to result—say in the case of a couple of sufficiently advanced age—then the "come together again" clause might not even apply.

Whether other reasons for abstinence are permissible is not textually clear. However, if we see the prevention of temptation as Paul's operating principle, we might suppose that other exceptions could be countenanced as long as an appropriate amount of effort were made to prevent temptation. Clearly one should not seriously endanger the life of another person in order to prevent a temptation, and so it would not be acceptable for a man to engage in sexual relations with his wife if pregnancy seriously endangered her life, at least assuming, as would certainly have been the case in the first century, that there were no reliable and morally permissible way to prevent pregnancy other than through abstinence. We need to avoid temptation, but there are circumstances where we need to brave it. It is not immoral for a person to become a bank manager even though it is likely that at some point in her career she will have at least a fleeting temptation to steal or embezzle.

Paul's temptation-based argument seems to be: "Marital sexual relations prevent temptation and are morally licit. There is a prima facie duty to prevent temptation by morally licit means. Hence there is a prima facie duty to engage in marital sexual relations." Reading the duty as prima facie, as applicable unless something overrides it, coheres with Paul's introduction of the discussion, where he talks about how each should have his or her own spouse (1 Cor. 7:2). This is clearly not a command meant for everyone, since Paul himself does not have a spouse and praises the idea of celibacy (1 Cor. 7:1,7), so Paul is aware that considerations of sexual temptation do not imply an absolute duty.

Paul grounds a particular aspect of the couple's duty to engage in sexual relations with the other in the nature of marriage. The husband must give his wife her due because she is the one who has authority over his body. The context makes it clear that what is due is some kind of sexual right, indicated euphemistically by the word *opheilê*,[67] simply meaning a debt or obligation. Again, we are not told that the duty is absolute. After all, our authority over our own bodies is not absolute, since Paul taught earlier in the same epistle that "your body is a temple of the Holy Spirit within you, which you have from God[.] You are not your own; you were bought with a price" (1 Cor. 6:19–20). For this reason, a wife's authority over the body of the husband (or vice versa) would not be absolute either, since ultimately the husband's body is a temple of the Holy Spirit. Nonetheless, it is clear that Paul thinks that there is at least a strong presumption in favor of yielding sexual rights to the spouse, though of course one might withhold oneself sexually if, say, health or other very serious considerations required it, since one must keep one's body a fitting temple of the Holy Spirit. Human authority is always limited by the divine authority from which it flows.

The philosophical account of marital union as a whole-person extension of the one-flesh union of sexual intercourse not only coheres well with but also gives a reason-based grounding to these Pauline ideas. We have seen in section 4 above that commitment extends the sexual union temporally. One aspect of an organic union is each part's responsiveness to the rest of the organism; there is some sense in which the rest of the organism (or the other part, in a two-part organism like the couple) has authority over the part. This responsiveness extends, through commitment, to times when the couple is not in bed, and hence there needs to be a committed willingness by each partner to engage in marital relations with the other.

This means that a good reason would be needed for a spouse to resist the entreaties of the other. And there *can* be good reason. Insofar as the spouses are responding to one another voluntarily outside of the marriage bed, the union is at a voluntary, not biological, level. Under some circumstances, a negative response to sexual overtures can, in fact, serve the *interpersonal* union which is what is at issue then. If the death of one of the spouses would result from sexual intercourse, the effect would also destroy the interpersonal romantic union. Similar though less extreme considerations apply in other circumstances. Thus, there can be room for refusal.

However, matters would be rather unsatisfactory for an organism were its functional parts *never* to engage in the cooperative activity that defines the notion of an actively functioning organic unity. While one's eyes would still be united to one's brain were one to insist on keeping them always closed, doing so would be appropriate only under particularly rare circumstances. Generally speaking, keeping the eyes closed for all of its life would be contrary to the good of the united organism of which the eyes are a part. For it is good for a biological organism for its parts to be actually functioning together. Nonetheless, rare circumstances can occur in which it is better for the parts not to actually function together, and there could be cases where such circumstances hold for the length of the marriage.

Finally, note that even a literalist reader of 1 Corinthians 7, who insists that it is only for the sake of prayer that a couple can engage in abstinence, should realize that serious health problems, difficulties in getting enough food for one's other children, and the like, also make serious inroads on one's time, thereby reducing the amount of time available for prayer. Hence, the "prayer exception," even if one holds it literalistically to be the only one, allows abstinence when sexual union would cause problems that would limit one's time.

19. OFFSPRING

The Anglican marriage vows include no mention of children. Obviously, it cannot be a part of the marriage commitment that the couple have children, since they may, in fact, be incapable of having children. On the other hand, it is clear biblically that children are always seen as a blessing. In the Hebrew scriptures, children and grandchildren are paradigmatic blessings in life (e.g., Ps. 128:6). Moreover, it appears that, biblically, marriage is the normative setting for having children.

But there is a significant Christian tradition that goes a little further in holding that the procreation and education of children is one of the primary goals of marriage, if not *the* primary goal. Catholic canonical practice goes so far as to count as invalid marriages where the couple is determined not to produce offspring, no matter whether the planned means involve "artificial" birth control or a method of regulating conception that is considered intrinsically acceptable, such as periodic or total abstinence.

This extreme canonical conclusion would indeed be correct if one could show that procreation is one of the primary goals of marriage. Let us suppose for the sake of argument that x is one of the primary goals of marriage, and a couple firmly intends to exclude x from their relationship. Then the relationship they seek is one that explicitly differs from marriage in at least one of its primary goals, and hence it is reasonable to say that what the couple seeks is *not* marriage. Imagine a person who came into a hardware store and said: "Could you sell me one of those objects with a wooden handle on one end and a sharp toothed sheet of metal on the other end? I do *not*, however, mean an object which has cutting as one of its purposes." While the first part of the description makes it plausible that the person is seeking to purchase a saw or a knife with a serrated blade, the second part of the description makes it clear that the person wants something else, indeed quite likely something that the hardware store does not stock, and maybe something for which English lacks a term. The primary purposes of something enter into its definition. A knife isn't just an object with a wooden handle on one side and a sharp sheet of metal on the other: it is an object for cutting.

Consequently, if one expressly wishes to exclude a primary goal of marriage, then one is not intending marriage but either something else or something quite impossible. But the marital commitment needs to be entered into voluntarily. Hence, someone who wishes to exclude *x*, which happens to be a primary goal of marriage, is thereby *not* entering into the marital commitment. But is procreation a primary goal of marriage?

Before attempting to answer this question, let us think some more about a couple that excludes procreation from marriage. Marriage is an interpersonal cementing-together of a one-flesh union, constituted, in its active form, by a mutual bodily striving for reproduction. It would be strange indeed if the relationship were constituted through active engagement in a mutual bodily striving for reproduction, or at least through a willingness to engage in this, and yet reproduction were something that the couple intended to exclude during the relationship. This would imply a schism between the biological level and the voluntary level in the couple, and this would be opposed to the wholeness of the union of persons in marriage.

Observe that a similar division is not present if the couple simply does not wish to have children *now*. I have argued that sexual union always includes a mutual biological striving for reproduction, but this striving does not always succeed. And it is quite natural biologically that it not always succeed—the ovum is available only for about twenty-four hours in a cycle and the sperm can survive in the woman's reproductive system for only about a week. A lack of a desire that the act should succeed in reproduction, as long as there is an at least implicit desire that the bodies should *strive* in the direction of reproduction, does not imply an innate contradiction, as we have already seen from sports analogies: it is possible to play chess with one's child, thereby intentionally striving for victory, while hoping that one will be beaten by the child. There need be no *opposition* to the wholeness of the union of persons in a case where the couple hope reproduction will not occur. We have discussed the question whether unitive integration requires the willing of procreation already in section 13 of the previous chapter.

However, if the couple intends that their sexual intercourse should *never* result in children, things seem to be somewhat different. In intending this, the members of the couple are changing the personal significance of sexual intercourse for them, so that it is no longer seen by them as a reproductive and integrally unitive type of act—for if they still see it as reproductive, then they must oppose it and hence cannot intend to be fully united as persons through engagement in it. And in changing the personal significance of sexual intercourse, they are ensuring that what they seek is something else than the act that consummates the marriage of a couple that is willing, at least, to have children *at some point* in their married life.

For this argument to be applicable, we have to be dealing with a couple for which the intention not to have children is quite firm. The case of a couple that has a good reason not to have children but that would be quite willing to have children should the reason be taken away, is different and unproblematic. Take, for instance, an ethnically Jewish couple living in a Nazi area where pregnancy is punishable by death, and so the couple naturally does not wish to have children. Even if the members of the couple pessimistically suppose that the Nazi regime will always be there, their commitment not to have children is only a conditional one: they do not wish to have children while the objectively pressing reasons not to have children are still present. To make the matter even clearer, one expects that the couple wants the reasons not to have children to disappear. The same is true of a couple with reasons generally seen as more permanent, like a couple that knows pregnancy would endanger the woman's life due to an incurable disorder. Again, even though the disorder is incurable *now*, the woman may well wish for it to be cured in the future, and be willing to strive to have children should a cure be found.

The above arguments do not, however, decide the question whether children are a primary goal of marriage or not, even if they do suggest that a couple that wishes to utterly exclude procreation from their relationship is not interested in *marriage*. However, the hypothesis that children *are* a primary goal of marriage can be argued for in the following way: Marriage is, as has been emphasized, the way to cement in the deepest personal way possible the one-flesh union of sexual intercourse. The deepest way to cement such a union would be to cement it in a way that integrates the union as a whole into the relationship. If the union is constituted by activity the goal of which is reproduction, then it is best integrated into a relationship that has reproduction as one of its primary goals. But at the same time, because the personal and the biological need to be intertwined in a truly human enterprise, this cannot be merely biological procreation: it must include in the goal the education and bringing up of the children as whole persons.

This does not imply that procreation and the education of children is the *only* goal of marriage. On the contrary, our account centered on romantic love makes it clear that the fulfillment of romantic love is directed at *union*, and this is clearly a primary goal of marriage. The procreative/educative and unitive goals are closely interrelated since the union occurs at the biological level only in and through a mutual bodily striving for the procreative goal. And there may well also be other goals, some more immediate and some more ultimate. For instance, love is the goal of *all* human life, and gives all human life its meaning. Hence an increase in love might be said to be one of the ultimate goals of marriage, though perhaps it is better to talk of love as the norm or meaning of marriage instead.[68]

There is, however, a powerful objection to the above ideas. If what romantic love seeks is the deepest personal way to cement a sexual relationship, a way in which the biological and the personal are intertwined as closely as possible, then it seems that romantic love would call for a relationship where children are *always* sought, since sexual intercourse always tends toward reproduction. But the result is absurd: it implies a duty for married couples to reproduce as often as they physically can (indeed, perhaps even to make use of fertility awareness techniques to ensure that they maximize the chance of conception in each act of intercourse by timing the act appropriately and ensuring that no ovulated ovum is left without sperm to seek it). What makes this result particularly absurd is that even when marriage was seen by the Christian Church predominantly in terms of the goal of procreation, no duty to maximize procreation (or correlated prohibition on abstinence) was believed to be present.

There is a response to be made here. Romantic love is, first and foremost, a form of *agapê*. As such it cannot be directed at something that would clearly be uncharitable to the spouse. The extreme procreation-maximizing conclusion is, thus, unjustified, because *agapê* by the man for the woman would be incompatible with it. Romantic love seeks a practically maximal union *in love*.

However, the objection is not so easily taken care of. For now we can formulate a more constrained principle: "A married couple should strive to reproduce whenever this is compatible with love toward one another." It is harder to deny that romantic love calls for this conclusion, if romantic love is to involve an integration between the will and the biology in the context of love for one another. Yet it seems that even this more constrained principle leads to unacceptable conclusions. For instance, it seems to imply that the married couple should have more children even when this would cause very serious harm to persons outside the immediately family, such as the couple's own parents who might be dependent on the couple for support.

But no human being is an island. To impose an undue burden on another person is not really to be acting in love. If I love someone, as Aristotle observed, the welfare of that person is in some way a part of my welfare: the friend is "another self."[69] Even if I do not know that my beloved has been harmed, through my beloved's being harmed, I am worse off. If all of Fred's friends died horrible deaths of torture, we would not consider Fred to be someone whose life was enviable, even if Fred did not know of these deaths. But we should love everyone. Insofar, then, as our romantic beloved loves the third party on whom we are imposing an undue burden, we are acting contrary to love for our beloved.

Of course, our beloved may not, in fact, care about the person we are harming. That he or she is *obliged* to love that person does not imply that he or she does. To respond, note that we should charitably assume the person we love does fulfill the duty to love neighbor as self. And if there is conclusive evidence to the contrary, so that we are unable to make this charitable assumption, we can still say that it would be *good for our beloved* to love neighbor as self. Thus, in that case, we ought to wish for our beloved that he or she come to love neighbor as self. And should our beloved do so in the future, then we will have harmed our beloved through having harmed this neighbor, for now our beloved will care, at least implicitly. But perhaps most importantly, observe that in harming this neighbor we will have acted in a way contrary to the desires that our beloved *should* have, even if he or she lacks them. In doing so, we have identified our beloved with a vice, and we have benefited him or her in respect of this ignoble aspect. This is not what love does. Thus imposing undue harm on others for the sake of one's beloved is contrary to love for one's beloved.

Theologically, too, we may note that true love of any human being is a love of the person *as a child of God, as an image of God*. Therefore, it is contrary to love for one to fail to simultaneously love God, since then one cannot really be loving the human beloved in the way that the beloved ought to be loved—in a way conditioned by who the person *really* is. But insofar as we love God, we love his children—this is one of the central points, already noted, of the First Letter of John. In loving any one person as an image of God we are actually, in some way, loving all persons who are united with her as co-images of God. This does not mean we love them all *equally*, but it does mean that love for one person does not allow us to impose an *undue* harm on other persons. Paul put it best in a passage we have already quoted: "Love does no wrong to a neighbor; therefore love is the fulfilling of the law" (Rom. 13:10). And it is not only true that love for x does no wrong to x, but also that love for x does no wrong to y, and especially not for the sake of x. Cases of injustice done "out of love" are cases of a distorted love that does not love the beloved as the beloved truly is, as an image of divine goodness.

Therefore, the "maximal" account of marital commitment implies no duty to procreate beyond any reasonable bounds. But it does imply that procreation is one of the primary goals of marriage, a goal one can only set aside at the cost of entering into a *marriage*, into that relationship which fulfills romantic love. While the Anglican vows cited above do not include this explicitly, if it is *marriage* that the couple desires, they implicitly desire procreation, at least in the absence of serious reasons against it. Thus, the *Book of Common Prayer*, in the priest's preface to the couple, also says:

> First, It [matrimony] was ordained for the procreation of children, to be brought up in the fear and nurture of the Lord, and to the praise of his holy Name.
>
> Secondly, It was ordained for a remedy against sin, and to avoid fornication; that such persons as have not the gift of continency might marry, and keep themselves undefiled members of Christ's body.
>
> Thirdly, It was ordained for the mutual society, help, and comfort, that the one ought to have of the other, both in prosperity and adversity. Into which holy estate these two persons present come now to be joined.[70]

20. "LOVE . . . , COMFORT . . . , HONOUR, AND KEEP . . . IN SICKNESS AND IN HEALTH"

Perhaps the most important part of the marriage promise is to unconditionally love, comfort, and honor the beloved. This is the most important part because it is what makes the romantic love be a form of *love*. What I have hitherto discussed is the sexual nature of romantic love. Even what was said about commitment applied to the love as sexual, since the commitment of the love as love is even more unconditional: *agapê* withstands death, Christians believe.

However, even though this is more important, I will not focus on it much. For this is something that romantic love has in common with *all* loves. Insofar as one loves persons, one seeks to comfort them, one honors them for being who they are, and one strives to keep them in one's love, no matter what may befall them. In fact, the obligations of love simply as love, i.e., as *agapê,* that obtain in marriage are no different in kind from the obligations of love we have to everybody else. We are to see Christ in everyone. The only potential difference is of degree.

Yet, there is room for different degrees of love. The fourth Gospel talks several times of the disciple whom Jesus loved (John 19:26, 20:2, 21:7, 21:20). The degrees of love could perhaps be apportioned to the worth of the beloved, but need not be. It is one of the themes of the Hebrew scriptures that God has a special love for those who are of little significance, including Israel. God chose to make a covenant with Israel and, having made that covenant, he lavished particular love on the people he chose, though we learn from the New Testament that he is love itself (1 John 4:16), from which it seems to follow that he loves everyone. And it is clear that, likewise, the marriage covenant presses on one a particularly strong duty to love the other person.

We cannot, however, say that marriage obligates one to the strongest possible degree of love. Love does not come in a simple hierarchy, but there are different aspects of different loves. Thus, a soldier should love a commanding officer in respect of authority. But one's spouse need not have the same kind of authority over one,[71] and thus one should not love the spouse *in that respect.* Thus, there is some respect in which Private Jones loves Captain Smith, in which respect he does not love his wife, as his wife does not have the authority that Smith has over Jones—an authority that commands near-instant *obedience* in things that are not immoral. More trivially, Private Jones may love Captain Smith for her skill as a baseball pitcher, a skill that his wife might entirely lack. At the same time, Private Jones should love his wife for her sexuality, in a way in which it would be wrong for him to love his commanding officer, and he needs to love his wife in and through the particularly strong duties of long-term care that he has with respect to her.

Now, we may feel we should say that, in some overall sense, Jones should love his wife more than he loves Captain Smith. But it is not clear how that sense can be made completely precise. For it is not clear that it makes sense to compare different kinds of love. Does it make sense, for instance, to ask whether Private Jones takes more care of Mrs. Jones than he obeys Captain Smith? After all, in the ideal case, Jones will be willing to do both to a heroic degree. He will obey Captain Smith even at the cost of his (Jones's) life, and he will also be ready to sacrifice his life to care for Mrs. Jones. It is just not clear that different kinds of love can always be compared in degree.

The maximality of romantic love is a maximality insofar as what we have is both romantic and undistorted love. It is thus a constrained maximization—constrained by the romantic form of love. If Mr. Jones loved Mrs. Jones in all those respects in which he loves Captain Smith his love would express a misapprehension of his wife, and hence would be distorted.

In fact, even though, strictly speaking, loves cannot be compared, one can imagine cases in which an ideal nonmarital love would generally be said to be greater than an ideal marital love. For instance, if someone were in circumstances where it would be appropriate to give up her life for a stranger, and her husband's life were not in danger, and she did, in fact, give up her life for that stranger out of *agapê*, then we might well say that her love for the stranger was the greater love. One might think that since she would, in the ideal case, be *willing* to give up her life for her husband, therefore her love for the stranger does not exceed that for her husband. However, love should be seen as more than just a willingness: love is exhibited *in act*. That is why, as we have seen in section 1 of chapter 2, the aorist tense is not infrequently employed for love in scripture, apparently signaling an act of love rather than a disposition. In fact, if we accept plausible theses about free will, a mere *willingness* to sacrifice one's life for one's husband is quite compatible with not making the sacrifice when the issue comes up: we can change our minds when faced with pain, and it is the action that is decisive.

Even if we do not accept the thesis that love is found particularly in act, we still have some reasons to suppose that ideal nonmarital love might exceed ideal marital love in some cases. The Desert Fathers and Mothers would insist that the greatest kind of love on earth was that between a spiritual father or mother and a spiritual child. After all, that love was most purely ordered to the glory of God, and mirrored the love between Christ and his disciples. Again, this is not due to a shortfall in marital love: a marriage where one spouse were a spiritual parent to the other would probably be inappropriate, indeed spiritually incestuous. While on the same theme, the ancient Greeks may have been right that one's primary duty, even superseding that to one's spouse, is to one's parents. It may, likewise, be a theologically significant fact that honoring one's parents is positively mentioned in the Ten Commandments, while honoring one's spouse appears only negatively, to the extent of prohibitions against adultery and lust for another's wife. And one loves one's parents in respect of a gratitude for their having conferred on one the greatest gift possible in the natural realm: existence. Further, if one's parents are Christian, one may love them for having told one about the Gospel, whereas it is more likely that one and one's spouse were both Christian before meeting.

All that said, romantic love is *one* of the deepest forms of love.

21. DIVORCE, SEPARATION, AND THE STATE

It would appear to follow from all we have said that divorce is utterly immoral, since it is directly contrary to the duties of love. Yet, perhaps surprisingly, the Christian tradition has not held that divorce is immoral. Rather, it has held, following the wording of Paul's and Jesus' statements closely, that, at least in the case of Christians, divorce *followed by remarriage* is wrong. Nonetheless, as we saw in section 13 above, some of the Church Fathers held that divorce was acceptable in cases of adultery, and there were even some who thought it obligatory. It is just that *remarriage* would be adulterous.

As noted before, we can formulate this in the language of validity. A divorce from a valid marriage is not a valid dissolution of the marriage. If we wish, we might justifiably make a qualification that was made in the Catholic tradition and is compatible with the text of scripture: a divorce from a valid *consummated* marriage is itself invalid. For Jesus talks of a union *as one flesh*, and we have seen that this kind of union is connected with intercourse.

If a divorce from a valid consummated marriage, at least, is invalid as a dissolution of marriage, then the couple that underwent the divorce is still married. Their divorce does not, thus, literally sunder the marriage. Of course, if there were an intent to remarry, then, barring polygamous inclinations, the divorce would be an *attempt* at sundering what God has joined. But if there is no intent to remarry, and if the couple understands that the divorce is invalid as a dissolution of marriage, there might be no attempt made to sunder the marital union in the divorce. Rather, the divorce might be an attempt to obtain certain legal consequences that protect one's own and one's children's legitimate interests. It is a civil act, without consequence for the question whether there is a real marriage there or not.

Whether civil divorce is ever morally permissible depends, thus, on the way that conjugal love is related to these legal obligations. First of all, there is no absolute duty to maintain the legal existence of the obligations. Let us suppose that Nazi Germany went to the extent of legally dissolving all marriages between ethnic Jews and non-Jewish Germans, and let us suppose that Helga and Friedrich were, respectively, a Jewish and a non-Jewish German, married and living in England. It would surely not be immoral for them to sneak back to Germany in order to help some friends escape, even though while they were in Germany, the obligations of their marriage would be legally nonexistent, though, of course, they would still have moral obligations. That conjugal love does not require one to have such obligations as legal obligations can be seen when we reflect that surely it ought to be possible for Christians to marry in a location where the marriages of Christians are not legally recognized, either due to a repressive regime or due to the region having no laws at all.

These examples, while suggestive, do not, however, settle the question, because the couple going to Germany is not going there *in order to* annul the legal consequences of their marriage vows, and the couple marrying in the region where the marriages of Christians are legally unrecognized is not trying to *avoid* such recognition. The example, thus, is compatible with the claim that the deepest form of romantic love prohibits one from intentionally trying to remove the legal obligations, and that it calls on one to *try* to establish such legal obligations.

There is good reason to suppose that love calls on one to strive to make the obligations binding in law if this is reasonably possible. We are social creatures. An obligation binding in law is a union of us considered as creatures in a community under a law. Insofar as love calls for a union on all levels, it calls for this legal union. However, the law at best is a blunt instrument, a poorly made law can be a bludgeon rather than an instrument, and legal obligations can stand in the way of moral ones. We are well aware, from many areas of our lives, that it might not be desirable for certain moral obligations to be legal obligations. While I ought to keep a promise to a friend to meet him at noon tomorrow by the clock tower, it would not be desirable for there to be a law that would punish me for failure to do so. My friend's disappointment ought to be sanction enough.

Nor are we necessarily going against the integrity of the person in expressing the desire that, in some special circumstances, moral requirements of marriage should not be legally binding. Rather, we are expressing the centrality of moral obligations.

This allows, at least, for the *possibility* that there might be times when one would do better not to have the marriage legally recognized. And, if so, there could be times when it would not be contrary to love to seek a legal divorce. As a somewhat far-fetched example, let us suppose that a new law is expected to be passed next month banning adultery, and you know for certain that an enemy of yours will testify in court that you are an adulterer. Both you and your wife know that he is a liar, but you also know that the court would believe your enemy. If the penalties for adultery are severe enough, you and your wife might conceivably choose to seek a legal divorce before next week if only married persons can be accused of adultery, because your going to jail would end up sundering the union even more.

Now such far-fetched cases are not the ones that the Christians who thought divorce without remarriage to be permissible had in mind. The paradigmatic case they had in mind was divorce as a response to adultery, though the Christian tradition, even in its Catholic form—which has historically been strictest with respect to divorce—has eventually come to recognize that divorce might be permissible in other cases, such as cases of abuse. In these cases, the legal divorce seems to be taken on in order to *avoid* the legal obligations of marriage, such as obligations of mutual financial support or of living together, and not simply in order to avoid unjust punishment as in the outlandish example in the previous paragraph. Whether divorce in cases of adultery or abuse is permissible, then, is connected with the question whether obligations of financial support or of living together are absolutely binding given the nature of conjugal love. If not, then it could be that one remains faithful to love even while severing the legal force of such obligations.

Now remember that conjugal love, like any form of love, is directed at union and the good of the beloved. There may be times when two people are closer when they are not living together. After all, if living together results in one person abusing the other, treating the other in a way not consonant with human, not to mention marital, dignity, the couple might be less disunited if they live apart. Just as love is exhibited in acts, so is hatred: acts of hatred are at least partially constitutive of hatred. In living apart, acts of hatred are decreased through lack of opportunity, which, in turn, implies a movement toward the ideal of love, even if it does not advance far. (To stop beating a spouse is progress in love, though it does not get one very far.) Living apart need not be directly contrary to conjugal love's call for union, since it may decrease instances of abuse that are directly contrary to that call. This living apart may be temporary or permanent, depending on the actual situation, and it is quite conceivable that for practical reasons it may require a removal of the legal bonds that marriage involves.

Moreover, continuing financial support of the abusive party by the innocent party may not be morally obligatory, for instance, if such support would be at the expense of the children, or if such support would be harmful to the abusive party, as by supporting a drug or alcohol habit. In such a case, severing financial support is not contrary to conjugal love, since the raising of children is one of the primary goals of conjugal love. In fact, it appears that the potential and actual complexity of abusive situations is such that we cannot lay down many hard and fast rules, just as we cannot lay down hard and fast rules for dealing with abusive people outside of marital relationships.

Indeed, *all* loves include an obligation of financial support under *some* circumstances—any stranger is someone whom we may potentially be obliged to help financially—but we cannot realistically expect to give rules to specify the circumstances. When is it a duty to give money or food directly to someone, and when should one, instead, refer the person to an agency and give money to the agency, among other options? We cannot say precisely ahead of time, though there are clear cases: The alcoholic expressly asking for money for alcohol should not be given cash by anyone, though other forms of help are appropriate; on the other hand, a financially needy but otherwise untroubled friend unable to pay the rent in a given month typically should be given (or lent, if, say, this better supports their dignity) cash upon request. But slight changes to the cases introduce murkiness. If my friend does not ask for help, for instance, then I need to weigh whether my offering him cash might not unduly encroach on his feelings of dignity.

Similarly, we can ask about what circumstances there may be during which sexual activity is inappropriate. In cases of ongoing adultery, marital activity on the part of the adulterous spouse could be a kind of deceit, while marital activity on the part of the betrayed spouse could be a sign of tacit approval, contrary to an *agapê* that calls on one to make clear to the spouse the need to change. Likewise, if marital activity is a consummation of romantic love, while it can be appropriate to engage in marital activity when the love has not yet fully matured—otherwise, marital activity would never be appropriate— surely the activity is expressively inappropriate in cases of hatred.

So there *are* realistic cases where a legal divorce followed by living apart can be acceptable. Nonetheless, the case of adultery is actually more complex than it seemed to those of the Church Fathers who thought (legal) divorce to be the answer. Granted, if the adulterous spouse persists in the relationship despite having been encouraged to do the right thing, then continuing marital cohabitation, whether physically living under the same roof or engaging in sexual relations, may count as condoning the adultery, and might be detrimental to the true good of the adulterer. But what if circumstances were such that the couple could live together in a way that would not imply that the adulterous relationship is condoned? After all, that it is not condoned could, perhaps, be made adequately clear through other means.

Of course, it is clear that if forgiveness has been asked for sincerely, it must be given by a Christian, though there could be constraints of prudence on the precise course of action taken after giving forgiveness. It is, however, less clear whether one must give forgiveness when it has not been asked. In the Lord's Prayer, we ask to be forgiven as we forgive, and we could perhaps be satisfied with only being forgiven by God when we ask for God's forgiveness. Thomas Aquinas, for instance, thought that while we had a duty to offer forgiveness when forgiveness was asked, to offer forgiveness when forgiveness was not asked was needed only for perfection,[72] which I take to mean that it was supererogatory.

Still, the fact that those who marry enter into an unconditional commitment to each other makes it very hard to maintain the view that it is permissible to withhold forgiveness in a Christian marriage, even when forgiveness is not asked. However, offering forgiveness is compatible with withdrawal of financial support and living apart financially, geographically, and sexually, as long as the good of the beloved—say, the desire to bring the beloved to repentance—is kept firmly in view.

Note that no such argument could justify the innocent party's remarriage, for several reasons. First, a divorce is not a firm commitment not to be together—talk of "irreconcilable differences" should surely be understood as "irreconcilable *in the foreseeable future*." Even if the spouse expects no change in the situation, change is always possible, especially by God's grace: a guilty party may seek counsel from wise persons, repent, and so on. Since the two are still validly married, in fact—the divorce merely affects certain legal features—they can come back together at any time, though of course it would be desirable then, if possible, to undo the legal effects of the divorce if it is clear that the problems have been overcome. An attempt at marriage with another person, however, would be an undertaking of a commitment incompatible with coming back to the first commitment. This attempt at marriage, if sincere and made in a monogamous setting, would be directly opposed to the marital unity of the first marriage.

Second, observe that divorce primarily acts to prevent a guilty party from continuing to act wrongly in certain ways (for instance, by preventing further abuse, or by making the betrayal in adultery less, since the less trust there is, the less betrayal there is), and hence benefits the guilty party by slowing the accrual of further burdens on his or her conscience. Of course, it also protects the innocent party, but given the Socratic and Christian principle that, in an important sense, it is worse to do evil than to suffer evil, the guilty party benefits more. That there is benefit to the ill-doer is even true if, say due to mental illness, the person is not culpable. For it is a serious harm to one to do bad things, even when one has an exculpatory defense. We should surely prefer that if we became insane, we would do so in a way that did *not* involve wicked activity, even wicked activity exculpated by the insanity. Divorce, thus, can be justified by love for the person being divorced. But remarriage is focused on another person, a new relationship, and is a definitive forsaking of the earlier committed romantic love (or else one is not truly faithful to the person one is marrying).

And, of course, besides all this we have the simple fact that, as part of the unitive consummation of romantic love, the persons had once entered into a relationship not dissoluble by anything other than death. The relationship would have been qualitatively different if remarriage were possible, or if divorce had any validity other than the merely legal. The impossibility of dissolving a marriage is needed to maintain the appropriate character of Christian marital relationships. A view on which divorce is valid—really dissolves a marriage—but immoral would be one where immoral behavior is rewarded, and where the temptation to divorce is significantly increased.

22. ARRANGED MARRIAGE

A common objection to seeing marriage as linked not just to sex and reproduction but also to romantic love is the prevalence of arranged marriages in many non-Western countries at present and in many Western countries in the past. Sometimes the two spouses barely meet prior to the wedding, and since love requires knowledge of the other, it does not seem possible that the couple marry out of romantic love. Given that there does not seem to be anything morally wrong with such marriages or with sex within them, it follows that sex in the absence of romantic love is morally acceptable and that marriage is not linked with romantic love.

Of course, one might object that such marriages are morally wrong. In fact, insofar as entering into a marriage is an undertaking of serious commitment, those arranged "marriages" where either party does not consent are not really marriages—they are invalid for the same reason that coerced "contracts" are nonbinding. But it is also possible for the members of a couple to freely undertake to please their parents or to entrust to their parents the choice of their marriage partners. After all, we might reasonably think that often others close to us understand us better than we understand ourselves, and so we might reasonably allow that our parents might make a wiser choice than we would, assuming they share our values and can be counted on to make the decision in light of considerations that we would endorse. So it is certainly possible for an arranged marriage to be consented to freely.

On the permissibility of sex without romantic love, it is worth noting that I did not argue that sex without *fully matured* romantic love is impermissible. Romantic love finds its consummation in sexual union, but romantic love normally continues to develop past its consummation. The union as one flesh may be complete, but the interpersonal union needs to grow in other respects. A requirement that one marry only when romantic love is fully developed in every respect would prohibit almost every, perhaps every, marriage that has ever taken place.

At the same time, love is always a duty, and love needs to be appropriate to the relationship. Thus, it is one's duty to love the person whom one is to marry, and it is a duty to love the person in the way appropriate to the person whom one is to marry. Of course, if one does not know anything about this person, the love cannot be very specifically developed. But it can involve the three aspects of all love: one has a ready disposition to benefit this person (should one find out what the person needs), one appreciates the other at least as a person, a creature of God, a fellow human being, and someone with whom one can engage in sexual activity, and one intends such a union with this person. (The sexual aspects of this union may be the easiest to intend for a young person!) All the while, one can remain open to the mystery, the surprise of the other person. And in this way, the arranged marriage is not so different from an unarranged "love match." In a love match, too, one must remain open to the enfolding mystery of the other person, traditionally including a lack of sexual knowledge of the other person. In any case, marriage and sex themselves can change people in unpredictable ways, and some of the knowledge of the person prior to marriage is likely irrelevant. Every love must involve a willingness to adjust its form to changes in the beloved and in the relationship, and must remain open to new things.

It is not so much wrong to marry someone that one does not love, as it is wrong not to love the person one marries. Love is required of us always, under all circumstances. It is wrong not to love the person with whom one shakes hands, the criminal one sentences to two years in jail, the homeless person one gives a meal to, or the person one marries. Of course a different form of love is required in each case. However, what primarily distinguishes the different forms of love is the type of real union toward which the love is directed and the aspects under which the beloved is appreciated. If one marries, one ought to have a directedness toward sexual and personal union with the other person, and an appreciation of the other person insofar as this person can be united with. But for this one needs only to know the other person as a fellow human being of the opposite sex with whom one can unite sexually.

There is an interesting objection to the latter requirement. There apparently still are cases where people enter into a marriage without any knowledge of intercourse—one hears of counselors being told: "We are sleeping together, but can't seem to make a baby," with it being only literally true that the couple is *sleeping* together. It would seem implausible to say that such couples are not really married, so that if they should one day learn about intercourse and engage in it, they would be fornicating. Yet seeing marriage as tied to sexuality and seeing consent as requiring knowledge of that to which one consents seems to push one in this direction.

One answer to this objection would be a view on which the couple, after finding out about intercourse and its connection to marriage and procreation, has a decision. They could go their separate ways, saying: "This isn't what we agreed to." Or they could extend their agreement to include the sexual aspects of the relationship of which they were previously unaware. Such an extension could then effectively be the completion of their marriage vows.[73]

23. INVALIDITY AND ANNULMENT

Recall that "invalid marriage" is like "fake money": it looks like marriage, especially in the eyes of the law, but it is not really marriage. There are obvious and uncontroversial cases of invalidity. For instance, the parties could turn out to be brother and sister, separated in early childhood. Or perhaps one of the parties had been tricked into participating in the ceremony by being told that it is just a scene for an amateur film production, so that the victim of the trick is only "mouthing the words" rather than making vows.

Or, rather more commonly, one of the parties might be still married to someone else at the time of the wedding ceremony. This could happen either clearly innocently, as when one erroneously but on good grounds believes one's spouse has died, or clearly guiltily, as in cases of deliberate "bigamy." But a much more common case in our society is when one or more of the parties was previously married to someone else and has had a civil divorce. Since Christian marriage lasts until death, that party is still married despite the civil divorce, and hence the new "marriage" is merely an invalid marriage.

Furthermore, marriage requires a genuine and sincere exchange of commitment, and such an exchange of commitment needs freedom. A contract signed under duress is both legally and morally null and void, and likewise a marriage "vow" made under compulsion is not a genuine vow. Similarly, some mental illnesses can make free consent impossible. Moreover, a commitment requires a sufficient understanding of what one is committing to. This means that either compulsion and ignorance at the time of the exchange of commitment can result in an invalid marriage.

Because marriage between Christians is a lifelong union while sexual relations outside marriage are wrong, determining whether a valid marriage took place can be a very important task. Granted, if a couple innocently but incorrectly believes themselves to be married, they are not culpable for their sexual relations being nonmarital, just as a camper who shoots at a shape in the dark while innocently believing that the shape is an attacking bear is not culpable if it turns out the shape is a fellow camper. But we should avoid wrongdoing, whether culpable or not, and we should help others to avoid it as well. Even inculpable wrongdoing can be harmful to one's moral life.

Two kinds of cases can come up where a determination of the validity or invalidity of a marriage needs to be made. In one kind of case, the couple wish to be married to each other, but are worried that they were never validly married in the first place. In such a case, it can be important to determine whether or not the couple is validly married. If the couple *is* validly married, their peace of mind can be restored. If they are not, then the next question will be whether they can *now* validly marry. If it turns out that now they *can* be married— perhaps one of them was previously married and the spouse has died, or perhaps they had insufficient understanding of the marital commitment, but that has now been remedied—then they can now have a genuine marriage ceremony, though for reasons of privacy they might make this ceremony be discreet. On the other hand, it may turn out that the couple is still incapable of marriage, for instance if they are siblings or if one or both of them is validly married to someone else. In such a case, they need to stop engaging in their (alas) nonmarital sexual relations and, typically, go their separate ways to avoid temptation. However, there are cases where children are involved in which such an unmarried couple chooses to live together chastely. Whether such a heroic decision is appropriate depends on how strong the temptations to sexual activity are and whether the couple would be giving a bad example ("scandal") to the community.

In the second kind of case, the couple wish to go their separate ways, and often to be free to marry another, and it needs to be determined whether they in fact had a valid Christian marriage to each other. If they had, then while under some circumstances they could get a civil separation or even divorce and live apart as discussed in section 21 above, neither can marry again until their present spouse dies. But if it is determined that they did not in fact have a valid Christian marriage, then as long as the condition that prevented the validity of their marriage does not apply again, they should be able to marry another.

Figuring out exactly what level of compulsion invalidates a marriage and what exact understanding of the marital commitment is needed is a difficult question, and goes beyond the scope of this book. But even this very short discussion shows that the determination of the validity of marriage can be a difficult task. After all, even leaving aside the conceptual issues, there is a difficult historical question: When the couple underwent the marriage ceremony, did they freely and with sufficient knowledge make their commitments, and were there then any conditions, such as a previous marriage, that precluded a valid marriage? To answer this, an investigation into the conditions at that time is necessary. Furthermore, the determination of the validity of one marriage may require a prior determination of the validity of others. If Sam and Sally are Christians who "attempt to marry" (i.e., go through a marriage ceremony with the intent to marry), and then have a civil divorce, and Sam and Samantha then attempt to marry, then to determine whether Sam and Samantha's putative marriage is valid, one may first need to determine whether Sam and Sally's putative marriage is valid.

Figuring out questions of validity can be a difficult matter, calling for specialized training on the part of the investigator. There is a value to there being established procedures and institutional structures for such determination, to help prevent constant individual speculation about the validity of one's marriage (or gossip about the marriages of others) and to assure peace of mind. Moreover, just as marriage is typically a community affair, there is a value in the procedures and structures being established by the community. At the same time, in a modern secular state, one cannot expect a representative of the state to perform the determination by means of standards that are both theologically and philosophically sound.

Therefore, there is good reason for Christian communities to have procedures and structures for determining the validity of marriages, as well as specialized training for those making such determinations. For instance, in the Catholic Church, these structures are marriage tribunals, whose primary task is to provide a determination whether a valid marriage had been entered into. When a negative answer is arrived at, the tribunal issues an "annulment," i.e., a declaration that there was no valid marriage.

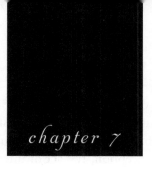

chapter 7

Contraception and Natural Family Planning

1. POSITIVE CONTRACEPTION

It does not follow immediately from the account of sexual union in terms of a joint bodily striving for reproduction that contraception is wrong, as I noted earlier. We have seen, after all, that sexual union appears compatible with neither person's intending reproduction. The question of contraception, however, is more difficult. It is not merely a matter of the person's not intending reproduction, but of the person's intending that there be no reproduction, and acting toward this negative goal.

I will divide the question into two. First, in this chapter we will consider whether it can ever be morally acceptable for a person engaging in intercourse to be acting so as to ensure that that act of intercourse should not result in reproduction. Such action I will call "positive contraception." More precisely, I will say that a sexual act has been positively contracepted provided one has intentionally acted so as to make the act be such as not to result in reproduction. *How* one has acted is irrelevant to the definition, and it is also irrelevant whether one's action succeeded in preventing conception or was even at all likely to succeed. Thus, if a man believes that the consumption of carrots decreases sperm motility and he ate a carrot before intercourse in order to prevent conception, the act of intercourse was positively contracepted by him, even though the probability of conception did not change at all.

If the man who believed in the contraceptive effect of carrots ate carrots to improve his eyesight and did not intend the contraceptive effect, he would not be engaged in positive contraception in the above sense, though his action would have a contraceptive consequence. Likewise, if someone refrains from having sex, and does so in order to ensure that there be no reproduction, this abstinence is not a case of positive contraception (one might call it "negative contraception"). Finally, it is not positive contraception by this definition if someone fails to take fertility-enhancing medication, even if the reason the person fails to take the medication is because the person does not desire to have children.[1]

In the media, one hears of the Catholic Church as having a prohibition on "birth control" or, at times, "artificial birth control." Terminologically, both options are unsatisfactory. First of all, "birth control" by itself is unsatisfactory, since abstinence can be a form of "birth control," and the Catholic Church has no objection to using abstinence to control conception, as long as one has sufficient reason to do so. Second, the term "birth control" fails to distinguish between contraception, which is the prevention of conception, and abortion, which is the destruction of the conceived embryo or fetus, both of which control what births occur. Third, the term "artificial" suggests technology to our ear, even though the term, as used in the context of Catholic moral teaching, is not meant to include that. Pope Paul VI's 1968 encyclical *Humanae Vitae* would presumably prohibit eating carrots to prevent conception just as much as it does using hormonal contraception. And indeed, traditionally, the paradigmatic example of artificial birth control is coitus interruptus, which does not involve any technology. The word "artificial" in this context is, rather, meant to suggest (positive) artifice, whether technological or other. But this is not the primary sense of the word "artificial" as it is commonly used in our day, and so I will use "positive contraception" instead. For brevity's sake, I will also at times use just the word "contraception" as short for "positive contraception."

The second question will be about the permissibility of orgasmic acts that are intrinsically different from intercourse, such as oral sex. These will be considered in the next chapter.

2. THE CONDOM

Before moving on to the general case of positive contraception, however, consider what appears to be one particular case of it—the condom. At this point, as in much of the rest of the book, the discussion is going to have to be markedly more graphic, due to the nature of the subject.

Intuitively, condoms are anti-unitive. They literally place a barrier between two persons. Granted, there can still be a great deal of direct physical contact between the couple. They may hold hands, their torsos may be in contact, they may be kissing, and so on. But full sexual union can occur without these physical contacts, and these contacts can occur, in turn, without full sexual union. The physical contact distinctive of sexual intercourse is intuitively missing. Any direct contact there may be is not that most intimate of contacts, since it is precisely there that the barrier was placed. Indeed given the physical barrier, the act does not appear significantly different from, say, an act of oral sex. The mere fact that the penis is surrounded by the vagina does not appear of much significance given that in between the two there is a latex barrier which significantly impedes their common functioning.

One may object that despite the barrier the parts *are* working together. But to see the limited nature of this cooperation, consider an example we might find in science-fiction. A well-meaning manufacturer of "marital aids" has decided to make things easier for married couples who have to be apart from each other for a significant period of time. The couple can purchase functional, anatomically correct, remote-controlled dolls that look just like the two of them. Each doll is set up in such a way that it transmits to the other doll detailed information about what the spouse in the same room as the doll is doing, and the doll then precisely mimics these motions. Each spouse then has the doll that looks like the other spouse and they can simultaneously engage in sexual relations with the dolls. Each doll's movements are precisely controlled by the spouse that the doll resembles. Consequently, each spouse physically feels just as if he or she had sex with his or her spouse. When Bob affectionately strokes the head of the Jane doll, the Bob doll consequently strokes the head of Jane, and so Bob's movement causes Jane to feel a pleasant stroke on the head. This also happens in respect of the sexual organs. Bob's sexual organs interact with Jane's through the mediation of the two dolls.

Thus, the kind of causal cooperation is in place here that exists when a condom is used. But surely something is missing. I am not arguing at this point that the use of this kind of surrogate for sex is immoral, but simply that it *is* a surrogate, that it is something significantly less than full sexual union, and yet that it is not something intrinsically very different from the condom if we imagine the couple using doll-based sex as a 100 percent effective contraceptive.

However, it is not the mere lack of physical contact that seems to be at issue. Imagine intercourse with a condom whose tip was cut off. It is possible, I suppose, that intercourse could go on without any physical contact between the penis and the vagina. But the organs would be working together properly. The vagina would be eliciting—through the mediation of the latex—the emission of semen into the female reproductive system. The emission would actually happen now in the way in which it was directed to happen by the sexual organs' cooperation. It would not be impeded. In this case we clearly have a full sexual union as one flesh. A functional union as one flesh does not actually require immediate physical contact but only physical interaction of the right sort.

The uncut condom's anti-unitive effect is not due merely to the removal of physical contact, but due to its severing of a crucial functional channel in the process of reproduction. This severing prevents the denouement of sexual intercourse from being coordinated appropriately, just as it would not be if the penis were somewhere else than within the vagina. Again, this is not yet an argument that the use of the condom is morally *wrong*, but simply that it results in something less than the consummation of romantic love.

3. FIRST ARGUMENT AGAINST POSITIVE CONTRACEPTION

But we do now have the ingredients for an argument showing that positive contraception is always wrong. The first version of the argument is quite simple in outline. Through contraception, as we have already seen in the case of the condom, one is intentionally transforming sexual intercourse into something other than sexual intercourse, something that does not have the physical unitiveness of sexual intercourse. In doing so, one is intentionally acting against union, and hence against that which romantic love seeks. And this is wrong, as it is contrary to love.

The weakness here is that the argument would seem to imply that abstinence, too, is always wrong for a couple in romantic love. But that view would clearly not be in line with either Jewish or Christian tradition. Judaism requires abstinence while the woman is menstruating, Paul apparently allows for abstinence for the sake of prayer, and Christian tradition has included seasons of fasting that have a requirement of sexual abstinence. Besides, the view would be absurd. Taken to its full extent, it would imply that the couple must engage in sexual relations whenever they physically can. Thus, if an anti-contraception argument implies abstinence is wrong, this implication constitutes a fatal objection to the argument.

In defense of the argument, however, remember that ethics often requires a distinction between doing something and refraining from doing something. A paradigmatic example is the distinction between killing and letting die. Suppose that you are imprisoned in a cell across from that of a person sentenced to death tomorrow, a person that everyone knows to be innocent. You, however, are scheduled to be released in a week. In Case A, the prison governor tells you that if you do not agree to execute the innocent prisoner today, you will be killed today—and the prisoner will still die tomorrow. In Case B, the innocent prisoner is dying of thirst, in addition to being sentenced to execution tomorrow. In fact, he will die today if he does not get something to drink. You have in your cell a number of small bottles of water. You could toss them over to the prisoner. However, you have been told by the prison governor that you will be executed as soon as one of the bottles of water goes missing from your cell. But the water would save the life of the other prisoner for a day.

In both cases, you are choosing between actions that have approximately the same effect. One option results in your death and the other prisoner living for another day, and the other results in your survival but the other prisoner dying now. However, there is clearly a moral difference between the cases, particularly if the prisoner in Case B is not asking you for the water. It does not seem that tossing the water bottle is the right choice. It gains a benefit for the innocent prisoner, but at a quite disproportionate cost, given that he is still going to die tomorrow. We need to act prudently.

On the other hand, in Case A, you are asked to do something that is morally wrong. You are asked to set your will directly against the good of your neighbor, to will something that is intrinsically evil, namely, an unjust execution. Love and hatred express themselves primarily in actions. When we act, we give our assent both to the goal and to the means of our action, because both the goal and the means are achieved by us. Thus, in Case A, if you kill the prisoner, you are giving assent to his death, and thereby bringing it about that you are actively hating him—that your will is set into the shape of hatred rather than that of love. It does not matter that his death is but a means to your survival—it is still true that you have assented to it. In Case B, on the other hand, it is a matter of not giving an assent of will to a particular good, the good of saving the other prisoner's life. Since we cannot always will every possible good to everyone we love, to refrain from willing a good is permissible. In Case A, one would be killing the prisoner. In Case B, one would merely be letting him die.

Likewise, abstinence is not an *action*, in the sense of positive action, but a refraining from an action. In abstinence, the couple refrain from acting in favor of one-flesh unity, but they do not act against it.

Thus, the abstinence is nonunitive, while contraception would be anti-unitive, just as not giving the water in Case B can be said to be "nonloving" while executing the prisoner in Case A would be "unloving." Arguably, on an ethics of love, it is always wrong to be unloving, but one may sometimes be nonloving in some respects. For instance, if instead of saving one drowning person I save another, in a situation where I can save only one, my action is *nonloving* to the person I do not save. If, however, to save one drowning person I need to push another one off the lifeboat, my action seems to be *unloving* with respect to the person I pushed off.

But what if the couple not only refrains from sexual activity, but does something positive to help ensure abstinence? For instance, supposing the couple decide to abstain for a month for some good reason, and in order to make the abstinence easier, the couple invite company over during as many evenings as they can, or sleep in separate beds.[2] It seems that in this case they are doing something *positive* in order to keep themselves from uniting as one flesh. By the above criteria, this appears to be an anti-unitive action, and hence wrong. Yet surely it is not wrong.

An answer can be given to this objection as well. The couple's inviting of company is an action whose purpose is to help the couple exercise self-control. Now, self-control is a good thing. The positive component of the action is, thus, directed at a good thing: at resoluteness in sticking to a rationally made decision. Whether this line of argument can be defended is not completely clear. It depends on whether one can distinguish between "resoluteness in sticking to a rationally made decision" and "resoluteness in sticking to the decision to abstain."

Moreover, speaking realistically, it is probably incorrect to think of the inviting of company as a means to abstinence. Rather, the inviting of company is what is done *instead of* sexual relations. It is a positive action insofar as it is an inviting of company, but insofar as it is one's way of abstaining from sexual relations it is a negative action, a refraining. This appears a better response here.

However, it is not clear that even this kind of an answer could apply in all cases. For instance, suppose that a married man deliberately does something positive to make himself less sexually attractive.

Maybe his wife finds that the shoes he wears to work make him irresistibly handsome, and so he removes the shoes outside the door, a positive action. It seems that the action plan is: "Remove shoes in order to be less sexually attractive, in order that sexual relations not occur." This would appear to be an anti-unitive intention. But with this the defender of abstinence can agree. Yes, this intention seems to be anti-unitive. However, there is a better intention that the man could have, which would justify the action. His action plan could be: "Remove shoes in order not to be sexually irresistible, in order that my wife be better able to make a rational decision whether to engage in sexual relations or not." And this last action plan has the advantage that it is more faithful to the mutuality that Paul wants decisions about abstinence to have.

Note, however, that even if the present anti-contraception argument can be defended, it could be that coitus interruptus escapes the argument, as the essence of that seems to be a nonaction, a discontinuation of intercourse. Since, intuitively, there does not appear to be a significant moral difference between coitus interruptus and, say, the use of a condom, and it would boggle the mind if coitus interruptus were morally permissible while a condom was not, this strongly suggests that the present argument, even if sound, is missing something of the essence. On the other hand, maybe coitus interruptus should be read as an *active* and positive interruption of "what comes naturally," as a *withdrawal,* and hence really does fall within the scope of the first anti-contraception argument. In any case, it will fall within the scope of other arguments.

4. SECOND ARGUMENT AGAINST POSITIVE CONTRACEPTION

While defensible, the first argument had its weak points. It depended on fine details of the distinction between acting and refraining, and required careful analysis of the kinds of actions that abstinence involves. There is a better argument. We have a number of moral intuitions, all centered on a sentiment that both doing something and not doing it, both setting out on a road and then stepping back, is morally unsatisfactory. In the Gospels, Jesus says to the man who wanted to say good-bye to his family, "No one who puts his hand to the plow and looks back is fit for the kingdom of God" (Luke 9:62). A Polish proverb has it that "the one who gives and takes back wanders in hell." In Acts 5, we read of Ananias and Sapphira being punished by God with death for handing over to the Christian community only a portion of the proceeds of a sale of property. Something like this attempt to have one's cake and eat it too is a part of what makes treason so despicable that Dante put the traitors in the lowest circle of hell. And even a run-of-the-mill lie is something of the same sort: in speaking, one is acting to communicate the truth, and so the liar acts against the truth precisely while acting in a way communicative of it. Likewise, a person who says "I love you. . . . That's a joke!" is acting odiously, raising a hope and then puncturing it.

The moral sentiment here may be prima facie puzzling. Is it any worse to give and take back than not to give at all? Were not Ananias and Sapphira doing a better thing by giving a portion of the proceeds than those people who gave nothing? Is it not better to put one's hand to the plow and look back than not to plow at all? Granted, in some of these cases there is more going on than just the inconsistency in one's actions. Ananias and Sapphira deceived the community. The person who takes back a gift is a thief. In individual cases, thus, the misdeed may involve other kinds of underhand behavior besides the forward-and-back movement. But we can look at this kind of associated underhand behavior as a fruit of the lack of internal integrity that the "giving and taking back" action reveals. The lack of consistency in one's action can be a failure to be honest with one's conscience, and that in turn leads to dishonesty with others. Peter rebukes Ananias and Sapphira not for deceiving the community, but for lying "to the Holy Spirit" (Acts 5:3; cf. 5:9). Given the indwelling of the Holy Spirit in the conscience of the Christian, we can see this as an instance of not being honest with one's conscience—telling oneself that one is doing something better than one is.

Considerations of integrity may help us understand what is behind the idea that giving and taking back reveals a bad character. Such persons lack integrity, i.e., wholeness. They act, in part, in one way and, in part, in the very opposite way. If we were Kantians, this lack of integrity, this contradiction in one's own will, would suffice to show the wrongness of the deed. But the ethics that I assume is not that of Kant but of the Gospel. Morality should follow from the duty to love.

Inconsistency by itself is a sign of the moral problem, but is not its essence. If inconsistency were the issue, there would be little difference between the son who said he would do the work but then didn't, and the son who said he wouldn't, but did (Matt. 21:28–31). One reason we should say that more integrity is displayed by the son who says he won't do the work but does, is because we identify people more with their better selves, so that the son came back to acting as "who he really is," his father's son.

If we look at things in terms of love, in cases of going forward and turning back, one acts in either an actually or an ostensibly loving way, but then one holds back that real or purported love, keeping the actual or apparent act of love from having full effect. Such an act is opposed to love. If the love is really there, the act stifles love, and if we see Christian love as the indwelling work of the Holy Spirit, it opposes the Holy Spirit—though hopefully not in a way that is unforgivable. And if the love was never there in the first place, then the act fakes love. Intuitively, the better or more holy the thing faked, the worse it is to counterfeit it. Aristotle notes that to pretend to a different kind of friendship than the friendship one actually has is worse than to counterfeit money.[3]

Now, intercourse is the expression par excellence of erotic love as *erotic* love. To prevent intercourse from attaining that which gives the reproductive striving its meaning, to oppose one's body while the body strives for love's consummating union, is to go back on that love. Thus, positive contraception is a sin against erotic love.

The obvious objection is, of course, as in the previous section. Is not abstinence equally a sin against erotic love? Does not abstinence require one to hold oneself back from sexual desire, from a desire for one-flesh union, and in doing so, is not the abstinence itself a going back on love?

Many a seducer, no doubt, has used this argument. And thinking about seducers suggests a disanalogy between abstinence and contraception. Abstinence acts against the goals of *libido*. Contraception, however, sets one against the activity that is the consummation of *erotic love*. Love normally comes with a desire for union[4] and in this case it is a desire for *sexual* union. However, love's desire for union is not just libido (see section 4 of chapter 3). On the contrary, in love one strives for interpersonal union and the other's good, and it does not go against love to abstain from sexual union when such union would not be good for the other or for the couple. And in cases where, say, having another child would endanger the ability to fulfill parental obligations to existing children, potentially reproductive sexual union would not be good for the couple, since it is not good for one to be placed in a position where one cannot fulfill one's obligation. Libido itself is not an act of love, though love may lead to libido and libido may enhance love. Love does not seek libido except perhaps as a means to engaging in sexual intercourse in a fully participating way.

Moreover, we can argue that the striving for reproduction in intercourse is there at a biological level, and insofar as the organs strive for reproduction, they do not do so through the concurrence of volition (for instance, the members of the couple do not have to specifically will that seminal fluid be emitted and accepted),[5] though generally a choice is needed in order to initiate and perhaps continue the physical activity of intercourse. Intercourse is a bodily, biological striving for reproduction that leads to its effect through biological, nonvoluntary means.

But engagement in intercourse is voluntary. Desire in persons does not act through overpowering the person and forcing him or her to act. If that happened, then we would say that the person did not really act as a person. It would, in fact, be rather like the person's being "raped" by his or her own desires, in that the sexual act would be nonconsensual and forced upon the person by desire, since voluntary consent requires will, choice, or intention, not just desire.

Desire, thus, does not *directly* strive for intercourse, and so the couple does not go against sexual desire in refraining from intercourse. Desire strives merely to incline the will in the direction of intercourse. A physical desire[6] that actually overcame the will and left one with no choice to make would be disordered, a psychological compulsion. If we identify the proper functioning of desire with desire's striving for its goal, then we will see the goal of desire not as the final action as such, but as either informing or inclining an act of choice in a particular direction. Consequently, one is not acting directly against the nature of sexual desire when one chooses to abstain or even when one takes measures to reduce the sexual desire—say, by having company until one is tired late at night. In fact, in such a case, one is acting in support of the sexual desire's function of *influencing a rational choice*, by ensuring that a rational choice actually occurs.

The present argument works well against the pill, the condom, and coitus interruptus. Each of these methods goes against the striving that constitutes love's consummation, and hence is wrong. But abstinence does not act against the striving that constitutes love's consummation, and hence is not forbidden by the argument.

The argument applies, too, when the love that I have argued contraception to oppose is nonexistent. For the married couple still has an objective normative *commitment* to conjugal love. And this commitment also includes a commitment to acting on that love: one is committed to both having the love and acting as if one had it. A husband who finds himself not loving his wife is not, on that account, excused from caring for her when she is sick. On the contrary, if he does not love her *and* does not take care of her, he has two wrongs on his conscience, while if he does not love her but does take care of her, there is but one. Not that one can really push this distinction very hard, because love is innately tied to the acts of love, and so love is already present in loving actions done.

5. THIRD ARGUMENT AGAINST POSITIVE CONTRACEPTION

For a third argument, consider first the case of a soccer player who wants the other team to win, because her best friend, who has lately been feeling rather down, is on that team. If she is actively trying to impede her team's victory while playing the game, she is a woman divided. Insofar as she is playing the game, she is striving for victory.

Insofar as she is deliberately impeding victory, she is acting contrary to the playing of the game. Now while the situation does smack of treachery, it is not completely obvious that under all possible circumstances something like this is wrong. The game, after all, is not something deeply holy. If someone's life depends on the other team's victory (it is possible to imagine a totalitarian state executing an unsuccessful athlete), such activity may be acceptable. A game is not intrinsically an expression of love.

But hold on to the idea that such a player is a divided woman. Not only is she not in the game with her whole heart, but her heart is set against the game. For it is with what we strive for, with our intentional actions, that we most effectively define where our heart is. That is why there is the tight link between obeying God's commandments and loving God that we see in the First Letter of John.

In the case of contraception, the same is true. The person's body is striving for reproduction. But on a voluntary level, the person is actively set against it. Thus the biological striving is not reflective of the person as a whole. On the contrary, the person as a whole is crucially disunited from the body. But if in the sexual act the two persons are supposed to be united *through* their bodies, then in being disunited from their bodies, the persons are thereby disunited from each other. Hence the deliberately contracepted sexual act fails to unite the persons as persons, since it disunites the persons from the act by which they are supposed to be united.

One way to complete the argument at this point is to note that then the members of the couple either have an illusion of unity without the reality—and illusion in matters of love is inappropriate—or else they are clearheadedly intending to engage in intercourse without thereby uniting as persons, or their sexual act is not a form of intercourse.

Now, for the couple to clearheadedly intend intercourse without full union is wrong for some of the same reasons that premarital sex is wrong. In engaging in the thorough union of bodies without uniting thoroughly as persons, a couple is devaluing that thorough union of bodies, not treating it as the act of uniquely unitive consummation of romantic love. With positive contraception, one acts against the body, and this alienates one from the body. But to alienate oneself from one's body in the context of sex is a way of failing to make intercourse be innately expressive of oneself as a person, and that makes intercourse less of an expression of oneself even on later occasions where contraception might not be *not* used. For, in the case of a couple open to the use of positive contraception, intercourse is expressive of union of persons only because the couple specifically chooses to intend it to be such. However when a couple that never contracepts (or that had contracepted in the past but now have firmly rejected positive contraception) has intercourse, it is expressive of union of persons not only because they specifically chose to intend it to be such, but also in virtue of the habitual connection between union and intercourse. This means that the contracepting couple makes even their uncontracepted intercourse shallower, and thus acts against the consummation of their love. (One can also adapt this consideration to yield another reason to refrain from premarital sex.)

Moreover, even if the couple is clearheaded about what they are doing, the sexual feelings for the sake of which they are most likely acting (after all, they are acting for the sake of neither reproduction nor full union) are feelings of closeness and union, feelings contradicted by a reality of striving against the act that generates these feelings.

But there is one more option. Perhaps the contraception turns the act of intercourse into something other than an act of intercourse. If the couple knows this, they are perhaps not devaluing intercourse by engaging in this act. In such a case, we have something that is perhaps not best understood as positive contraception that renders an act of *intercourse* infertile, but as a change of sexual activity. And in that case, different arguments need to be made, namely, the arguments in the next chapter against orgasmic acts outside the context of intercourse. That said, there are few defenders of contraception who think that contraception transforms intercourse into something else, so the present argument will still work ad hominem. And in any case, the only two kinds of birth control in which it could be argued that intercourse is not really what takes place are coitus interruptus and barrier methods such as condoms.

A final way to finish the argument would be to accept the premise from the Catholic tradition, as reiterated in Vatican II, that the two legitimate purposes to sexual intercourse are reproduction and union. If we take "union" here to be the full union of persons, then the contracepting couple is either deceived about what is going on, unaware of the lack of union, or else they are pursuing some third goal, such as pleasure, at the expense of reproduction and union.

6. SCRIPTURE AND HISTORY

Christian tradition, as far back as we can trace it, has unhesitatingly taken both positive contraception and engaging in orgasmic acts other than intercourse to be immoral. The earliest example, dating from the second century, is the presupposition in the Letter of Barnabas that Christians take oral sex to be wrong. Fancifully, Barnabas says that the weasel is not kosher because "this animal conceives [*kuei*] with its mouth,"[7] and the prohibition in the Old Testament on eating weasels was a sign that one should not "[b]ecome such a person—such men as we hear committing lawlessness in their mouths through impurity [*di 'akatharsian*]; nor shalt thou cleave to women who are impure and who commit lawlessness in their mouths."[8] Obviously, Barnabas is presupposing a prohibition on oral sex. The word "cleave [*kollêthêsêi*]" recalls the Septuagint translation of Genesis 2:24, which says that a man "shall cleave [*proskollêthêsetai*]" to his wife. Barnabas's bizarre biology and anachronistic Old Testament exegesis are beside the point, since we are only using the text as an early witness to the existence of a presupposed Christian prohibition on oral sex. What Barnabas is trying to do in his letter is to explain puzzling prohibitions from the Torah as symbolizing sensible doctrines and moral rules. Thus, we were told we should abstain from pork, because we ought not associate with swinish people.[9] Barnabas's task requires that the community to which he addressed himself would accept, or at least find plausible, the doctrines and moral rules that he took the Torah to symbolically express.

Now, there seems to be significant similarity between oral sex and, at least, intercourse using condoms—in neither case is seminal material directed into the female reproductive system. Furthermore, I do not know of any contemporary defenders of contraception who do not also think intercourse using condoms and oral sex are permissible. It seems that all of these issues are linked.

In general, the Patristic tradition has universally condemned abortion and contraception. Apparently the first unambiguous discussion comes from the first half of the third century. Hippolytus criticizes Callistus for allowing certain illegal marriages or concubinages to unmarried women, and then says:

> For this reason women who were reputed to be believers began to take drugs to render themselves sterile [*epicheirein . . . atokiois pharmakois*], and to bind themselves tightly so as to expel what was being conceived, since they would not, on account of relatives and excessive wealth, want to have a child by a slave or by any insignificant person. See, then, into what great impiety that lawless one has proceeded, by teaching adultery and murder at the same time![10]

As Noonan[11] notes, the structure of this text is such that Hippolytus is criticizing the relationships of the women as "adultery," and their use of contraception and abortion alike as "murder." There may be some hyperbole here—the women are not married to anybody else, and their consorts are presumably not married, and so the literal "adultery" is too strong. Likewise, the use of "murder [*phonos*]" may either be hyperbolic, or else Hippolytus sees the prevention of conception as being anti-life in the same way that abortion is.[12] From that time on, a number of patristic authors condemn contraception, notably including St. Clement of Alexandria, St. John Chrysostom, St. Jerome, and St. Augustine. As far as one can determine, every patristic author who deals with contraception ends up by condemning it. Some but fortunately not all of these authors go so far as to condemn all intercourse (e.g., in old age) that cannot achieve conception.[13]

The condemnation of contraception was accepted by the Protestant reformers, such as Luther[14] and Calvin,[15] and continued largely unabated until, in 1930, the Anglican Church at Lambeth decreed the matter up to the conscience of the individual. For Catholic and Orthodox Christians, and any others who believe that whatever the Church as a whole has historically taught about morals or theology is guaranteed by the Holy Spirit guiding the Church, this should be a conclusive argument against contraception. Or, more precisely, against *positive* contraception, since there is no traditional prohibition against abstinence.

But even for those who do not believe that the Church as a whole does not err in its teaching, the above should provide a strong argument. It seems an eminently reasonable Christian position that we should accept the teaching of an unbroken Christian tradition, as long as the teaching does not contradict either scripture or reason. After all, the Holy Spirit surely does guide the Church (John 16:13) so that the Church is "the pillar and bulwark of the truth" (1 Tim. 3:15). Now, the teaching that positive contraception is wrong does not contradict scripture. And it does not contradict reason.

The latter point bears further discussion. After all, many people think the view that contraception is impermissible is most unreasonable. But in fact there is a paucity of good arguments, or at least good arguments that are plausible on Christian grounds, for the permissibility of contraception. In fact, in general, there are very few moral arguments for the permissibility of anything. Most arguments for the permissibility of something are responses to arguments *against* the permissibility of a thing.

Specifically, in the case of positive contraception, the main *positive* arguments for its permissibility are based on utilitarian or other consequentialist premises that Christians must reject, arguments that proceed from the claim that contraception is in some way beneficial to the claim that it is permissible. Such arguments cannot be conclusive, since wrongful acts are sometimes beneficial, the standard case being the one where you are asked to shoot one innocent person to save several others. Given that I have given at least plausible positive arguments for the impermissibility of positive contraception earlier in this chapter, once one adds a strong presumption in favor of Christian tradition, we get a very strong case indeed.

Furthermore, and this contradicts intuitions that some people in our culture hold, we should take Christian tradition (as well as scripture) to be particularly reliable in sexual matters. Why? Because Christianity is a religion of love, so that the teaching of how to live a life of love is at the center of Christianity, and sexual matters are closely tied to how one should live one of the main human types of love. Nor will it do to say that what is central to Christianity is *agapê*, not erotic love, because as we have seen (in section 2 of chapter 2), erotic love, like every genuine kind of love, is a form of *agapê*, the word "*agapê*" simply meaning "love." And indeed erotic love is one of the central kinds of love in human life.

Moreover, a specific scriptural case—though one not perhaps up to the exegetical standard of relying only on major themes or truly seminal texts—can be made based on the story of Onan, at least against coitus interruptus. Tamar's husband was slain by God for his wickedness, without leaving any progeny. In fulfillment of the levirate duty, her brother-in-law Onan married Tamar: "But Onan knew that the offspring would not be his; so when he went in to his brother's wife he spilled the semen on the ground, lest he should give offspring to his brother. And what he did was displeasing in the sight of the LORD, and he slew him also" (Gen. 38:9–10). Now there are two interpretations of this text. The more traditional Christian interpretation is that it prohibits Onan's practice of coitus interruptus. Given that if coitus interruptus is wrong, it is plausible that so are other kinds of positive contraception, this would support the thesis of the impermissibility of positive contraception. We need, thus, to consider the main alternative interpretation, and it is that the text presents Onan being killed by the Lord not because the coitus interruptus was wrong, but because it was employed for a wrongful goal, the avoidance of the levirate duty to raise up children on behalf of one's dead brother.[16]

However, there are three considerations against the alternative interpretation. The first is that the text expressly says that what Onan *did* displeased God, which somewhat favors the anti-contraceptive reading. The next observation is that this story is set at a time prior to the giving of the Law at Sinai. Thus, while levirate practices may well have been a *custom* at the time in which the story is set, it is neither clear whether the custom had the status of a divinely sanctioned law, nor whether the author thought it did. And it would seem unreasonable if God killed Onan for failing to fulfill a mere custom. But most seriously, observe that even the Mosaic Law does not appear to consider violation of the levirate law a capital offense. Its punishment is not death but public shaming, through having one's shoe removed and face spat upon (Deut. 25:7–9). In fact the interpretation that seems to fit best with the severity of the punishment is to see Onan as employing immoral means to a bad end.

It has also been argued that the *pharmakeia* prohibited in Galatians 5:20 and other places, although translated by the RSV as "sorcery," is in fact the use of a contraceptive potion. This interpretation, while not required by the text, is possible, and coheres even with the RSV translation, since contraceptive potions might well have been one of the most popular "magical" wares. This further is consistent with the use of a cognate term in the second-century Christian text known as the *Didache:* "thou shalt not steal; thou shalt not use magic; thou shalt not use philtres [*ou pharmakeuseis*]; thou shalt not kill a child by means of abortion, nor slay it after it has been born."[17] A prohibition on the use of contraceptive potions would fit logically between a prohibition on magic and a prohibition on abortion. But a weakness of this interpretation is that if a Greek-writing Christian author wished to be explicit about contraceptives, this was quite possible. Recall Hippolytus's discussion of women whose loose ways led to their using *contraceptive* potions (*epicheirein . . . atokiois pharmakois*).[18] On the other hand, the use of *pharmakeia* on its own may be euphemistic. But even if a reading of *pharmakeia* as contraception were correct, it would only increase the probability of the wrongness of contraception but would not prove it, since it would still not be clear from either Galatians 5:20 whether what is wrong in *pharmakeia* is the presumed magical efficacy, the contraceptive intent, or both.

A conservative Protestant adherent to *sola scriptura* might, then, offer a theological objection to the idea that positive contraception is wrong. Let us suppose that this Christian rejects the traditional interpretation of the Onan story in favor of the account that it was merely violation of the levirate duty that brought down divine punishment, and is not convinced about speculations on *pharmakeia*. Then, the Protestant Christian might argue, scripture nowhere prohibits positive contraception, either explicitly or implicitly. But what scripture does not prohibit, either explicitly or implicitly, is permitted. Call this the "liberty thesis."

But first note that the liberty thesis can be trivialized by the observation that scripture often prohibits all "wickedness," and hence if an action *A* is wicked, then *A* is implicitly prohibited by scripture even if scripture never alludes to *A*. Thus, the liberty thesis on this understanding is of no help, since it is quite compatible with contraception being wicked.

Obviously, the liberty thesis is not intended in such a trivial way. But now observe that on a nontrivial reading which requires pretty much explicit mention of a prohibition, the thesis is false. For instance, necrophilia is clearly immoral but not prohibited by scripture.[19] Nor is cruelty to animals in general prohibited by scripture, even though it is immoral.[20]

Of course one might say that cruelty to animals is wrong because it does not exhibit proper love for the Creator, and hence the prohibition is implicit in scripture, while necrophilia is an instance of sexual immorality, *porneia*, and prohibited as such. But once one says that, then the *sola scriptura* argument for the permissibility of contraception evaporates. For it would need to be established that contraception does not go against proper love for one's spouse, which is biblically commanded, whereas I have argued that it does, and it would also need to be shown that contraception is not an instance of sexual immorality, whereas the opponents of contraception think it is.

The liberty thesis is either false or not very helpful. It might be, though, a guiding rule. If an activity is not explicitly condemned in scripture, and we cannot use reason to show how a prohibition on the activity follows from more basic principles in scripture, we should at least assume the activity to be permitted for the time being. This modified liberty thesis, however, does not provide an argument for the permissibility of contraception. Moreover, I think this thesis is unsatisfactory, for instance, because it seems likely that the moral teaching of the apostles as exhibited in their day-to-day pastoral work went beyond the summaries in scripture, and it is plausible that this teaching is embodied in the tradition of the Church.

7. CONSUMMATION AND THE FRUITFULNESS OF TRINITARIAN LOVE

Recall that Augustine had explored, but ultimately rejected, the notion of the family as an image of the Trinity, with the Holy Spirit's procession from the Father and the Son being seen as analogous to the generation of a child by the parents.[21] There is something right about this rejected analogy, though it is imperfect, since (except perhaps in the case of Adam and Eve) neither the husband proceeds from the wife nor the wife from the husband in the way the Son proceeds from the Father. But even without pressing the analogy, we can learn from the doctrine of the Trinity that unitive love is innately fruitful. And, if so, to act against this fruitfulness seems wrong.

8. NONMARITAL POSITIVE CONTRACEPTION AND NATURAL LAW ARGUMENTS

The arguments above are essentially made in terms of positive contraception's being directed against the deepest form of romantic love, the kind of form to the existence of which a married couple is committed. This leads naturally to the question of the permissibility of positive contraception in nonmarital contexts (here I deem rape, even within marriage, a nonmarital context, since insofar as a spouse is committing rape, the spouse is not acting *as a spouse*). Since in these contexts there is, at least as yet, no commitment to mature romantic love, and in fact there may even be no duty to have that kind of a commitment (one shouldn't marry everyone with whom one falls in love), the above arguments do not appear to apply. If there are no further arguments against contraception, then it is not immoral in nonmarital contexts.

Of course, given that I have argued in the previous chapter that intercourse outside of marriage is wrong and that I shall argue in the next chapter that orgasmic activity other than intercourse is also wrong, the question is not whether the person engaging in nonmarital intercourse is doing wrong, but whether engaging in contraception while doing so puts an additional burden on the person's conscience, much as breaking a window and entering someone's house adds an additional burden over and beyond that which one would accrue by just breaking the window.

We can classify philosophical arguments against positive contraception into three categories. The category of which this book is to some extent representative, and which is also currently very prominent in the Catholic milieu in large part due to the prominence of the work of John Paul II, is "personalist" arguments based on the meaning of marital love. These arguments apply primarily to marital situations, though one might perhaps imagine some nonmarital cases in which the love is sufficiently deep that contraception could be argued to do wrong by introducing disunity (and where the couple should get married given the depth of their love, and should do so prior to engaging in intercourse).

In fact, on the basis of personalist arguments, contraception in many nonmarital contexts could well be a good, in that it acts against a one-flesh union that should not be present. On such views, contraceptive nonmarital sexual activity would be wrong, indeed seriously wrong, since it would still be an attempt to engage in something that feels like one-flesh union without the reality, but noncontraceptive, nonmarital sexual activity could sometimes be *more* wrong since there is a greater one-flesh union there. What kinds of social implications this has vis-à-vis counseling the use of contraception to unmarried persons is not clear. We do not counsel potential bank robbers how to rob banks in safer and less immoral ways—say, by wearing bullet-proof vests and not beating up the customers. Rather, we tell them not to rob banks. At the same time, if Felicia is firmly set on robbing a bank and beating up the customers, and if we have failed to persuade her not to rob the bank, we might individually try to persuade her not to beat up the customers, at least.

The second class of arguments has been worked out by Grisez, Boyle, Finnis, and May (GBFM),[22] and is centered on the principle that one may not perform any "contralife" act, i.e., any act characterized by a "contralife will." What makes contraception contralife is the intentional prevention of the coming into existence of a new human life. The contraceptors "imagine that a new person will come to be if that is not prevented, they want that possible person not to be, and they effectively will that he or she never be."[23] We thus have a basic principle that it is wrong to act against the good of human life (or at least innocent human life), either by preventing the coming into existence of the life (contraception) or by terminating this life once it has come into existence (murder). Contraception and murder are wrong for the same reason, in that they involve a willed opposition to life.

The GBFM approach appears to imply that *all* positive contraception is immoral, including in nonmarital cases, and even in the case of rape. Given the strong intuitions we might have that use of contraception is acceptable in cases of rape, intuitions not contradicted by the teaching of any major Christian body,[24] this consequence is likely to make one sceptical of the principle. Note, too, that none of the arguments I offered based on the nature of one-flesh union would make contraception wrong in cases of rape—in fact, it seems that it can be a positive good to act against this unconsented-to one-flesh union.

However, GBFM also have an elegant response to the objection that their view prohibits contraception in cases of rape. It is permissible for a woman to resist the continuation of a rape, e.g., by forcing the attacker to withdraw. Conception is "the ultimate completion" of the act of rape. The victim is justified in striving to prevent this completion of the act of rape, perhaps by using a contraceptive measure. In doing this, the victim is opposed to the process of conception itself rather than the new life that is the outcome of the process of conception.[25]

According to GBFM, the victim's use of contraception is justified by the Principle of Double Effect (PDE), which says that one may do something that is, in and of itself, morally neutral or good and which has a bad result, as long as the bad result is not intended either as an end or as a means, and as long as there is sufficiently good reason to act. The PDE in one formulation (difficult questions about details of the formulation will not matter in this book)[26] says that it can be permissible to perform an action that has both a good and a bad effect, provided that (a) the action is intrinsically morally neutral or good, (b) the bad effect is proportionate to the good, and (c) the bad effect, or "side-effect," is not intended, either as a means or as an end. The PDE is frequently used to defend military actions against legitimate military targets that can be expected to have some civilian deaths as an unintended but not reasonably preventable side effect.

In the rape case, then, it can be argued that the victim intends to stop the completion of the act of rape—by flushing with a spermicide, for instance. The victim does not intend to prevent the coming into existence of new life, which new life comes from that completion. If the victim did in fact intend to prevent the new life, the victim's action would be unjustified.

This response, though, will not take care of the following case. Suppose that a nonconscious robot running an unlikely but entirely randomly produced program enters your house at night, ties you up, and cultures some of your skin cells. It then takes some of the cells that result from the culturing process in a Petrie dish and leaves (it does not actually take any skin cells that are yours but rather takes genetic copies of your skin cells). It will use these cells to make a hundred clones of you, which it will then torture. There is only one way to stop it. You pick up a small paperweight and throw it at the Petrie dish in its hand just as it is leaving. (You can't usefully throw the paperweight at the robot—it is too well armored.) Your intention is to prevent the robot from creating a hundred clones of you who would then be tortured, or maybe to prevent the torture by preventing the existence of the persons who are going to be tortured. This seems to be a clear case of a contralife intention. But on the other hand, the action looks like it is morally quite justified.[27]

It appears that the GBFM approach goes wrong by shifting our intuitions about respect for beings that can exemplify goods such as *human life* and about respect for these goods as possessed by such beings into the context of a respect for the abstract values themselves. We need to respect the persons who have life, and we need to respect the life they have, but it does not follow that the abstract value of life itself calls for a similar kind of respect. In murder, one has acted against a particular individual being,[28] by depriving this being of the good of life. But when contraception—or the smashing of the Petrie dish in the above example—is successful, there is no individual being who is deprived of a good.

Perhaps here is a place where an ethics of love departs in an important way from other ethical theories. Plausibly, love is only properly directed at concrete beings (including future ones), and the duties that derive from love or from the duty to love are duties to concrete beings. But the GBFM approach seems to make us owe a duty not to a being, but to a value. To some extent this formulation is unfair. GBFM can, after all, escape the criticism by saying that one owes it to oneself or to God that one should respect the value of life. But the criticism will, I think, make the GBFM argument less plausible.

The third, and most traditional, category of arguments consists of those based on "natural function" arguments. The traditional versions of these arguments insisted that contraceptive sex is wrong because it contradicts the natural telos of the sexual organs. Now, an argument that simply claimed that contraceptive sex used these organs for a purpose *other* than their natural one would be quite weak. Let us suppose that medical technology finds a way to make one kidney take over the secretion of bile from the liver in a patient whose liver is not functioning. Even though secretion of bile is not a natural function of a kidney, extending its functionality in such a way seems a good thing. And this seems true even if the cost of this operation is that that kidney can no longer engage in the waste expelling and water balancing functions that are normal for a kidney. (There is another kidney for that.) If so, then there is nothing wrong in general with using an organ for something other than its natural purpose, even if using it for that purpose is incompatible with the original use.[29]

However, the case of making the kidney produce bile is disanalogous to the case of contraception in at least four ways. The most obvious is that there is another kidney. Thus the functions of a kidney are *still* fulfilled, albeit no longer by *this* kidney. But contraception seeks to destroy an organ's striving for an end that cannot be successfully fulfilled by another organ. It would not typically be an act of contraception to deactivate only one of the two functioning testicles or ovaries. This particular disanalogy, however, can be overcome. Take an organ that serves some minor function. There does not appear to be anything wrong with adapting it to serve a more important purpose when the organ that serves the more important purpose is not working, even if this means that the less important purpose will not be served at all. Thus, if a patient had serious damage in her visual cortex but neurosurgery could make the portions of the brain responsible for olfaction take over visual perception instead, this would surely be acceptable. Hence, the first disanalogy does not help the natural function argument against contraception.

The second disanalogy is that in all the fictional medical examples above, there is no *intention* to deprive an organ of success at fulfilling its function—that deprivation is just a sad side effect of the treatment, tolerable by the PDE. But in positive contraception, there is a positive intention to deprive the reproductive system of success. This is a morally significant difference. In the far-fetched medical cases, one merely happens to act against a human body's functioning, while in the case of contraception, one is intentionally impeding good functioning.

Note, however, that the contraceptive intention is typically to deprive the reproductive system of success only *temporarily*. This is morally significant. For it seems plausible that it would be acceptable to temporarily deprive an organ of its natural function. Thus, there would not appear to be anything morally wrong with performing a neurological experiment that "turned off" olfactory processing for a few minutes (and it would be strange if there was some cut-off, such as that it is acceptable to turn off olfactory processing for three hours but not for three days). Again, the disanalogy does not damage my objection to the "natural function" argument against contraception.

There is a third disanalogy, and it is probably the most important. When one adapts a kidney to do the liver's work or the olfactory processing facilities to do the visual cortex's work, while one is frustrating the immediate goal of the organs in question, one is not frustrating their more ultimate goal, which is the proper functioning of the human body as a whole. Thus, it might be claimed that it is wrong to frustrate the functioning of an organ except for a higher purpose subserved by the frustrated functioning itself. And this claim still makes contraception wrong. For, let us take a case where pregnancy is avoided precisely because it would endanger the woman's life—if we can show that contraception is wrong even then, surely it is always wrong. Now, the reproductive system is unique among our bodily systems in that it does not subserve our own survival, but that of our species. The reproductive system is directed to a goal outside of us, the existence of a new human being. It is this goal that is intentionally frustrated by contraception, but this goal does not itself subserve our own survival. The new human being is not a means to anything, except maybe the greater glory of God (and one still can say that the human being is a *constituent* of the greater glory of God, rather than a *means* to that glory). Thus, when the reproductive system's functioning is frustrated, it is not for the sake of any further purpose of that reproductive system. And so contraception still falls under the prohibition here, again by its being irrelevant whether this is a case of nonmarital sex or rape.

But now note that this defense of the "natural functions" argument does not overcome the objection from the neurological experiment that turns off olfactory data processing. For that need not be done to further any goal of olfactory data processing. The brain receives olfactory data so that the individual whose brain it is might gain knowledge. The neurological experiment is done so that the medical profession should gain knowledge. The experimental subject's knowledge need not subserve the knowledge of the medical profession. Hence, the modified principle about frustrating natural functions is violated: the subject's olfactory data processing is shut off, and not for any purpose normally served by olfactory data processing. But it seems plausible that there is nothing unethical about an experiment like this.

Now one might defend such experiments and the natural function principle on the grounds that, both in the individual and in the medical profession, the value of knowledge—whether olfactory or medical—is as a means to the increase of knowledge on the part of society as a whole. This is a dubious claim, but let us leave it for a moment. This broader context lets one suspend the olfactory data processing for the sake of society's epistemic betterment. If one accepts such broader context analyses of the functions of organs, one might by parallel defend nonmarital contraception. For one might think that it is our function to reproduce in the context of the family—in the context of committed marital relationships—rather than just to reproduce *simpliciter*. The sexual organs' natural purpose is not just to produce more human beings, but to produce the fruit of a committed relationship. This natural purpose is not purely biological, but has both a biological and an interpersonal component. This is a deeply plausible view, if one thinks, as traditional natural law theorists do, that nonmarital sex is unnatural. But given this view, the purpose of the reproductive systems need not actually be frustrated by nonmarital contraception, since nonmarital contraception need not prevent the production of the fruit of a *committed* relationship.

Thus, it appears that each of the leading arguments against positive contraception either (a) does not prohibit all cases of nonmarital contraception (as in the case of the personalist arguments and some variants of the other two kinds of argument), or (b) rests on premises implausible for other reasons (such as the GBFM argument),[30] or both. Still, while nonmarital contraception might not add to the wrongfulness of nonmarital sexual activity, it highlights that activity's nonmarital nature, thereby drawing attention to the fact that there is something wrong with the activity in the first place.

9. ABORTION AND ABORTIFACIENT EFFECTS

All of the above assumed that we were dealing with contraception and not abortion. If contraception is wrong in a given context, surely so is abortion. But the converse is not true, since abortion could be wrong not only because it is a form of birth control, but also because it is homicide.

Abortion is not primarily a matter of sexual ethics. Granted, the embryo or fetus subject to abortion is typically begotten in sexual intercourse, but neither is the question of the appropriate treatment of prisoners of war a matter of sexual ethics, even though prisoners of war are typically begotten in sexual intercourse. It is, thus, beyond the scope of this book to examine whether abortion is homicide or not. It is clear that abortion in the context of marriage is wrong for *at least* the same reasons that contraception is. There is also a weighty argument from the Christian theological tradition for the claim that abortion is always an immoral form of homicide, and many have argued that this claim can be sustained on philosophical grounds.[31]

But one issue *is* to the point. There is evidence that hormonal contraceptives, whose primary way of functioning is by preventing ovulation, sometimes work by preventing the implantation of the already conceived embryo. In somewhere between 1 percent and 43 percent of cycles, depending on chemical formulation (the high 43 percent number is for "traditional" progestin-only pills), hormonal contraceptives fail to prevent ovulation.[32]

For the contraceptives to have the high method rate of effectiveness that they do, as high as 99 percent or more, despite the relatively frequent failure to prevent ovulation, there must be secondary mechanisms that prevent pregnancy. Two kinds of mechanisms operating prior to a potential fertilization have been proposed: "alterations in cervical mucus that limit sperm penetration, and changes in the endometrium and fallopian tube that may impede normal sperm transport."[33] In regard to the mucus changes, it should be noted that research shows that while the transport mechanism of spermatozoa may be disrupted by thick mucus, the female reproductive system is still capable of transporting particles through the cervix despite the mucus.[34] There is some reason to think, thus, that pre-fertilization mechanisms are insufficient to produce the high effectiveness rates of contraception.

However, there is also evidence that there are post-fertilization mechanisms of hormonal contraception, i.e., mechanisms that ensure that, although an embryo has begun its life, a pregnancy is not successfully established, and the embryo dies. These mechanisms probably involve changes to the uterine and/or fallopian environment, making the environment less favorable for life[35] and thereby preventing uterine implantation.

Noteworthy circumstantial evidence for an anti-implantation effect is given by the fact that ectopic pregnancies are significantly overrepresented among pill users' pregnancies, by a ratio of 4.5:1 for combined pills and a ratio of 13.9:1 for progestin-only formulations as compared to pregnant controls.[36] This is precisely what we would expect if one of the major modalities by which the pill worked was by preventing uterine implantation, since that modality would work only against uterine and not ectopic pregnancies, and thereby increase the ratio of ectopic to uterine pregnancies.

Similarly, there is evidence that postfertilization effects make a significant contribution to what one might call the "effectiveness" of intrauterine devices (IUDs).[37]

Thus, if abortion is always wrong because, from fertilization, the embryo or fetus is a human being to whom we owe love and respect, the use of these contraceptives is wrong not merely on account of the nature of sexual love, but also on account of duties to one's conceived children, and especially the duty not to act in ways that endanger the lives of one's children. And this argument, unlike the marital love argument, applies just as much in nonmarital cases as in marital ones, though only to some contraceptives.

10. NATURAL FAMILY PLANNING AND PERIODIC ABSTINENCE

Modifying either the way the sexual act is done, as in the case of the condom or coitus interruptus, or the way the reproductive system is functioning, as in the case of hormonal contraceptives, is not the only way to bring it about that conception is unlikely or impossible. One can also abstain. A major scientific discovery of the twentieth century has been that sexual relations, under most circumstances, can only result in pregnancy for about eight or nine days in the woman's cycle.

Therefore, abstinence on these eight or nine days will just about en-sure that conception does not occur. Thus, one can achieve the same goal of avoiding reproduction over, say, a period of a year through (a) modifying how the sexual act is done, (b) preventing the biological functioning of the reproductive system, (c) abstaining altogether from sexual relations, or (d) abstaining from sexual relations during the po-tentially fertile days of that year.

In practice, it is not possible to abstain from sexual relations only on the eight or so days of fertility because current methods are not able to precisely delineate these eight or nine days. The fertile time consists in seven days preceding ovulation, because that is how long sperm can survive in the female reproductive system, and then 24–48 hours after ovulation, since that is how long an ovum can remain vi-able for reproduction. For women with regular cycles, the fertile time occurs at approximately the same point in each cycle, and can be ap-proximately predicted solely by use of the calendar. Additional days of abstinence can be added before and after the estimated fertile time period for safety. Abstinence guided solely by such data is known as "calendar rhythm." When a modern version of the method is followed correctly by a woman with regular cycles of length 26–32 days, it will be 95 percent effective annually; i.e., 5 percent of women correctly using the method will get pregnant in a year of use.[38] The particular algorithm here was implemented through a simple ring of beads, ap-propriate for use by the illiterate.

However, in addition to purely calendric data, it is also possible for the woman to observe mucus secretions, changes in temperature and other symptoms, which, in turn, allow for an estimate of the po-tentially fertile stretch of time even for women whose cycles are not regular. These methods, collectively known as "Natural Family Plan-ning (NFP)," typically involve about one and a half to two weeks of abstinence per cycle when used to prevent conception, though at cer-tain times (e.g., toward the end of breastfeeding) significantly more. The efficacy of the method when used correctly depends on how much abstinence the users can tolerate, but effectiveness figures as high as 97 percent or even 99 percent or more can be achieved.[39] A re-cent German study found an actual use pregnancy rate of 1.8 percent per woman per 13 cycles, and for couples that used the method correctly, the pregnancy rate was 0.4 percent per woman per 13 cycles.[40] Actual effectiveness depends on the couple's motivation, including the commitment of both the man and the woman.[41] If one adds enough extra days of abstinence on both sides of the estimated fertile period "just to be sure," then the Natural Family Planning user can probably obtain even higher degrees of effectiveness.

For comparison, implantable contraception pregnancy rates are about 1.5 percent per five years for Norplant and Norplant II, and according to a survey by A. Glasier in 2002, no pregnancies have been reported with Implanon.[42]

Obviously, the effectiveness of periodic abstinence methods depends greatly on how motivated the couple is to follow the method. After all, the couple can always choose to engage in sexual relations during the fertile part of the cycle, in which case, by definition, conception is not unlikely. They can also make a mistake in estimating the fertile period. Stryder notes that a study of 19,843 "predominantly poor women in Calcutta" found a pregnancy rate of 0.2 percent per year per woman, with Stryder attributing the high effectiveness to "poverty motivation," while a study of Italian women found no pregnancies in couples desiring to have no more children, and a pregnancy rate of 3.6 percent in couples merely wanting to "space" their children.[43]

In third-world countries, Natural Family Planning methods have a practical advantage over other methods of preventing conception, in that they have minuscule ongoing costs. Most of the cost is the initial training, as well as the provision of a thermometer, beads, and/or preprinted charts.

I have argued that contraception is a betrayal of romantic love, but that abstinence can be morally acceptable. Where does periodic abstinence fit in here? On the face of it, we are pulled in two different directions. The modus operandi of periodic abstinence is *abstinence,* and hence if abstinence is permitted, so should be periodic abstinence on fertile days. On the other hand, periodic abstinence appears to be a method for "outwitting nature," whereby the users ensure that conception does not happen, without having the honesty to stop having sex, and thus it appears it should be wrong for the same reasons as positive contraception.

Unlike the case of positive contraception, the data in scripture and the Christian tradition appear not quite sufficient to settle the matter definitively. However, even before the twentieth century, the Christian tradition, with some reluctance from certain quarters, generally permitted sexual relations at times at which it was known that conception was very unlikely, such as during a woman's pregnancy or old age. There was apparently some speculation, in part accurate,[44] by women that the time of menstruation was an infertile time. Augustine condemned the Manicheans' use of periodic abstinence, but as Noonan notes, the Manicheans wanted to ensure that they had no children at all (rather than to delay or space children), and this may be the main reason for Augustine's attack.[45] We do not know how widespread this condemnation was in the Christian tradition. For instance, while Aquinas apparently condemned sexual relations during menstruation, his condemnation was based on a false empirical belief that conception during that time would result in a deformed child.[46] Evidently, Aquinas does not think that that time is infertile, and so we do not know what he would say if he thought that it was.

In the nineteenth century, methods of periodic abstinence for avoidance of conception were developed. As a matter of fact, these methods incorrectly estimated the fertile period, but of course this was not known at the time and hence did not affect the theological discussion. The main overt reaction on the part of Christians in the nineteenth century is an 1880 statement of the Sacred Penitentiary saying that the consciences of those using periodic abstinence methods should not be disturbed.[47] This suggests that the methods were not seen as obviously immoral. Finally, the research of Ogino and Knaus in the first part of the twentieth century[48] yielded a more accurate way of determining the fertile period, which made possible the rhythm method. In 1930, Pope Pius XI, in the encyclical *Casti Connubii*, after condemning contraception, wrote:

Nor are those considered as acting against nature who in the married state use their right in the proper manner although on account of natural reasons either of time or of certain defects, new life cannot be brought forth. For in matrimony as well as in the use of the matrimonial rights there are also secondary ends, such as mutual aid, the cultivating of mutual love, and the quieting of concupiscence which husband and wife are not forbidden to consider so long as they are subordinated to the primary end and so long as the intrinsic nature of the act is preserved.[49]

During the twentieth century, use of periodic abstinence to avoid conception in cases where there is a sufficiently good reason for such avoidance was generally accepted by Catholics of all stripes and at all levels of the hierarchy, including in Paul VI's famous 1968 encyclical against positive contraception, *Humanae Vitae,* and in John Paul II's statement that "[t]he choice of the natural rhythms involves accepting the cycle of the person, that is the woman, and thereby accepting dialogue, reciprocal respect, shared responsibility and self-control."[50]

Currently, it is the official position of the Catholic Church that positive contraception is wrong and periodic abstinence can be acceptable, though the position probably has different theological weight in the two cases: it is held to be an unchangeable ("irreformable" according to a 1997 *Vademecum for Confessors* from the Pontifical Council for the Family)[51] teaching that positive contraception is unacceptable, whereas the teaching about the acceptability of periodic abstinence seems to rest on the present-day agreement of theologians, hierarchs, and the flock, rather than on any tradition or teaching of comparable weight.[52]

The issue currently appears to be one of controversy among the Eastern Orthodox. Protestants, on the other hand, tend to accept positive contraception and, by implication, to accept periodic abstinence as long as the length of abstinence is not a problem vis-à-vis Paul's injunction for the couple not to separate.

The Christian tradition, thus, may leave some room for disagreement whether periodic abstinence is sometimes morally acceptable or is never acceptable. I will argue on philosophical grounds that indeed it *is* morally acceptable.

First, consider a scenario. Let us imagine Joanne who has internalized the detection of fertility in such a way that without any conscious effort, she just knows at any given time whether she is likely to be fertile or not. Anecdotal data suggests that experienced NFP users can do this because some of the fertility signs may be observed whether one wants to observe them or not. Note that even an opponent of periodic abstinence should admit that *learning* NFP is morally acceptable, because the signs of fertility are used not only for preventing conception but also for promoting it in couples of low fertility, and surely the use of NFP to promote conception is permissible.

Assume that Joanne, then, has, at any given time, a very good idea whether she is fertile or not. Let us suppose further that the initiative in sexual relations is always hers and not her husband's, and assume also that Joanne has such a good reason for avoiding pregnancy that we all agree that if total abstinence were the only way to prevent pregnancy, total abstinence would be morally justified. (For instance, Joanne might have health problems making pregnancy imprudent, while we may suppose that neither she nor her husband has particularly strong sexual desire, so that abstinence does not seriously endanger the relationship.)

Let us now suppose that on a given night Joanne is trying to decide whether to initiate sexual relations with her husband. She reflects on the fact that she has relevant health problems, and, as it happens, she can't remember any signs of fertility or infertility. She chooses to abstain. There does not appear to be anything morally wrong with this decision. We have assumed that the health problems were sufficient to justify total abstinence.

Two weeks later, Joanne is trying to make up her mind again whether to initiate sexual relations. She decides that she should probably abstain for the same reasons above. But then she remembers that her involuntary observations show her to be infertile. And so she says to herself:

Wait a second! I am actually infertile today. If I am infertile today, then my reason for abstinence no longer applies. The reason for abstinence two weeks ago was that sexual relations were likely to cause conception and thereby seriously damage me physically. Two weeks ago, it didn't occur to me to think about fertility issues. But now I know I am infertile. Since I am infertile, sexual relations would not lead to serious physical problems, and so I have no reason for abstinence.

This is surely sound moral reasoning. The argument is quite compelling, given that married couples should not abstain over a significant period of time, except when they have a serious reason to do so, and in this case there appears to be no reason to abstain.

But now if Joanne follows this reasoning on a day-by-day basis, she will end up abstaining whenever she is fertile, because then she does have a good reason to abstain, though she will not abstain on every infertile day, since those days are a period of time during at least some of which she lacks sufficient reason to abstain.

Why should Joanne have to engage in the same reasoning on a day-by-day basis? Surely it would be equally acceptable for her to sit down once and figure out ahead of time what conclusion her reasoning would yield: "Fertile day, abstain; infertile day, maybe have sex." And then instead of going through the reasoning on a day-by-day basis, she could apply the rule. Of course a certain day-by-day element might be required. We need to adapt to changing circumstances, and, for instance, she needs to monitor whether she continues to have the health problems that gave her the reason for abstinence.

Joanne's case does, however, miss one ingredient in the typical case of NFP. The typical woman using NFP, unlike Joanne, goes to some deliberate and preplanned effort to find out when she is fertile. She may buy a thermometer, fill out charts, and make deliberate mucus observations. She is not someone who "just knows." Let us suppose that Martha is such a person, and that she has just as good a reason to avoid pregnancy as Joanne. I will now argue that, given the moral permissibility of Joanne's actions, the permissibility of Martha's follows.

Joanne's decisions are rational given the information she has. It seems that to provide oneself with the information to make rational decisions is an intrinsically good thing, so long as one is not obtaining the information in a morally illicit manner, for instance, by stealing documents. It should be acceptable for Martha to act so as to gain the information that Joanne has instinctively. In fact, it seems that unless we are dealing with people's secrets, misleading facts, or irrelevancies, it is always better to have more information than less.[53] It should not be a secret to Martha how her body is functioning. Nor is the information irrelevant or misleading, given that it is the same kind of information as crucially affects the *rational* decisions that Joanne makes on the basis of the same information. The method for gathering the information—taking temperatures, checking mucus, and so on—is intrinsically morally neutral. Thus, Martha is not doing wrong.

The discussion of Joanne and Martha appears to yield a sound argument showing that if abstinence is permissible in a circumstance, so are standard methods of periodic abstinence. But now an opponent can try to turn this argument into that which I claimed is hard to come by: an argument for the *permissibility* of positive contraception. This argument would go as follows. Periodic abstinence is morally acceptable since abstinence clearly is. Both periodic abstinence and positive contraception are morally the same kind of thing: actions to ensure that sexual intercourse does not result in conception. Thus, positive contraception is also morally acceptable. This argument can be used to counter my argument for the impermissibility of positive contraception, or else to produce a paradox: there is a strong argument against positive contraception and now a strong one in its favor.

However, there is a crucial difference between the case of periodic abstinence and that of positive contraception. The difference is in regard to what can be said of the sexual acts performed. In the case of positive contraception, if a sexual act is performed at a given time, one can say that the couple did something to render *that act* sterile. They engaged in withdrawal, say, or used a drug that rendered the woman anovulatory. In other words, they tried willfully to frustrate the reproductive striving in that act.

On the other hand, in the case of periodic abstinence, one cannot say that the couple does anything to render that particular act sterile. Their abstinence from sexual activity at fertile times does nothing to make sterile the acts in which they do engage.[54] Their engagement in sexual activity during infertile times also does nothing to make the acts sterile: on the contrary, if they did not engage in sexual activity, conception would be *less* likely. Finally, the information gathering and recording does not affect fertility.[55] So nothing they do renders their act infertile, and hence they have not contradicted the innate reproductive striving of the act.

This may well seem like sophistry. After all, has not the couple moved their fertile acts to infertile times, thereby rendering the acts infertile? But this is a misunderstanding of the nature of actions. One cannot step into the same water in a river twice. Likewise, one cannot perform Monday's action on Tuesday instead: it will be a different action, though perhaps of the same type. The couple has not rendered a sexual act infertile, but they have abstained from one act, and engaged in another.

One may object, however, on the grounds that it is likewise incorrect to say that the contracepting couple made a contracepted act infertile. For if the act were not contracepted, there would have been a different act. Just as the couple engaging in periodic abstinence cannot be said to be changing a fertile act into an infertile one, so too the contracepting couple is not changing a fertile act into an infertile one. Instead, both couples are doing the same thing: they are *substituting* an infertile act for the fertile one that they would have done otherwise. This is a particularly sharp form of the argument for the permissibility of positive contraception from the analogy between positive contraception and periodic abstinence.

One response could be that if the couple engaging in periodic abstinence is *substituting* an infertile act for a fertile one, then they have a "contraceptive mentality" (a term sometimes used, typically without definition, in NFP circles). But substitution is not the only possibility. If the couple would have had sex twice every week if they were not trying to prevent conception, and, given NFP, they would have sex twice a week during infertile times and not at all during fertile times, then we cannot say that there is substitution. There is only abstinence from the sex during the fertile weeks. In practice, however, it appears likely, based on anecdotal data and human nature, that the sexual frequency of NFP users during infertile times is higher than the frequency that would have obtained had there been no use of NFP at all, especially at the beginning of an infertile period. Still, it is not clear how the alleged substitution is supposed to work. Let us say the couple abstains on Monday and Tuesday, but then has sex on Wednesday and Thursday, and let us even grant that they would not have had sex on Wednesday and Thursday had they not abstained on Monday and Tuesday. Is the sex on Wednesday a substitution for the sex on Monday? Or is it a substitution for the sex on Tuesday? It seems hard to make precise the notion of substitution that this argument requires in order to show a parallel between NFP and positive contraception.

A further response to the sharpened version of the analogical argument for the permissibility of contraception is that *to affect* and *to change* are not the same thing. In change, there is a relationship of temporal succession. First, things are one way, then, another. On the other hand, if Atlas from all eternity and for all eternity were to hold up the heavens, his activity would be *affecting* the position of the heavens—presumably, they are where they are because of his holding them up—but if he did his job right, the position of the heavens would never change.

It is incorrect to say that either couple *changed* a sexual act from a fertile one to an infertile one. To say so would imply that, at one time, there was a fertile act, and then, at another time, there was an infertile one. When we act, however, we *affect* things, and we can gauge the effect of our action by looking at the causes and explanations of things. In my variant on the Atlas myth, the heavens are where they are *because* of Atlas's unceasing activity. Likewise, it can be true that the lawn on Tuesday is neat *because* of Jones's mowing the lawn on Monday. Thus, Atlas's eternal activity affects the position of the heavens, while Jones's activity on Monday affects how the lawn is on Tuesday. Now, the contracepted act is infertile *because* the couple made it so. But in the case of periodic abstinence, the act is infertile *because* that is just what acts at that point in the cycle are like. The explanation of contracepted act's infertility involves the agency of the couple, and hence the couple have affected the act by making it infertile. But the explanation of the infertility of the sexual act by the couple practicing periodic abstinence has nothing to do with their actions, and everything to do with, say, the unavailability of an ovum, which unavailability the couple is not responsible for.

Compare the cases of Gertrude and Matthew, who are midlevel chess players, and each of whom is afraid of victory, because each believes that victory makes one haughty. But they still want to play the game, because they find it pleasant. They use different methods to ensure defeat. Gertrude's method is to refrain from playing anyone other than a grandmaster. Matthew will play anyone, but he takes a drug that clouds his mind. Let us suppose Gertrude played Kasparov and Matthew played someone close to his own level. We can now ask: "Why did Gertrude lose her game?" Surely the answer is that Kasparov was a great chess player, much better than Gertrude could ever be. On the other hand, the answer to the question why Matthew lost his game is that Matthew drugged himself. What Matthew did, namely taking the drug, negatively affected the success of his game. What Gertrude did, on the other hand, did not negatively affect the success of her game; we may suppose that she struggled valiantly against Kasparov, but victory was unattainable, and hence her modesty was safeguarded.

Granted, there is a sense in which Matthew would have played a different game had he not drugged himself, just as Gertrude would have played a different game had she played a weaker player. But the difference between the two cases is morally significant. Matthew was not really trying to beat the opponent against whom he was playing, because it was a part of his intention that he drug himself into defeat—assuming, of course, that he did not change his mind about that intention while he was playing.[56] Matthew threw the match; we might even say he was not really "playing the game." But Gertrude did not throw the match; she did nothing to decrease the chance of victory in the match that she played, though she did do something to ensure that, in general, she would not play in matches where she would have a decent chance of winning.

Matthew negatively impacted his striving. Gertrude did not negatively impact hers. In the same way, the contraceptive couple is positively opposing reproductive striving. The couple engaging in periodic abstinence is not engaged in such opposition.

If this response to the argument alleging a parallel between NFP and positive contraception fails, then NFP will still be disanalogous to positive contraception in the case where there is no "substitutive" mentality, where the couple does not choose to have sex on infertile days *instead of* on fertile ones. For, between such a case and contraception, the difference is completely clear. One kind of case of NFP that lacks substitutive mentality would be if the couple made a day-to-day decision whether or not to have sex, in light of the fertility information on that day and the reasons they had, if any, to avoid conception. It may even be that an approach of this sort is morally preferable to a substitutive mentality as the best way to safeguard spontaneity. Deliberately choosing to postpone sex to a later infertile day means that the decision to have sex is made ahead of time, and this may be seen as decreasing the spontaneity of the activity on that infertile day. The opposite case, that of choosing to have sex earlier, on an infertile day, instead of later on a fertile one, may seem unduly calculating, since it implies that the couple did not really have sufficient interest in the sexual act on that day to engage in it, were it not for the abstinence ahead. There is thus something to be said independently against the "substitutive" approach to periodic abstinence. Hence, the position that only "nonsubstitutive" periodic abstinence is permissible—where the couple does not reason in terms of "moving" their sexual relations from day to day, but rather in terms of making prudent daily decisions whether to engage in sexual relations, is not an implausible one—though I do not endorse it.

In all of the above reasoning, I have assumed that the couple engaging in periodic abstinence has a good reason, a reason that would have been good enough to justify total abstinence. That a good reason is needed is clear, since, in refraining from reproduction, they are refraining from cooperating in producing a great good, a new person in the image and likeness of God. To refrain from that good, especially in the context of a relationship directed in part towards that good (see section 19 of the previous chapter), surely does require powerful considerations to the contrary.

11. OBJECTIONS TO ARGUMENTS AGAINST CONTRACEPTION

i. Cost. The first, and rhetorically most powerful, objection to the argument against the morality of positive contraception is that holding positive contraception to be immoral has enormous social, familial, and individual costs. Poorer countries are becoming overpopulated. Many families and individuals are struggling to put food on the table for the children they have. Contraception is *needed*.

Before I dispute the claims about the costs, let me grant the claims for the sake of argument. Still, there is no contradiction between something being very costly and something being morally required. In the case of just about any absolute moral requirement, we can imagine circumstances in which adhering to the requirement is extremely costly. A classic example is the case in which one is asked to kill one innocent person and told that if one does not do it, ten people will die. Given that the killing of the innocent person would be murder and that Paul (Rom. 3:8)—and the Christian tradition with him—insists that we are not consequentialists, that we cannot do evil that good might come of it, we must entrust the cost to God, and not act directly against love of the innocent person. In the vocabulary I have used in this book, killing the innocent person is unloving. It is contrary to the love one owes that person, since it is an action directly opposed to his or her basic good of life; on the other hand, not killing the innocent person, which alas results in ten deaths, is not unloving but nonloving toward the people killed by others, since one does not take their deaths into one's heart as a goal. Any goal we pursue, even if we pursue it as a means to a further goal, is something that we make an object of our will, something we set our hearts on.

The early Christians understood this, and rather than bow down to gods they did not believe in, they were willing to allow both themselves and their families to die. Of course when the cost is so high, one does need strong confidence that one is doing the right thing. Thus, a variant of the objection is that given the high cost of refraining from contraception, one needs a confidence in the wrongness of contracep-

tion that is so strong as to be unavailable from the kinds of philosophical arguments I have given.

As a first response, I can dig in my heels. The arguments *are*
strong. Basically, the argument is that one-flesh and one-body union
is achieved through sexual intercourse, and sexual intercourse is, biologically, a mutual striving for reproduction—that just is the nature
of the act. This is clear, and hard to dispute. If a one-flesh and one-
body union essentially involves the biological, which is clear given
that we are talking of *flesh* and *body,* then acting against that which
constitutes the union is surely either acting against the union or is a
personal disclaiming of the union. Neither option is compatible with
romantic love.

But let me now relax the insistence on the strength of the philosophical arguments. Let me grant, for the sake of argument, that the
arguments are not absolutely conclusive, but only plausible. Nonetheless, when one combines the existence of plausible arguments in
favor of the thesis with the near-unanimous testimony of the first
nineteen centuries of Christian tradition, one gets an overwhelmingly
strong case. A Christian presumably believes that the Holy Spirit is
involved with guiding the Church "into all the truth" (John 16:13).
Moreover, since Christianity is a religion centered on love, the trust
should be particularly strong in the case of matters that are closely tied
to love. At the very least this creates a strong presumption in favor of
what the Church teaches, especially in sexual matters. To go against
this presumption, we would need a very strong argument. But on the
contrary, the weight of philosophical argument is in favor of this
teaching.

Now let us observe that the actual costs are not as high as adver-
tised. If my arguments in the previous section are sound, then NFP is
morally acceptable when pregnancy would cause undue harm. As we
have seen, NFP *is* an effective means of family planning. Thus, the
cost of refraining from positive contraception need be no greater than
the cost of engaging in periodic abstinence from sex. It has been alleged on anecdotal or intuitive grounds that such abstinence is apt to
be harmful to a relationship, but the allegations have little empirical
backing. In fact, if anything, there might be a weak piece of evidence

to the contrary: only 3 percent of NFP-using Catholics aged 21–44 have ever been divorced, while 15 percent of the general Catholic population in that age group has been divorced.[57] This evidence is suggestive, but could also be explained by a hypothesis that Catholics abandon NFP as soon as they become divorced. Moreover, use of NFP among Catholics may, for instance, correlate with a greater Christian commitment, and this commitment, in turn, with greater marital stability. Still, the correlation of a factor with Christian commitment, whatever the causality, would be a consideration in favor of the correlated factor, since there is good reason to posit the activity of the Holy Spirit in the lives of committed Christians.

In any case, we certainly do not overall have evidence that NFP is destructive of relationships. Moreover, NFP has been argued to promote intra-couple communication on difficult sexual issues. Among slogans popular in the NFP community is the following: "If you can talk about mucus, you can talk about anything." If it turns out empirically that NFP is more supportive of marital stability, then in light of the economic hardships to children and adults consequent on divorce, there could be poverty-based reasons to prefer NFP to positive contraception, at least within marriage.

Furthermore, if it is only specifically *marital* positive contraception that is morally prohibited as incompatible with the nature of marital love, then this prohibition on contraception does not have any clear implications for social policy regarding nonmarital sex. This does not immediately imply that counseling or distributing contraception to those engaging in nonmarital sex is morally licit. Given the wrongness of nonmarital sex, such distribution could be morally suspect: even if the contraception did not make the nonmarital sex morally worse, since such distribution could be seen as acquiescing to nonmarital sex. We do not distribute stun guns to potential bank robbers, in the hope that they'll use them instead of real guns. But this argument applies whether or not contraception is morally prohibited within marriage.

My arguments against marital contraception did yield one consideration in favor of nonmarital contraception, namely, that contraception decreases the amount of sexual one-flesh union in contexts where that kind of union is inappropriate. However, in respect of policies, there is an argument in the other direction as well: the habit of nonmarital contraception is likely to carry over into a habit of marital contraception. The policy question in regard to contraception and nonmarital sex is simply not settled by the arguments of this book, and without showing that the moral judgments force particular answers to the policity questions, it is not possible to make use of conclusions about the policy question in opposition to our above arguments against marital contraception.

ii. Moral progress. The moral views of Christians change with time, and in the case of contraception, like that of slavery, we have now seen that we used to be wrong. There is moral progress after all.

Indeed there *is* moral progress. But there is also periodic decay. Thus, while Christians from early on believed that it was wrong to exchange divine grace for money, in the middle ages the practice of "simony"—the charging of fees for sacraments and spiritual benefits—became entrenched in the Christian community. Granted, not everyone believed simony to be acceptable. The highest levels of the hierarchy spoke out against it in council. And yet it was practiced, and probably accepted by many as a matter of course. Likewise, the moral sensibilities of many Christians during late Roman times apparently became so weakened that a number would watch the blood sports in the arena, presumably little thinking that not long before it was the Christian martyrs who were being killed there.

Change of moral beliefs does not imply moral progress. The claim of progress in any given case needs to be supported by positive argumentation, either by direct argument in favor of the merits of the case or by an argument that the case looks more like cases of progress than ones of deformation. The "moral progress" argument, if it is not simply to be a rhetorical flourish added to positive argumentation for the permissibility of contraception, must show that the case of contraception looks more like progress than deformation.

But does the case of contraception look like other cases of moral progress, when we abstract from the question of the specific merits of the case? First, I claim that most, though far from all, cases of moral progress involve our coming to believe that something that we used to accept is, in fact, morally problematic. Moral progress problematizes the previously unproblematic. This is the direction of progress in simony, dueling, slavery, racism, and so on. There is good reason why the direction of moral progress tends to be from the less restrictive to the more restrictive. We humans are not very good at loving. Love is a hard thing for us to learn. As time progresses, then, we discover new things that love calls on us to do. Our love expands its scope, for instance, to include those we called "slaves" or those who have dishonored us. Love carries with it duties, and so we discover new duties. But duties are, of course, restrictive.

Moreover, arguably, conscience typically tells us what we ought or ought not do. Conscience is, as John Henry Newman put it, a "stern monitor."[58] It does not give permission, but commands and forbids, and the more one's moral character develops, the more conscience speaks:

> [T]he more a person tries to obey his conscience, the more he gets alarmed at himself, for obeying it so imperfectly. His sense of duty will become more keen, and his perception of transgression more delicate, and he will understand more and more how many things he has to be forgiven. But next, while he thus grows in self-knowledge, he also understands more and more clearly that the voice of conscience has nothing gentle, nothing of mercy in its tone. It is severe, and even stern. It does not speak of forgiveness, but of punishment.[59]

When we say: "My conscience says I am permitted do *A*," most likely all we have the right to say is: "My conscience does not object to my doing *A*." We interpret the silence of conscience as a permission, but the silence of conscience may simply be a sign of our insensitivity. The *argumentum ex silentio* is one of the weakest of arguments, and this is no less true when it is an argument from the silence of conscience. On the other hand, the argument from the voice of conscience is stronger than that from silence. Thus, in general, when two people disagree about whether something is morally acceptable, and the conscience of one has nothing against it while the other's conscience is opposed to it, it is prima facie more likely that the deed is unacceptable. For conscience is a way of perceiving duties, and when two people disagree about perception, one claiming to see something and the other claiming not to, it is prima facie more likely that one sees it and the other is insensitive to it than that the one who claims to see it is in fact suffering from an illusion. Perceptual insensitivity seems to be rather more common than perceptual delusion.

Thus, within the individual, moral progress tends to place greater restrictions on our actions, until the eschatological time when we will do everything for the greater glory of God, Christ acting through us. This movement toward greater restrictions is only a tendency—sometimes we make progress by dropping restrictions, such as on women's careers or interracial marriage—but it does make prima facie less likely the hypothesis that it was progress for many Christians to come to believe contraception is permissible.

Secondly, it is plausible that what John Henry Newman argued to be the case for doctrinal progress[60] is also true for moral progress within Christianity: in cases of genuine progress, rather than moral degeneration, one can find the later view growing organically out of earlier ones. It does not appear that the permission of contraception grows organically out of earlier Christian reflection on sexuality. On the contrary, the widespread acceptance of contraception seems to have developed culturally as part of a larger sexual revolution that rejected rather than deepened other aspects of traditional Christian views on sexuality, such as the traditional belief in the tie between sex and commitment.

iii. What if there is no sperm? It does not seem wrong for a married couple to have sex if the man is completely lacking in sperm. But sex without sperm appears not to be a reproductive-type act because a reproductive-type act requires the deposit of sperm in the woman's reproductive system. Hence, it seems, at least one sex act that is not of a reproductive type is morally permissible.

A simple response is to note that it is a reproductive *striving* that makes for biological unity. The man's body is still striving to emit sperm, but it emits seminal fluid empty of sperm because sperm production has failed. All the fertility available is being offered by the man, and genuine sexual contact is made because the man's semen, the primary purpose of which is to carry the sperm along, is indeed directed into the woman's reproductive system.

But other difficult questions abound in the neighborhood of this one. What, for instance, should we say about the case where the man has an ejaculation void of any fluid? One might argue that it is not wrong for such a man to engage in intercourse because he is striving, both voluntarily and biologically, to emit semen, although he may know from past experience or medical data that the striving is doomed to a failure. However, it also seems that the act in such a case is not completed. For a successful ejaculation seems to be essential to a reproductive-type act being engaged in. If the woman does not receive the semen because the act has been terminated prior to such ejaculation, it is not biologically an act of reproductive type (even if conception accidentally occurs due to sperm getting in by some fluid other than semen) since the fluid whose function is to carry sperm has not been employed. But if the woman's reproductive system has received the semen emitted by the ejaculation, an act of reproductive type has occurred.

On the other hand, one might say that the act is completed not by actual ejaculation into the female reproductive system, but by a spasmodic attempt at ejaculation directed at the female reproductive system. So, yes, there are further questions raised by the present account and not definitively settled by it. But that is true of every substantive moral view, and is no objection.

iv. Male-centeredness. The present account can be criticized for being male-centered, defining the essence of sex in terms of ejaculation or at least the attempt at it, which is held to be definitive of a reproductive-type act.

However, ejaculation or the attempt at it is only going to be *partially* definitive of a reproductive-type act. It is also necessary that the woman's reproductive system receive the semen or strive to do so. We should not think of the woman's role here as that of a receptacle. First of all, the reception of semen is typically but part of the functioning of a complex and active reproductive system, which secretes ova, produces mucus that significantly controls sperm migration, and may even actively move sperm along through the cervix in orgasm.

Second, just as the man typically emits semen, the woman has typically acted on the man to elicit the emission of semen. The vagina walls' exertion of frictional forces on the penis causally contributes to the ejaculation by stimulating nerve endings that are receptive to this stimulation, and just as one might say that biologically the man's reproductive system is causally active in the striving for the emission of semen, the woman's reproductive system is active, slightly earlier, in causing this striving.

The sexual act is defined in a way that requires the transmission of semen from the man to the woman, or at least an attempt or striving at this. In that sense, the act is asymmetrical, and this asymmetry cannot be eliminated. We cannot define sex in terms of the emission of ova, because the emission of ova is typically entirely involuntary. However, this asymmetry is not an objectionable male-centeredness. Note that in biological activity defined by its primary purpose, it is what enters into the *purposes* of the act that is more central. But the primary purpose of the ejaculation is not a state of the man's body, say a purgation of semen, but rather a particular state of the woman's body, the uptake of seminal fluid into the female reproductive system.

Of course, typically as a result of ejaculation, the man's body enters into a state of relaxation and the man receives pleasure. But these features are not essential to the act. The relaxation is clearly a contingent feature, and neither the man's nor the woman's having pleasure is essential to the act. Even if the man and woman have medical conditions that render orgasm nonpleasurable, we would say after an instance of reproductive-type intercourse that "they had sex." Marital sex does not require the man's pleasure any more than it requires the woman's (see also sections 7 and 9 of chapter 5). Nonetheless, the sex is unitive at more levels when the pleasure is present, and that means that the couple should strive to make the act pleasant, or, at least, not to impede its pleasure.

v. What if one does not know about the connection between sex and reproduction? As mentioned earlier, from time to time, one hears of legally married couples that do not know about sexual intercourse. And there are, or at least were, tribes where the connection between sex and pregnancy was not known. These cases present a problem for the present account. For it seems that people who do not know about the connection between sex and reproduction cannot engage in reproductive-type acts. But surely such people are not doing anything wrong when they have marital sex.

One answer would be that we need to distinguish between objective rightness and culpability. Thus, if it turns out it is wrong to engage in orgasmic activity except when intending it to be a sexual union induced by a mutual striving of reproductive organs qua reproductive organs, we can say that if these people engage in orgasmic activity, they do wrong. But because they are innocently ignorant of the fact that the pleasure of orgasm signifies a reproductive biologically based union, they are not culpable here. They do not do justice to the significance of the activities in which they engage with their reproductive organs, but their ignorance is an excuse.

But we might be able to avoid giving this somewhat harsh response. The main line defended in this book may not require that a couple intend a mutual striving of reproductive organs qua reproductive organs, but only that they do not oppose this striving, though one of the arguments in section 12 below will require something like a positive intention, and considerations of the maximality of marital commitment suggest something positive. But even a positive intention can be implicit. The couple engages in the mating activity of our species. They do not fully understand the implications of this mating activity, but in doing "what comes naturally," they implicitly accept and perhaps even endorse the natural consequences, including ones they do not fully understand. This is particularly true if they are open to accepting and raising children together, even though they are mystified by the process by which children come to be.

All married couples are in this boat to some degree: no one understands all the implications of sexual union fully. And the maximality of union in intercourse, while it requires significant engagement of the mind, does not require omniscience—that just isn't practically possible for humans. Likewise, Christian faith does not require explicit belief in all the details of Trinitarian and incarnational doctrine—an implicit acceptance of what the Church teaches is enough when that is all one is practically capable of.

vi. This is all about mechanics and legalism, while surely the moral life is about the spirit. Jesus spent much of his time deflecting people's concern for physical details of action, such as whether hands should be washed, and redirecting them into a concern about the "heart" from which actions come:

> Do you not see that whatever goes into the mouth passes into the stomach, and so passes on? But what comes out of the mouth proceeds from the heart, and this defiles a man. For out of the heart come evil thoughts, murder, adultery, fornication [*porneiai*], theft, false witness, slander. These are what defile a man; but to eat with unwashed hands does not defile a man. (Matt. 15:17–20)

A concern about positive contraception, coitus interruptus, and other "mechanics" of intercourse is legalistic and a misunderstanding of sexuality, which is about relations between *persons*—about the *heart,* in the broad Semitic sense that includes intellect and will—and not about biology.

There are three distinct objections here. There are two theological objections, first, that the discussion of contraception goes against Jesus' sayings about the importance of the heart, and, second, that the discussion is legalistic. Third, there is a philosophical objection here about the nature of sexuality.

Let us take the theological ones first. Jesus does not say that *only* what goes on in the heart defiles a person. "Evil thoughts, murder, adultery, *porneiai*, theft, false witness, slander" all defile a person. Murder, adultery, *porneiai*, and theft are all physical actions, though ones with deep interpersonal significance. Moreover, *if* contraceptive sex is immoral, then it is an instance of sexual immorality, i.e., *porneia.*

The point here is that what we do with our bodies matters precisely when it is relevant to the heart. If the members of a couple do not have it in their hearts to give themselves to each other *entirely,* but withhold their fertility in the very act of giving themselves to each other through the mediation of their reproductive organs, then this is certainly a matter of the heart. If we look at the objection to positive contraception, the objection was not to the physical state of infertility that it produced. Rather, the objection was to the *intention* to produce a physical state of infertility, since it is this intention that opposes the intention to unite as one flesh. Intentions are precisely matters of the heart. Murder, adultery, *porneiai*, theft, false witness, and slander are all acts coming from intentional acts of will, and in significant part defined by intentions. One is only committing theft if one is *intentionally* appropriating another's property without consent—driving home in the wrong car, because it is dark and one's keys happen to fit, is unfortunate, but not theft. Even the "evil thoughts," the *dialogismoi ponêroi*, are arguably intentional actions. The word *dialogismos* here suggests not a fleeting thought passing through the mind, but a sequence of reasoning, a (nefarious) plan of action, or a connected mental story.

The objection to positive contraception was based precisely on the intentions that are involved. In fact, the very notion of positive contraception was defined in section 1 of this chapter in terms of intention, and I have argued that such an intention disunites the person from the organs through which that person tries to unite with another.

Next, consider the charge of legalism. The *locus classicus* for the concept of legalism is in Jesus' harsh words to the scribes and Pharisees in Matthew 23:

> Then said Jesus to the crowds and to his disciples, "The scribes and the Pharisees sit on Moses' seat; so practice and observe whatever they tell you, but not what they do; for they preach, but do not practice. They bind heavy burdens, hard to bear, and lay them on men's shoulders; but they themselves will not move them with their finger. . . .
>
> Woe to you, blind guides, who say, 'If any one swears by the temple, it is nothing; but if any one swears by the gold of the temple, he is bound by his oath.' You blind fools! For which is greater, the gold or the temple that has made the gold sacred? . . .

Woe to you, scribes and Pharisees, hypocrites! for you tithe mint and dill and cummin, and have neglected the weightier matters of the law, justice and mercy and faith; these you ought to have done, without neglecting the others. You blind guides, straining out a gnat and swallowing a camel!

Woe to you, scribes and Pharisees, hypocrites! for you cleanse the outside of the cup and of the plate, but inside they are full of extortion and rapacity. You blind Pharisee! first cleanse the inside of the cup and of the plate, that the outside also may be clean." (Matt. 23:1–4, 16–17, 23–26)

Jesus begins by reiterating the claim that the scribes and Pharisees are to be obeyed (v. 3), thereby showing that his sympathies about the structure of authority lie with the nascent rabbinical Judaism, and locating his harsh criticism as coming from someone who accepts the rabbis' authority but nonetheless has a radical critique of the way that authority is exercised.

Jesus warns that the scribes and Pharisees impose burdens on people without helping to carry them (v. 4). This may show Jesus dissociating himself from the rabbinical practice of "putting a fence around the Law," i.e., introducing additional rabbinical regulations beyond the ones believed to be imposed by God. What is significant about this practice is that the rabbis honestly recognized that the additional restrictions were their own, but they nonetheless introduced them in order to make it harder to accidentally break the rules that God had put in place. This principle was in play in the first century and has continued through the later development of Judaism. Jesus does not question the rabbis' authority to introduce these regulations. (Just as the state can produce additional laws, so can the religious authorities, we might say.) However, Jesus does complain about the weight of the burdens, and especially about the lack of help offered.

We thus have two aspects of legalism here. One is the introduction of additional, onerous rules, explicitly recognized as not coming from God. To make this criticism against those objecting to contraception would be question-begging since those who think contraception immoral *do* believe that it is contrary to the nature of human beings as created by God.

The second aspect of legalism criticized here is a love of regulations without any positive attempt to help people follow them. This is not a criticism, however, of the rules but of those who promote them. The solution is not that they should stop promoting the rules, but that they should help others to keep them. Whether sufficient help *has* been offered by those objecting to positive contraception is an empirical question that does not bear on whether contraception is permissible. In any case, in the United States, the most vocal persons opposed to positive contraception are various lay Catholics. Many of these are involved in different capacities with lay-run organizations, such as the Couple to Couple League, that try to teach NFP as an alternative to contraception. If NFP can be morally acceptable, and I have argued it can, this teaching is a genuine help that is being offered. A further amount of help is given by those medical researchers who continue to try to produce more effective and easier to follow NFP regimens, particularly ones suitable for illiterate couples in the third world.[61]

Jesus goes on to give one example of legalism, a regulation according to which saying an oath by the temple is not valid but an oath by the gold of the temple is valid. The position he is attacking is not entirely absurd. It might, for instance, be based on the notion that it is the act of offering that makes something sacred, so that the gold of the temple is sacred because it is an offering by us made to God, while the temple itself is, perhaps, not such an offering. Nonetheless, Jesus insists that the gift is sanctified by the temple, a view with deep theological consequences for Christians who see themselves as members of the body of Christ, the new temple, and who are thus sanctified by that temple in which they are found. Jesus is no doubt right: after all, the holy of holies at the heart of the temple is surely best understood as sanctified by God rather than through its being offered by us.

But Jesus' main point is not just to engage the debate over what is sacred, even though he does just that through an argument that is brief and compressed like some in the Mishnah. Jesus is, rather, pointing to an attitude that allowed one to use the letter of the Law, as interpreted in a particular way, to go against the purpose of the Law. It is clear that the regulations against making false oaths are there to instill honesty. Finding a loophole in these regulations—based on poor reasoning, one might add—leads one to neglect the *point* of the Law, "justice and mercy and faith" (v. 23).

Thus, the third kind of legalism is that of using the letter of the law to undo the point of the law. An example would be a Catholic enjoying on Good Friday a sumptuously delicious soy burger made up to taste *exactly* like a hamburger and having the same nutritional content, claiming thereby to fulfill the obligation of fasting from meat. The letter is satisfied, but the point of the Law is penance, and if the burger tastes just like meat and has the same nutritional content, then no penance has been done. This kind of legalism involves a relaxation of the law. The spirit of the law requires more than the letter, but only the letter is followed. This is, of course, not at all what happens in the case of the prohibition of contraception. In fact, in hindsight, the early acceptance of the contraceptive pill by some Catholic thinkers may have been closer to legalism. Some believed that coitus interruptus and the condom modified the nature of the sexual act in an unacceptable way, and while accepting the Christian tradition's opposition to such acts, thought that they could find a distinction between these and the pill, so the pill could be permitted even though the "unnatural acts" unanimously condemned by the Christian tradition would still be forbidden. Once we see, as they did not, that the same considerations of marital union as mediated by joint reproductive striving prohibit the pill and condoms, we might see their position as *unconscious* legalism—as a way of using the letter of older prohibitions against unnatural acts in such a way as to find a loophole. It is gratifying to note that this odd position is now largely extinct among Christians.[62]

However, one might make the accusation of legalism against the permission to practice periodic abstinence. But that would require a sound argument to show why there is no morally significant difference between the permitted and the prohibited practices. In the previous section such an argument was examined and found wanting. The mere fact that two practices are in some way similar—say, by sharing the same goal—is quite compatible with the fact that a real nonlegalistic distinction can be made between them. The goal of elimination of poverty can be served by killing the poor or by finding meaningful work at just wages for them. Both activities have the same goal, but there is a nonlegalistic distinction.

The final kind of legalism that is condemned is that of neglecting "weightier matters of the law," in favor of minor things like tithes on herbs (v. 23). This is not, however, an objection to insistence on the less weighty matters; the more important matters "you ought to have done, without neglecting the others" (v. 23). Even if it is granted that avoiding positive contraception is a minor matter, it is still not something to neglect. Nonetheless, it is not clear whether anything that relates to a form of love as directly as sexuality and its reproductivity does to romantic love can fail to be a weighty matter.

None of the four kinds of legalism we find criticized in Matthew 23 is something that can be used effectively to attack the claim that positive contraception is immoral. An accusation of legalism is not typically a good stand-alone argument. Unless it is self-evident that the legalist made the wrong distinction, a further argument, such as Jesus' compressed argument about offerings and the temple, is needed.

This still leaves the philosophical critique that sexual love is not about the physical organs, not about the biology, but about the heart. Here the right answer is, surely, that there should be no opposition. Sexual love is precisely about *both*. That sexual love has to do with physicality is difficult to deny. We have discussed this already at length. There is a focus on appearance, on the sense of touch—and, phenomenologically, that which we can *touch* is the paradigm of the physical—and on the body in general. This is not a focus on the body merely as a collection of bits of flesh, as in Marcus Aurelius's quip about spasmodic secretions of slime. It is a focus on the body as an organized, functional whole. But in the end sexual love goes beyond that. It involves a focus on the body as an organized, functional whole that, by being such, is an expression of us as persons. Sexual love is supposed to be an integrated love, one that encompasses us as whole persons, both in our spirituality and in our concrete physicality.

Otherwise, it will either become spiritualized into something that is not sexual or physicalized into something that is not love. It is this integration that positive contraception attacks.

What we do intentionally with our bodies does matter. While an animal may engage in biologically the same acts, these acts lack the meaning they have for us because of a difference in intentions—or maybe even a lack of intentions altogether on the part of the animal. The man who says that only his arm should be jailed, since it is the arm that committed the crime,[63] is either joking or else is implying that his arm acted on its own—that it just twitched. But sexual activity is not just a twitch. It is a human activity, done by people willingly, and, ideally, in order to unite together through their bodies. And surely when we are trying to unite physically, it matters what we do physically. However much we may try to think that punching some-one in the nose will be intrinsically unitive, that is false. The physical is not infinitely elastic; it does not adapt to our wishes; it can be re-calcitrant. It is this combination of mental control and bodily re-calcitrance that gives sexual expressions of love much of their phe-nomenological richness. And this recalcitrance includes the fact that certain physical things have innate meanings. And they had better—otherwise communication could not get off the ground, since some gesture or sound had to have innate meaning in order for language to begin, in order to avoid the regress in which every gesture or sound is defined in terms of another.[64]

vii. Postcoital contraception. Arguments against contraception based on the importance of the unitive dimension of sexual union face the following difficulty raised by Lawrence Masek.[65] It seems that postcoital marital contraception is wrong if and only if precoital marital contraception is wrong. But imagine a couple that engages in uncontracepted marital union, believing themselves to be infertile, but a day later they realize that they were fertile. Consequently, they use a spermicide to neutralize any remaining sperm. But their past sexual union is, nonetheless, unitive.

This very interesting case shows the importance of the temporally extended aspects of marital union, as discussed in the previous chap-ter. Couples are not merely united when they are engaged in intercourse—the whole temporally extended marriage is a form of union. It is important that one not direct one's will against the striving that constitutes one's past union with one's spouse, whether that striving is in the future or in the past.

12. MEDICINAL USE OF CONTRACEPTIVES, CONDOMS, AND DISEASE PREVENTION

Physicians sometimes prescribe hormonal contraceptives for noncontraceptive purposes.[66] Our main arguments against contraception involved the idea that in contracepting the couple is deliberately opposing the reproductive striving that constitutes their union as one body. In using a hormonal contraceptive for noncontraceptive purposes, the couple does not appear to be deliberately opposing the reproductive striving.

There are, after all, presumably all sorts of activities that increase or decrease a person's fertility. For instance, there appear to be correlations between stress and infertility.[67] But it is clear that a married man or woman need not be at all opposing the reproductive striving by taking such a job. Granted, the decrease in fertility due to stress is lower than that due to use of hormonal contraception, but the difference here is merely quantitative. The arguments in this book against contraception focused on the couple's intentions. When the couple does something that they know to decrease fertility, but do not do so in order to decrease fertility, the arguments do not apply.

The distinction between what one expects to happen and what one intends is indeed central to moral thought. Suppose a police officer arrests Smith, a tax cheat. In doing so, the police officer increases the probability that Smith will commit suicide. The moral evaluation of the action depends crucially on what the officer intends and what the officer merely expects to happen. If the officer intends to drive Smith to suicide, or even just to increase the probability that Smith will commit suicide, the officer acts wrongly. But if the officer merely knows that tax cheats who are caught have a certain probability of committing suicide, but is not arresting Smith in order to increase the chance of Smith's suicide, the action is not wrong (assuming every other aspect of the action is in order).

The Principle of Double Effect (PDE) makes use of the distinction by sometimes allowing one to do something that is foreseen to result in an evil, but not intended (either as an end or as a means) to do so (see also section 8 above), as long as the foreseen evil is not disproportionate to the evil. Using contraceptive pharmaceuticals—or taking on a stressful job—for noncontraceptive purposes can fall under the PDE. A decrease of fertility is in itself a bad thing, but in a case like this, the decrease of fertility is merely expected, and is not intended, either as a means or as an end. Matters are more complicated, however, if the pharmaceuticals have a postfertilization effect—for instance, if they sometimes prevent the fertilization of the embryo, since then the pharmaceuticals endanger an embryonic human life (cf. section 9 above), which may require a couple to abstain from marital relations.

Likewise, recently, some Catholic thinkers have suggested that it is coherent to reject contraception and yet accept the use of condoms in marital intercourse for the sake of disease prevention, typically from the man to the woman.[68] The most notable figure here is Martin Rhonheimer.[69] (And note that in the case of the condom, there are no concerns about postfertilization effects.)

One argument parallels the above justification of the use of contraceptive pharmaceuticals for noncontraceptive purposes. Putting on a condom is morally neutral (one could imagine it done quite uncontroversially to protect the male reproductive system during a medical treatment). The good effect in this case is preventing the transmission of disease—the standard example is HIV/AIDS. The bad effect is the prevention of conception. The bad effect is not a means to the good effect. Given the lethal nature of AIDS, especially in the third world, proportionality holds.

Alternately, one might more simply say that contraception is defined by an intention that a child is not conceived, and hence the condom, when used to block HIV transmission, is not even a form of contraception. This is the approach Rhonheimer takes.[70]

It is indeed logically coherent to reject contraception and yet accept the use of condoms to stop HIV on the above grounds. However, whether this coherent position is correct depends on the right reason for rejecting contraception. If one rejects contraception solely because of the GBFM argument that it is wrong to deliberately interrupt a process aimed at life,[71] the PDE argument for the use of condoms to stop HIV is correct. But if the unity-based arguments earlier in this chapter succeeded, the question becomes more difficult, and indeed Grisez himself argues, on grounds similar to those that will be given below, that a married couple's use of a condom is incompatible with marital intercourse and hence wrong.[72]

Before considering the principled question whether the use of condoms to stop HIV is permitted, it is worth noting that one can have genuine *practical* worries about whether a particular policy of promoting condom use is likely to actually decrease the incidence of HIV. The problem here is the well-documented phenomenon of "risk compensation."[73] When a risky activity is made inherently safer, the behavior of individuals is likely to shift in a way that at least partly offsets the inherent safety improvement. A typical example is given by a study showing that drivers of taxis equipped with antilock brakes compensated for the improvement in braking technology by following more closely behind the vehicle in front.[74] It is thus very reasonable to worry that the availability of condoms, while unquestionably greatly decreasing the probability of HIV transmission in any one act, will increase the prevalence of risky acts in a way that partly or wholly offsets the gains in safety: "as with all prevention technologies, people might believe that they can engage in risky sex with impunity as long as they use (or plan to use) condoms. Evidence from Uganda has shown that such condom disinhibition is real."[75] How complete the offsetting is likely to be will no doubt depend on details of the intervention and the target population.[76]

But let us bracket the empirical question, and return to the principled question whether the use of a condom is permissible to a married couple. I have argued that it is wrong to act positively against the body's reproductive striving in sexual union, and that this makes contraception wrong. The defender of the PDE argument can say that the use of condoms to prevent HIV transmission has the frustration of the body's reproductive striving as merely an unintended side effect. There is no intention for the condom to stop the sperm but only the HIV virus. It is like the case of tuna fishing: one pulls in some dolphins along with the tuna, but does not intend to catch dolphins.

In my arguments above, I defended only the claim that the members of a couple uniting sexually should not *oppose* themselves to their body's striving, since that would be opposed to unity of individuals or couple. But one may instead argue that a lack of opposition is insufficient.[77] Rather, a couple needs to positively intend to engage in a reproductive-type act (perhaps implicitly, as discussed in section 11). Surely it is right to say that, for sex to be a union of whole persons, the sex must be *willed*. If the nature of sex is to unite the couple through mutual engagement in reproductive-type activity (see chapter 5), then to intend sexual union requires that one intend, at least implicitly, to engage in reproductive-type activity. It is not required that one intend to reproduce, however.

Human reproduction involves ejaculation by the male into the female. In order to engage voluntarily in reproductive-type activity, it is plausible that one needs to intend the semen to reach the woman's reproductive system, or at least one needs to intentionally *try* to have the semen reach the woman's reproductive system. After all, where the semen is being directed seems to be the crucial difference between one-body unitive intercourse and mutual masturbation or oral sex, and it is plausible that this directedness, crucial as it is to the distinction, should be intentional. Now, it may be possible for a condom-using couple to intend that the condom stop the virus without positively intending that the condom stop semen (imagine a couple that does not care where the semen goes, but cares very much where the virus goes). But it seems unlikely that the couple can positively intend semen to get through, or can even intentionally try to have the semen get through, while intending HIV not to do so.

To intend semen to get through while intending to stop HIV would be like casting a net into water containing trout and dolphins and intending that the dolphins should get out of the net while trout should be kept in. If one has made the net small enough to stop trout, then one isn't even *trying* to let the dolphins get out of the net. The general principle here is that if on some occasion I am trying to accomplish both *A* and non-*B,* then I need to be trying to do something different in regard to *A* and *B,* in a way that favors *A* over *B.* Suppose it is claimed that I am trying to keep all the trout in and let all the dolphins out. Then my action needs to treat the trout and dolphins differently, in a way that favors the keeping in of the trout over the keeping in of the dolphins. For instance, I might make some kind of special net that the dolphins, being smarter, have some hope of escaping, but the trout do not. Even if, in fact, I still end up catching the dolphins, because they don't succeed in slipping out, I can claim that I intended and tried to let them all out.

The couple that uses a condom is not doing anything different to the semen than they are to the HIV. They cannot, thus, claim to be trying both to contain HIV and transmit semen. To intend is not, after all, the same as to wish.[78] A couple can certainly wish for the semen to get through, but to *intend* it, they need to try to do something to promote it that goes over and beyond what they would do were they intending it not to go through. In other words, they need to treat semen differently from HIV, which they intend not to go through.

This reasoning is quite intuitive if we agree that there is no significant difference between intercourse involving a condom and a sexual activity where the ejaculation occurs somewhere other than into a vagina. The argument that during intercourse involving a condom, the semen comes to be in the condom, and the condom is in the vagina, and hence the semen comes to be in the vagina is a poor one. For given the view of sexual union defended in chapter 5, the relevant sense of "be in" needs to be one in which the semen's entry into the vagina is part of a mutual striving for reproduction. It is not enough for the semen to be contained in the spatial region surrounded by the vagina (the vagina is not the spatial region but the muscular organ surrounding it). It is not spatial containment but causal connection that matters. If the semen is not actually sent to *make contact* with the woman's organs, unitive intercourse has not taken place.

Sex with a condom is like oral or anal sex insofar as none of these are unitive. It might be objected that a handshake through a glove is still a handshake.[79] But the relevant kind of causal interaction in a handshake is the exertion of pressure on the other's hand, and in this, a glove is no impediment. Whereas the relevant kind of causal inter-action in the case of sex is the attempt at the transmission of semen, rather than the exertion of pressure, and to this a condom is an im-pediment. One is no longer engaging in a reproductive-type act.

The question whether a condom may be used by a married couple for disease prevention, thus, comes down to the question whether one is permitted to induce orgasm outside the context of intercourse, a question we shall consider in the next chapter, where I shall, at this point, I think, unsurprisingly, come to a negative conclusion.

13. DOES CONTRACEPTED INTERCOURSE UNITE AS ONE BODY?

I have argued that the use of contraception is wrong, primarily be-cause the couple oppose themselves to the reproductive striving that constitutes their union. But there can still be a reproductive striving present, despite the opposition.

Suppose that a third party slipped oral contraception into a woman's food without her or her husband's knowledge. In that case, she would be infertile, and her intercourse with her husband would be just as unitive as the intercourse of any other infertile married couple. But biologically, this woman's coitus is just like that of the woman who takes the same pharamaceutical product with contracep-tive intent. This suggests that a biological union remains despite the use of hormonal contraception for contraceptive purposes, even though the use of the contraception opposes the reproductive striving that constitutes the union.

Is this biological union sufficient for a union as one body, suffi-cient for the consummation of the marriage? This is a difficult ques-tion. In the preceding section, I suggested that the use of condoms, and by extension other barrier methods, is incompatible with sexual union. But hormonal contraception, though still morally wrong according to our arguments, seems to differ from barrier methods and for reasons like this some Catholic canonists say that intercourse by a couple who uses nonbarrier methods of contraception can consummate a marriage, while barrier methods prevent consummation.[80]

Such a distinction between barrier and hormonal methods can be defended. As we saw in the preceding section, the use of a condom in intercourse modifies the intentions of the couple in the act itself, and the point is particularly clear when the condom is used contraceptively. When a condom is used, there is no intention for the relevant kind of contact between the male and female reproductive systems (after all, if there were such an intention, the couple could have realized their goal simply by removing the condom), but only for a limited interaction across a barrier. On the other hand, just prior to and during the sexual act itself, the couple that makes use of hormonal contraception can have intentions for a sexual union mediated by their reproductive system very much like those had by an involuntarily infertile couple that is not presently pursuing reproduction.

Granted, the intentions during intercourse by the hormonally contracepting couple are in tension with their earlier contraceptive behavior—indeed, that is at least one of the things wrong with the contraceptive behavior. But it is the intentions in the act of intercourse that seem most relevant to determining whether there is a union as one body.

14. CONCLUSIONS

Positive marital contraception is morally wrong, as it is intrinsically opposed to the nature of marital love. However, there are some suggestions that condoms and coitus interruptus change the sexual act from an act of intercourse to something else. If so, then condomic or interrupted acts will need to be examined in the next chapter, not as contraception but as something else. In any case, such acts are not fully sexually unitive.

Whether or not positive contraception adds to the objective guilt in cases of nonmarital sexuality is not so clear. This lack of clarity is to be expected, because generally questions about what combination of immoral acts is worse than another are murky. Is it better or worse if Sherlock Holmes's worthy opponent Irene Adler actually has the incriminating picture over which she is blackmailing the king of Bohemia? If she has it, then presumably she is ready to blacken the king's reputation. If she doesn't have it, she is a liar. Which is worse? Who is to say? One is worse in one way and the other in another. Contraception makes the nonmarital sexual act look less like a marital sexual act. In doing so, it makes the act be further from the ideal. On the other hand, in doing so, it makes the act less unitive, in a context where there should be no sexual union.

At the same time the social fruits of the use of contraception appear negative. As far as we can tell, the increase in contraceptive use was correlated with a vast increase in the acceptance of nonmarital sexuality.[81] This is not surprising on the one-flesh model, since contraception lessens the significance of sexual activity, thereby making it less sacred, and making it seem less important in what circumstances exactly it is engaged in. The sacred, that which in Hebrew is *qadosh*, is something set apart. Sexual love is sacred in this way, in part because of its connection with biological strivings directed at the production of human beings, human beings who are, after all, in the image and likeness of God. The initiation of processes that are biologically aimed at the production of images and likenesses of God is surely not something to be taken lightly. But contraception is felt to remove the connection, allowing sex to be taken more lightly.

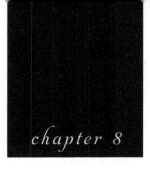

chapter 8

Sexual Pleasure and Noncoital Sexual Activity

1. A PLAUSIBLE THEORY OF SEXUAL PLEASURE

In the case of a typical pleasure, we are taking pleasure in something meaningful, be it food, conversation, camping, or a novel. Sexual pleasure, particularly the feeling of complete sexual satisfaction[1] in orgasm, is phenomenologically too important a contributor to the consummation of romantic love for it to be plausible that it is a meaningless pleasure. Thus, in sexual pleasure, the couple is taking pleasure in *something*. What is this *something*?

If the argument in chapter 5 (section 7) is right, this something must be good and important, because the value of a pleasure derives from the value of that in which pleasure is taken. Along this line, a plausible pair of theories about the nature of sexual pleasure are that it is a taking of pleasure either in a mutual striving for reproduction *or* in the one-body sexual union that this mutual striving constitutes, given that these seem to be the main goods in sex as such (at least when children do not actually result—but sexual pleasure is not the pleasure of having children, since most of the time, there are no children resulting from a sexual act, though intercourse always tends toward procreation). Pleasure is a way of seeing either this reproductive striving or this one-flesh union as valuable. Hitherto, I did not have to decide between these two accounts. But now note that there are considerations in favor of the view that the pleasure is taken specifically in the one-flesh union.

First, consider the case of couples that engage in sexual relations while not knowing that reproduction can result. They certainly receive pleasure. While it is possible to experience something without knowing quite what one is experiencing—when I feel heat I experience molecular kinetic energy, but when I was a small child I did not know this—it appears to be preferable to suppose that people *do* know the meaning of what they are experiencing unless there is an argument to the contrary. Now, we can easily imagine such a couple seeing themselves, implicitly or explicitly, as taking pleasure in *union,* and this is a consideration in favor of seeing union as the good in question.

Second, the perception of union account of sexual pleasure is better able to explain the integration between sexual pleasure and romantic love. This integration is deeper if the pleasure is taken directly in the consummation of romantic love, for then the pleasure is itself unitive, because it is a perception of union, and a perceived union is a deeper, more personally integrated union than an unperceived union. It is phenomenologically plausible that pleasure is important to sex, and important in a unitive way. The union account of sexual pleasure does justice to this phenomenology.

The better account, thus, has it that in sexual pleasure the one-flesh sexual union is perceived as valuable. When sexual pleasure occurs without a one-flesh sexual union or without the one-flesh union being valuable, the pleasure is not veridical, just as one's vision is not veridical when one sees a pink elephant and either there is no elephant or there is only a blue elephant there. However, just as the vision of a pink elephant is meaningful in the absence of the pink elephant, so too, sexual pleasure is meaningful in the absence of a valuable one-flesh union. They are meaningful in exactly the same way that a false claim is: a false claim is like a true claim in having meaning, but unlike the true claim in that the false claim's meaning does not match reality.

2. SELF-DECEPTION AND MASTURBATORY PRACTICES

On the view of pleasure as a perception of an apparent good (see again section 7 of chapter 5), those who intend pleasure without the good to which it is tied are intending something that is, in fact, a self-deception, though of course they may not be explicitly aware of this. Such self-deception is either successful, in that it makes one actually come to believe that there is a valuable one-flesh union where there isn't, or else it produces a division in the person where, in one way, the person feels that there is a valuable one-flesh union, while being aware, in another way, that there isn't one. When the self-deception is successful, this is clearly a bad thing. And even when a self-deception in an important matter is not successful, it introduces a division in one's self, a division contrary to the value of our integration as human beings.

Therefore, the deliberate induction of sexual pleasure without a one-flesh sexual union, or only in conjunction with some variety of union that lacks the full value of a sexual one-flesh union (e.g., holding hands), is morally wrong. It follows that masturbation, oral sex, and anal sex, at least when done for the sake of sexual pleasure outside the context of unitive intercourse, are wrong. These activities divorce one from sexual and interpersonal reality by making one or one's sexual partner feel what is not there, just as the "satisfaction pill" discussed in chapter 5 divorces one from the reality of one's actions.

Note that while the argument works best on the proposed theory of sexual pleasure as a perception of the good of union, it also works on the alternate theory that sexual pleasure is a perception of the good of reproductive striving.

On theories of pleasure that do not make pleasure the apparent perception of a good, one can still argue against these acts by analogy with the case of the "satisfaction pill," the taking of which is wrong, being contrary to one's personal integrity.

3. VISUAL ILLUSIONS

There is, however, a powerful objection to these plausible arguments. We enjoy looking at visual illusions in books and museums, and surely that is not immoral. But a visual illusion is precisely something that induces a nonveridical visual perception. Thus, self-inducing non-veridical visual perceptions is not wrong. Why should inducing non-veridical sexual pleasures be wrong?

This argument is most plausible in the case where the sexual pleasure does not actually deceive either member of the couple into thinking there is a one-flesh union. For there is good reason to think that it would be wrong to deceive oneself or the other, and that such deception would be contrary to one's dignity as a rational being. Let us, then, consider the case where both persons see through the illusion. Someone induces sexual pleasure. This pleasure is a perception of a one-flesh union as valuable, but there is no one-flesh union there. Nonetheless, the person does not for a moment entertain the idea that there is a one-flesh union—just as we may know the trick of a visual illusion so well that even though it appears to us, say, that two lines are not straight, we firmly and continually know them to be straight.

But there is a crucial disanalogy between the pleasure and visual illusion cases. Pleasure is an apparent perception of a *normative* state of affairs, indeed of a good. But the good is not just something for abstract intellectual consideration: it is something that guides our actions and informs our wills. In fact, the good is the object of our love. For when we love something, we love it as being good, and conversely when something is good, it deserves our love, since insofar as it is good, it is a reflection of God who alone is good in the fullest sense (Mark 10:18). When something is presented as a good to us, it is thus presented to our will as an object to be striven for. This is a part of how pleasure motivates: it presents something as valuable, and so of course we are motivated in favor of it, since the good is what is to be pursued. A nonveridical pleasure in something that is not good—or is good in a different way from the way the pleasure presents it—pulls us in the direction of either loving something we should not love or loving something in a way we should not love it.

Now, granted, one may feel pleasure at something without loving it. A person who chose to fast but is compelled at gunpoint to eat might well feel pleasure at the taste of the food, but might not love the food. Nonetheless, the pleasure pulls one directly toward love. When something is presented to us as good, it is natural for us to love it; not to love it requires holding ourselves back. Recall the example from chapter 5 of the option to watch an oncology ward for all one's life and *enjoy* the sight. What is so repellent about this option is that by enjoying the sight, one is, at the very least, pulled in the direction of loving that which in itself is not lovable, namely suffering. We could imagine a form of brainwashing that ensured we would feel pleasure at the suffering of others. Such brainwashing, despite the literally pleasant consequences, would surely be something to be avoided, since to be pulled to love evil is a terrible thing.

To feel pleasure at something not good, or not good in the right way for this kind of pleasure, is to tempt oneself either to love something not lovable or to love something in a different way from the way it is lovable. This temptation can perhaps be resisted, but it is quite difficult to do so, given that it is natural to love something when one feels pleasure at it, and to love it as having the value that the pleasure represents. This does not mean one has to explicitly recognize what kind of value the pleasure represents its object as having: one may love something indefinitely and implicitly, "insofar as it has the kind of good that the pleasure represents it as having," without knowing exactly what kind of good is present. The temptation to love incorrectly is indeed a temptation to an evil: to acting in a way not consonant with the reality-centered nature of love. And to deliberately place oneself in the way of temptation, to induce the deceitful pleasure that constitutes the temptation, is itself wrong.

Now, we are sometimes morally permitted to place ourselves in circumstances where we will be tempted, providing we have sufficiently good reason for this. We may get a job at a bank while knowing that this will cause temptations to greed, as long as we are confident that with God's grace we will resist. To defend such activity one might apply the Principle of Double Effect: there is a bad effect, namely the temptation, and a good effect, the valuable employment. The bad effect is not a means to the good effect, and if we have confidence that we are unlikely to succumb, the bad effect is proportionate to the good.

However, pleasure is intrinsically attractive in such a way that it may not be possible to intend to feel pleasure at something without intending to be tempted to love it. Pleasure presents apparent goods as *attractive* goods, goods worth having. This seems to be at the core of the notion of pleasure. Hence, to will a fraudulent pleasure is to will to be attracted to something in an inappropriate way. Moral growth consists not just in avoiding evil outward action. It also consists in improvement of character, and an essential part of having a good character is being attracted only to genuine goods. We can use the Principle of Double Effect to tolerate unintended danger to our characters, but in the case of the empty or fraudulent pleasure, by willing the pleasure we have willed an instance of poor moral functioning.

Even if one is not convinced about the argument about the general wrongness of intentionally self-inducing pleasures that are illusory, one may argue that there is something particularly problematic with having the pleasure of a deep interpersonal good, indeed a good consummation of love, in the absence of that good. For to do that is to distort oneself in respect of that which is central to human life—our loving relation to others. And the self-induction of orgasm in the absence of sexual union would be precisely such a distortion. For the same reason, one should not take pills that give one the satisfying feeling of having acted generously when we in fact had not acted in this way, as that distorts one in respect of love. In respect of interpersonal relationships, truth is central.

4. CHEATING AND USING

There is an intuitive sense in which masturbation and other sexual acts different from intercourse "cheat" the body into yielding a false pleasure, by providing the body with sensations relevantly similar to those received in intercourse. Can we make an argument against non-coital orgasmic acts simply out of this insight? The difficulty with giving such an argument, however, is that normally we feel free to manipulate our bodies in various ways. To lose weight, one must have a lower caloric intake than output. Our bodies send us signals of dissatisfaction with our caloric intake when this intake is lower than the output, but it does not seem problematic to suppress these signals with drugs in order to make dieting easier. Likewise, with analgesics, we suppress pain signals that may be correctly informing us about a malfunction.

The weight-loss case is easy for the defender of the "cheating" argument to answer. The signals of dissatisfaction carry normative information—they say that we are not eating enough. But under the circumstances, we *are* eating enough, even though our output exceeds our intake. Hence, the signals are inappropriate, and in suppressing them we are not cheating ourselves or our bodies. The case of analgesia is a bit more difficult, because the pain we have may be *correctly* signaling something wrong with the body. But it is clear that pain distracts us from valuable activities (certainly it tends to distract us from pleasant and good thoughts), and this may generate a prima facie reason to remove pain. Note that suppression of pain is not a self-deception, anyway. Replacing the pain with a pleasure would be a self-deception, but suppressing pain is no more a self-deception than closing one's eyes is.

Nonetheless, I think there is something to be said about the idea that we have a certain authority over our bodies that permits the use of drugs which mimic various natural hormones in order to achieve our ends. This suggests that the "cheating" argument cannot be good. But I am going to argue that in sexual contexts we need to hold ourselves to a higher standard of integrity in the treatment of our bodies and of each other than in many other activities.

Kant said it is wrong to use other people as mere means. But there seem to be cases where it is permissible to make use of another person in ways that Kantianism does not allow. Suppose that you are waging a just war and are raiding an enemy base. The base commander, seeing that defeat is imminent, has set a time bomb. The time bomb has a fingerprint-based security system that can only be bypassed by placing the commander's finger on a scanner. The commander is currently lying unconscious, near the bomb. Only a few seconds are left. To save your life and the lives of your comrades, you drag the commander's body to the scanner and put his finger on it.

It seems clear that you *used* the commander's body as an instrument for defusing the bomb. Yet the use is permissible. Nothing hangs on the commander's unconsciousness, either. If he were conscious, it would be permissible to take him by force and place his finger on the scanner.[2]

Now, we might say that the commander, were he rational, would consent to the use of his finger for this purpose, and we only need to respect the autonomy of people insofar as they are acting rationally. But the sense of "rational" that would be needed to take care of all cases like this one is a very strong one. If the commander were fighting on a just side in a just war, he could be morally justified in setting such a time bomb (if we are worried about the fact that this would be suicide, we can imagine that he hoped to escape before the bomb went off). Moreover, he could be quite rational in being willing to die rather than defuse it—the cause of a just war is, by definition, worth dying for. To count the commander's resistance as necessarily irrational, we need to assume that he is fighting in an unjust war and that it is not rational to fight in an unjust war, even if one is innocently unaware of its injustice, as indeed the commander might be. The sense of "rational" in the claim "He would consent were he 'rational'" has to be the strong Kantian sense of the word, where one is acting rationally if and only if one is acting morally rightly. But the idea that we only need to respect the autonomy of people insofar as they are acting rightly would allow for very strong paternalism, of a rather un-Kantian sort. It would endanger Kant's idea that we may not lie even to evildoers.

In any case, an unrestricted thesis that it is wrong to use people or their bodies does not seem defensible. But, I suggest, the sexual sphere is different. It is wrong to compel someone sexually, even if one is compelling the person to fulfill a duty. Suppose that Bob and Jane are married, and Bob promises Jane that they will have sex in the evening, which Jane very much wants, but then Bob, for morally insufficient reasons, chooses to go to sleep early. It would still be wrong, indeed an instance of marital rape, for Jane to compel Bob to fulfill this particular promise or to use Bob's body for sex without his consent while he is asleep. In some nonsexual cases, it is acceptable to compel someone to perform a moral duty, or to use the person's body for a purpose that the person would be morally obligated to share (the case of the enemy commander above is such—the commander morally ought to help defuse the bomb). But not so in sexual cases, even if great goods are at stake. It would be wrong of Jane to compel Bob to have sex with her even if both knew this was their last chance to have a child together.

One explanation for the higher standard in sexual behavior could be given in terms of love. Sexual activity is about uniting with another in a way proper to erotic love, not just as bodies but as persons. Were Jane to compel Bob to have sex with her, he would not be uniting with her as a human being possessed of free will.

An account of sexual union that is biologically based also implies a higher standard for the involvement of the body in sexuality. In sexual union, a couple is uniting through their bodies. To cheat the body in that context is to oppose oneself to one's body, in a context in which one is trying expressly to unite with someone through that same body. In order for the biological union to be the basis for personal union, one must live the sexual union in an embodied manner, at least in respect of the sexual faculties. These faculties need to be functioning in a way that is both voluntary and biological.

This implies the value of inculcating habits which treat one's sexual faculties with respect, in a way that unites the biological, the emotive, and the intellectual, and provides a prima facie argument against all activities that "cheat" one's sexual faculties—say, by simulating the sensations of intercourse—since in doing so, one is inculcating in oneself a habit of dissociating oneself from one's sexual faculties.

One might object, however, that for the same reason, one would need to inculcate a habit of not resisting sexual desire, so as not to become dissociated from the desire. This, however, does not follow. For when two people are to unite sexually, they are uniting in the way that erotic love calls for. The interpersonal is the controlling element here. We are, as individuals, organic wholes, but an organic whole can be hierarchical. It is one thing for parents to be telling their children what to do, and another for them to be lying to the children in order to get the children to do what is needed—the latter is contrary to familial unity, in that it gives up on a unity of purpose. Likewise it is one thing for the will to set the direction for the desire, choosing one among several appropriate objects for the desire, and another for the will to manipulate one's sexual faculties to give one pleasure in a context in which the faculties are failing to engage in the activities the pleasures of which are being induced.[3] The direction-setting is the exercise of the hierarchical integrity of the person, while the self-deceitful manipulation is contrary to one's development of the virtue of acting as an integrated human being.

5. PORNOGRAPHY AND AROUSAL

It is not intrinsically immoral to look at pictures of nude persons of the opposite sex; after all, there is nothing wrong with a male medical student studying for a gynecology exam. Neither is it always wrong to look at pornography, even pornography of the worst kind. Police officers, after all, need to look at child pornography in order to rescue the victims and capture the perpetrators. These two examples show that there is a difference between looking at sexually explicit images or even pornography, and *consuming* pornography.

Likewise, the production and limited distribution of sexually explicit images is not intrinsically immoral. Someone who is witnessing a person being raped by a well-known politician might do well to make a video to give to the police and, if the police failed to act, some carefully chosen, respectable media outlets. This video would not be an instance of pornography, even though it could, in fact, be visually indistinguishable from a pornographic snuff film.

The institution of pornography involves two aspects: pornographic production and pornographic consumption. The two aspects are related. Pornographic production is the production of materials for pornographic consumption. If there were nothing intrinsically wrong with pornographic consumption, there would probably be nothing *intrinsically* wrong with pornographic production. However, even though there is a relation between production and consumption, it is nonetheless possible to consume pornographically something that was not pornographically produced (e.g., an anatomy textbook), and it is possible to look at something that was pornographically produced without engaging in pornographic consumption (e.g., the child pornography viewed by the police investigator).

Let us start with the consumption, since the production is defined in terms of the consumption. As we saw, to *consume* something pornographically is not the same as to view a certain kind of image, and, for the same reason, it is not the same as to read a certain kind of text. Nor is actual sexual arousal or titillation either a necessary or a sufficient condition for pornographic consumption. To see that it is not sufficient, observe the fact that arousal can be purely involuntary and unexpected. Think of the police officer investigating child pornography and being involuntarily aroused through some aspect of the imagery by which the officer is intellectually revolted. This arousal would be good reason to hand the case over to someone else, but if that is not possible, it might be necessary to endure the involuntary reactions as unintended side effects of one's worthy activity, applying the Principle of Double Effect. To see that actual arousal or titillation is not necessary for pornographic consumption, take a long-time user of pornography who has become inured to the sexual allure of most images, and who surfs the Internet looking for images that are more and more outré. This user might have a session of consuming pornographic images without succeeding in being aroused or titillated.

It seems, thus, that the central aspect of pornographic consumption is the intention to be aroused. But, I shall argue, it is wrong to intentionally arouse oneself except at one's spouse, and it is wrong to intentionally arouse another unless that other is one's spouse and is being aroused at one. If so, the consumption of pornography is wrong, except perhaps in a conjugal context. Moreover, even the consumption of pornography involving arousing images not of one's spouse would be wrong in a conjugal context, since then the arousal would be not at the spouse, but at someone else. Whether the use of sexually explicit images of a spouse for arousal is permissible is a question we will consider later.

Why is it wrong to arouse oneself except at one's spouse? One might start to argue for this by noting that an aspect of arousal is a desire for sexual union coupled with a degree of psychological and physical readiness for it. But it would be intrinsically wrong to engage in sexual union with anyone but one's spouse, as has been argued in this book, and to induce in oneself or another a desire for an intrinsically wrongful action is to direct one's own or the other's will away from the good and right. The virtuous person desires what is intrinsically good and right, and hence the intentional induction of desires for that which is intrinsically wrong is morally bad. Moreover, virtuous persons do not ready themselves physically for an activity that would distort the nature of a relationship—and sex would distort the nature of a nonmarital relationship in an inappropriate direction.

There might still be cases that fall through the cracks of this argument. Suppose Patricia and George are not married, but would like to have *marital* sex with one another. Since marital sex is a good thing, could they not legitimately induce in themselves a desire for marital sex, and hence arouse each other?

In response, one can first question the "hence." It is possible for a married or unmarried couple to desire marital sex without being at all aroused. For instance, the couple may believe that marital sex is good, and simply desire this good without any physical component to the desire. In fact, a couple might desire sex, and *therefore* desire arousal, without actually having arousal. So it is possible for Patricia and George to come to have a desire for marital sex, without arousing each other. Moreover, while arousal involves a yearning for sex, it has an urgency and immediacy to it. It does not involve a yearning for sex *later when one is married*. It involves a yearning for sex here and now, and if the arousal is *at* someone or something, then it is a yearning for sex here and now involving that person or thing as one now experiences that person or thing.

A married couple can legitimately intend mutual arousal, even if they cannot have sex immediately, because the arousal involves a yearning for something that, in their case, is intrinsically good—sex with this person here and now, a person who is experienced as a spouse.[4] The members of the unmarried couple who are aroused at each other are each aroused at someone who is experienced as existing within a relationship that is nonmarital. And, certainly, in the typical case of pornography, the consumer is not aroused at a person experienced as his or her spouse, but at a stranger.[5]

The consumption of pornography is, thus, wrong (leaving aside the question of sexually explicit images of the spouse) because it is an intentional induction of nonmarital arousal. At the same time, it would not be a case of pornographic consumption to consume an arousal pill, though it would be wrong for the same reason. To have a case of pornography, the cause of the arousal needs to be something representational and it needs to be intended to arouse by virtue of what it represents and/or how it represents it.

There are gray areas with regard to the representationality, but fortunately they rarely give rise to any moral questions, since the intentional nonconjugal arousal suffices for moral wrongness, regardless of the presence of representationality. Nonetheless, it is worth saying a few things about the representationality. A case of viewing a stripper involves consumption of a representation insofar as the stripper is engaging in a *performance,* which is a representational activity—the stripper *plays the role* of a sex object, rather than genuinely disclosing herself or himself to the audience.

On the other hand, seeing one's spouse in a mirror while engaging in marital union need not involve the consumption of a representation, since the phenomenology of viewing in a mirror can be that of viewing *through* the mirror. On the other hand, if the arousal is not at the *spouse* seen through the mirror but at the spouse *in the mirror,* with emphasis on the mirror, then representation enters in.

Given the earlier argument, the only case where we do not yet know whether pornographic consumption is wrong is the one where the arousal is at one's spouse. If the representation by which one is aroused is not that of one's spouse, it will be the case, at least to some extent, that one is being deliberately aroused at someone other than one's spouse. This is always wrong, but particularly wrong for a married person since that arousal directs one's heart, to some extent, away from fidelity.

The remaining question is one where the representation by which one is aroused is that of one's spouse. The question here is difficult. One feels that there would be something creepy about someone self-publishing something that looks, at first sight, like an ordinary pornographic magazine but where only one copy is printed and all the pictures are of the publisher's spouse. Nor does one's concern about this stem merely from worries about other people finding the copy. On the other hand, it does not appear wrong for someone to think sexual thoughts about the beloved spouse, to remember past sexual activities while doing so, or to look at a wedding picture and think about how sexually attractive the spouse looks in it.

However, because sexual love, like all love, is centered on reality, it is plausible that any arousal should be *at the spouse as he or she really is*[6] rather than at the *representation,* or at the spouse as he or she is not. The self-published magazine is creepy precisely because of the context in which it represents the spouse, and the fact that it is a representation would, one assumes, be phenomenologically central to its power and manner of arousal. But presumably the person who looks at the wedding picture of his or her spouse is aroused at the spouse rather than at the fact of the spouse's being pictured. The unitiveness of sexual perception requires that the perception be, as much as possible, of the other as he or she is. Thus, looking at the spouse *through* the mirror is morally preferable to looking at the mirror as framing the spouse. The focus should be the spouse rather than the representation or the context. Moreover, the spouse needs to be seen, as much as possible, as a person and hence as an *agent.*

In a picture or even a film clip, there is a danger that the spouse is "tamed," encapsulated, and made inert for the benefit of the viewer. Scruton emphasizes the perniciousness of something like this taming in the case of sexual perversions, such as bestiality, which allow one to escape from the terrifying personhood of the other.[7]

Normally, Westerners do not particularly worry about this danger of taming and making inert when taking family pictures, though some cultures are more circumspect about depictions of persons, and we can see that there is some reason for circumspection. A higher standard is needed vis-à-vis objectification in sexual contexts than in other contexts, since sexuality is closely tied to one of the basic kinds of interpersonal love, and objectification in a context tied particularly closely to love is going to distort people's loves. Likewise, a higher standard is needed for sexually explicit photographs than for ordinary snapshots. For in being intentionally aroused by the depiction, the viewer is likely to be interacting sexually with the spouse *as* encapsulated, and, particularly if the depiction is expressly sexual in nature, *as* reduced to the sexual aspect. Physical appearance is the primary focus in the depiction, and being aroused at the appearance divorced from the rest of the person contributes to a sexual focus on the purely physical. In this situation, the connection between the libidinous aspects of the relationship and the personal is damaged. Granted, an artistic photograph or painting can go beyond that, but insofar as it is used for purposes of arousal, it is not likely that these deeper aspects are of the essence in the experience.

The above considerations suggest that even in the case where it is the spouse who is represented in a medium, pornographic consumption is morally problematic, unless it is a case of seeing *through* the medium—for instance, if the wedding picture is but a memory aid that leads to recollection of that stressful but joyful day. It is worth noting that being aroused at *memories* of one's beloved is different. For memory does not reduce a person we know well to an appearance. In memory, we can bring to mind the whole of the other person as we know him or her, not merely in regard to the senses, but in a way that is rich with emotional and cognitive content, and that content includes a vague or precise recognition of the other's character. In fact, in remembering a person, there can be a kind of mutuality, in that we can come to recognize aspects of a person that we did not recognize on the original occasion we remember, so that there is a continuation and deepening of the earlier interaction. There is, however, a danger in memory as well—the danger of reducing the other to what we have observed of the other or what we can plumb out of these observations, and of neglecting the need for dynamism in love.

If the intentional remembrance of sexual aspects of one's beloved is self-centered—focused on arousing oneself as an end in itself, rather than on appreciatively remembering the beauty and goodness of the beloved spouse—then one is making sexuality into something selfish, and in doing so one is acting contrary to love. As soon as the primary focus is on one's own state of arousal, even if the activity does not reach the point of masturbation, this becomes a nonmutual sexual activity, and hence a kind of infidelity to one's spouse, by being a sexual activity where the focus is on someone other than the spouse. An interesting corollary: sexual selfishness in general can be a kind of infidelity, in that it places one's sexual focus on a person other than one's spouse—namely, on oneself.

Nonmutuality and subjugation of the other to oneself are general problems in pornographic consumption, whether the object of the pornography is one's spouse or not. We can now, in fact, give a speculative argument why being aroused by a representation, in virtue of what or how it represents, is a kind of morally objectionable objectification. For in being aroused by a representation in virtue of what or how it represents, the object of arousal is not a person as he or she exists in himself or herself—it is, at most, a person *as represented,* with a focus on the fact of representation. However, arousal is properly supposed to be an arousal *at a person,* since arousal is a way of seeing the other as particularly fit for the consummation of romantic love. Thus one's aroused state brings something nonpersonal, the being-represented, into one's sexual perception. This is one way to justify Andrea Dworkin's claim that pornography intrinsically harms all women[8]—for, to some degree, pornography makes a man relate to an image as to a woman, and hence distorts the man's sexuality in such a way that he relates to women, to some extent, as images. This is particularly clear when the pornographic depiction is of someone with whom one has a romantic relationship, such as a spouse. For then one is both sexually interested in the other *and* in the other as represented, and one cannot keep the latter relation from affecting the former.

Earlier I said that intentionally being aroused by a representation in virtue of what and/or how it represents was a necessary condition for something to be a case of pornographic consumption. In fact, it seems that the necessary condition is also sufficient. And it appears that a negative moral judgment of pornographic consumption is appropriate whether or not the context is conjugal. The case of the person with the creepy magazine filled with nude pictures of his or her spouse shows that in some conjugal cases pornographic consumption may be even worse, in that it may be an offense against the dignity of someone whose dignity one has a special duty to uphold.

Pornographic production is the production of artifacts for pornographic consumption. While it is not wrong to produce artifacts that *can* be used wrongfully (e.g., knives), it is wrong to produce artifacts *for* a wrongful use. Hence, the production of pornography is wrong.

Nor will it do for a pornographer to say that inappropriate arousal is unintended—that an aesthetic experience is all that is intended. For in pornography the representations are optimized in such wise as to produce not *just* an aesthetic experience (if there is any attention paid to the aesthetic at all). A pornographic magazine will not fill its pages with photographs of sunsets and mountains, even if the editor finds that a collection of these photographs is more beautiful than that month's lineup of nudes. The reason is simple: the business plan of a pornographer who sells pornography depends on the arousal, as the items are bought *for* the arousal. If, on the other hand, we genuinely had a photography magazine, one that sometimes carried beautiful nude photographs and at other times beautiful scenes of snow-capped mountains, then we would have to pay attention to the possibility that the magazine is *not* pornographic, and that arousal is unintended. There would still be considerations of prudence in publishing the nudes, since even if the magazine is not pornographic, consumers could consume the nude photographs pornographically. It is not wrong to sell sharp knives some of which are used for crimes, but if one expects the criminal use to be very common, it may be contrary to prudence to sell the knives.

We can now define *pornographic media* in three ways: as media produced pornographically, as media consumed pornographically, or as some combination of these. The term "pornography" as usually used in our culture is a combination of these, together with a requirement of sexual explicitness. It seems that an artifact is generally counted as pornographic if it is sexually explicit and produced with the intention of being consumed pornographically, though maybe only if the intention is somewhat successful. However, sexual explicitness is not the defining feature if the term is to be morally useful. A book of pictures of shoes produced by a shoe-fetishist for shoe-fetishists would certainly be a work of pornography in the morally relevant sense.

Finally, it needs to be noted that in Western countries, the most readily available source of pornography is currently the Internet. The availability of this source appears to have affected pornographic consumption in ways that are relevant to its moral description.

For it is now much easier to obtain pornographic materials. This ease lowers psychological barriers there might be to going into, say, a poorly lit store full of other people seeking pornographic materials. It can be difficult, especially for a young person, to see as morally significant something that involves "merely a few clicks." Redescription of an activity is one of our main ways of self-justification. A plagiarist once redescribed to me the plagiarism as just "leaving out a footnote." One might also redescribe killing someone with a gun as a contraction of the forefinger.

What is easy can become routine, and what is routine is indeed likely to be seen as unproblematic. The ease with which pornography is available provides an additional moral reason to refrain from its consumption. If there were only one shot of heroin left in the world, one would still have a decisive reason to refrain from using the heroin, since doing so would still mean acting contrary to the good functioning of one's intellect, though the reason would be strong in a case where more heroin is available, since the latter case makes long-term addiction possible.

Unlimited availability and ease of access to something pleasurable tends to lead to satiation. This, in turn, can push one to seek more intense versions of the stimulus. Interviews conducted by Pamela Paul[9] suggest that this sometimes happens with pornography: a heterosexual man might start by arousing himself with "tasteful" nude pictures of women, but eventually move on to seek more sexually explicit or degrading material, which he would initially have judged to be morally inappropriate.

A further phenomenon that Internet pornography facilitates is the search for "perfection." The perfection sought may involve maximal beauty, or maximal sexual explicitness, or extremes of degradation. Because the quantity of the material is virtually unlimited, it is possible to click through hundreds in the search of an ideal instead of focusing on one particular image. In doing this, one is not just treating the objects of sexual attraction as *objects* to be used for one's purposes, but as objects that typically do not measure up. This can, in turn, lead to an attitude where one pursues, say, physical perfection or the willingness to engage in some particular act in one's sexual relationships.[10]

In fact, even if one does not think it is wrong to view sexually explicit imagery for the purpose of self-arousal, one has a good reason to abstain from the viewing of pornography because of the ease with which such viewing might move one toward enjoying images that are degrading to (typically) women, or might distort one's approach to sexuality. We cannot predict with full confidence whether we will fall into a particular moral danger when exposed to it, and a belief in one's immunity to a moral danger increases the vulnerability. Moreover, we can predict that at various difficult times in the future we will be likely to find ourselves emotionally vulnerable in ways that are now unpredictable, thereby potentially exacerbating moral dangers.

A person might, of course, set down a line beyond which he or she will not go. Thus, one might resolve not to look at images that involve anything other than two persons portrayed as loving. However, in the case of Internet pornography, such limits do not seem practically possible. In searching for an image within bounds one may well come upon images outside of the bounds, and there is a moral danger that one will then come to enjoy them. Moreover, there is a continuum of types of images, and one can end up each time pushing the envelope a little more. A somewhat easier line to hold in practice might be to refrain from pornography on the Internet, and limit oneself to print or film media of a particular genre. However, it is difficult to be confident ahead of time that this is a line one will not cross, given the easy availability of electronic forms.

The easy availability of pornography, thus, gives one additional good reason to abstain from all use of pornography. We can go into situations of significant moral danger when we have very good reason to do so, but we cannot court moral danger for morally insignificant reasons. If I know that I have a violent temper after drinking two beers, it is wrong for me to drink the two beers for the sake of pleasure, but it might be acceptable (depending on just how violent the temper and whether I could take at least some precautions) if a qualified doctor prescribed the beer for a serious medical condition. The pleasure of being aroused by pornography is clearly not a *significant* good, if it is a good at all.

Aristotle thought that we should act like the perfectly virtuous prudent agent. He was wrong. If Jennifer were an Aristotelian perfectly virtuous agent, she would not be vulnerable to moral danger, having all the right dispositions for the right occasions. She could thus enter into situations where she is tempted to commit significant evils even though entering into the situations would produce but a minor benefit. But we cannot morally act like Jennifer. We must forego some morally licit goods in order to avoid moral danger. Even if some pornographic consumption were morally licit, which it is not, the addictive nature of the consumption provides one with good reason to avoid it entirely.

6. PRIVACY AND MODESTY

In the above, I took the salient features of pornography to be representationality and the intention of arousal. Nonetheless, it is worth considering whether there is not something right about considering sexual explicitness as at least a morally relevant feature of an objectionable work. For sexual union is appropriately expressed in a certain privacy, because the erotic appears to be the only form of love to which the exclusiveness of a one-to-one relationship is essential. If so, then a sexually explicit pornographic production may be wrong not just on account of being arousing, but on account of violating that privacy of sexual union. In fact, this suggests that there is something at least problematic about any sexually explicit portrayal, even the ones that are morally unobjectionable, such as images in a medical textbook.

However, the romantic relationship can be entirely exclusive without total privacy being accorded the sexual act, and hence the imperative to privacy is only prima facie. There would be no duty for a dissident couple to abstain from marital sexuality if they thought that the secret police has installed a hidden video camera in every room. And there are cultures where privacy is not available.

Privacy, anyway, is often a matter of degree. It is acceptable for a couple to talk about their sexual activity to a doctor or a confessor in as much detail as is medically or morally relevant. Married couples do not need to hide the fact that they engage in marital activity—after all, the existence of their children is typically a sign of the parents' having had sex. Modesty is important both in order to avoid even unintentionally arousing others and in order to signify the privacy of the act. But the amount of effort to which one must go in order to avoid observation—whether visual or auditory—by others is surely not infinite, as we can see from the case of the dissident couple potentially under surveillance. A prudent judgment is needed.

Furthermore, standards of modesty are in part culturally relative, though in part they may be absolute. To deliberately reveal one's *reproductive* organs to all and sundry seems opposed to the privacy of the romantic relationship, to the consummation of which these organs are ordered. But one can *nonintentionally* appear completely naked in a public setting—say, when running out of a burning building (the Principle of Double Effect applies: running is intrinsically good or neutral; the intention is to escape from the building; public nudity is not intended either as a means or as an end).

The appropriate standards of dress depend crucially on what the culture considers to be sexual in nature. In a culture where shapeless brown sweaters for men are seen as intensely sexual and are found deeply arousing by the women, it would be wrong for a man to appear in public deliberately wearing such a sweater (of course, if he was escaping from a burning building in winter that would be a different matter). In so doing he would be contributing to the arousal of others outside of a conjugal context. The contribution might be nonintentional, but if less suggestive clothes are available, that is no excuse (Double Effect does not apply if there is an unproblematic alternative). Moreover, by behaving in an overtly sexual manner, the man would be signifying a lack of respect for the privacy of sexuality, and hence for the exclusivity of the romantic bond.

7. FANTASIES

In a mental fantasy, a person deliberately imagines living through an experience. A fantasy, in the technical sense in which I want to use the word, is, however, not just any case of imaginatively living through an experience. It is a case where one deliberately guides the thought process for the sake of enjoying the imagined as if it were real, thereby affectively blurring the line between the imagined and real. One might imagine what it is like to receive the Nobel prize, in order to better describe the event in a novel about a great scientist. That is not a fantasy in our technical sense. But it would be a fantasy for a person to imagine going through the ceremony for the sake of the pleasure proper to the recipient. It is essential to the pleasure received that, at some level, one be treating the imagined ceremony as a real ceremony, that one be letting it move one's heart the way a real ceremony would.

Fantasies, then, can be sexual or not. If the sought-after pleasure involves sexual arousal outside of a marital context, the arguments in section 5 above show the fantasy to be morally wrong. Likewise, fantasizing about doing something that is wrong is very different from merely thinking about wrongdoings (police investigators and moral philosophers have to do that!). In fantasizing, one deliberately enjoys the imagined activity, and when the activity is vicious, one is thereby taking pleasure in vice, which is contrary to virtue. The virtuous person, as Aristotle insists, is one who takes pleasure in virtue and is repelled by vice. To deliberately take mental pleasure in vice is, thus, wrong. Of course, one might find oneself having a thought of a vicious action and a flicker of pleasure associated with that thought. As long as no free action has occurred, one is not culpable for any wrongdoing. But, apart from cases of mental compulsion, one then has a choice—a choice whether to continue that line of thought or not.[11]

It is interesting that there is a general argument against a large class of fantasies, including many sexual ones, and some nonsexual ones as well, that does not depend on the production of inappropriate arousal or even on the fantasized action being wrong. Often, fantasies are about specific others behaving a certain way with regard to us. Sexual fantasies are one species of the genus I am interested in, but the genus is wider than that. There can, for instance, be fantasies about the recognition of our excellences, about others doing something humiliating, about climbing Mount Everest with one's best friend, and so on. It is many such fantasies—in some of which the fantasized situation is not actually a bad one—against which I will offer an argument,.

The problem occurs when the fantasy does not respect others as autonomous persons. The fantasizer is, after all, in charge of the situation. Like a film director, the fantasizer tells this actor to do this and that actor to say that. But unlike a real film director who does this in cooperation with actors who have read the script and agreed to act according to it, the typical fantasizer is arranging the persons in the mind without any cooperation, all on his or her own. Herein lies both the attraction and the danger of the fantasy. In creating the fantasy, the fantasizer is, in a sense, more powerful than God in creating the world. For while arguably God cannot make a person freely do something, the fantasizer can.[12] It may, for instance, be a part of the fantasy that some persons freely fawn on the fantasizer. This attitude of being in charge of others is not a virtuous one.

Granted, there is a certain respect of autonomy if the behavior of the characters in the fantasy is constrained by the real-life behavior or commitments of the persons. If I have had a number of delightful conversations with George, there may be nothing wrong with fantasizing about another, since, in doing so, I am constrained by George's actual character, and, thus, he is to some extent autonomous, even as found in my mind. If I do this well, I might even find myself rebuked by fantasy-George in the course of the fantasized conversation. I am not more-than-God-like in ordering his life around. Likewise, if a friend has undertaken a commitment to go for a hike with me, it does not seem problematic to look forward vividly to that hike. Again, the actual person has had a moment of autonomy in the creation of the fantasy.

But the more the fantasizer is in charge of arranging the behavior of the characters in the fantasy for his or her own gratification, the more problematic this fantasizing is, as it is a failure to respect the fact that others are independent persons and not subordinate to one's pleasure.

One obvious objection to my argument is that I am confusing fiction and reality. The student who fantasizes about me saying that his hastily written paper was the best I have ever read is not actually making *me* do anything—he affects his thoughts, but not me. This is true, but he is, in an important way, using me for his own gratification. His fantasy gets its life from my reality. That I am not actually, physically affected by the fantasy does not mean that I am not being used—certainly, a voyeur's victim is being *used* by the voyeur even if the victim does not find out.

It is true that when sane people fantasize, they can typically distinguish fact from fiction. But at the same time, what gives pleasure in the fantasy is a deliberate mental relaxing of the distinction, a willing suspension of disbelief. The more clearheadedly one takes the fantasy to be a mere hypothetical, the less one is going to have the pleasant feelings the fantasy was going to induce. In fantasizing about being praised by a professor, the student is trying to induce the feelings that attend *real,* and not merely hypothetical, praise. But to treat the characters that inhabit one's fantasies as pawns to be moved in accordance with one's desires, for one's gratification, is seriously problematic, and it develops a disrespectful habit of the mental treatment of others. Even if this habit will not overflow into controlling behavior—and how can one be sure of that?—the mental attitudes are themselves morally bad.

8. MENTAL UNDRESSING

Nonmarital fantasies engaged in for the sake of sexual pleasure can be criticized because it is wrong to mentally enjoy wrongful pleasures.

And fantasies, sexual or not, that involve real people can additionally be criticized as a way of using people. Mental undressing of strangers that a person is sexually interested in is a closely related case.

Here is an argument against such a practice. Consider that it is generally agreed that voyeurism is wrong. It would be wrong for a heterosexual man to peep into a women's shower room through a hole in the wall for the sake of sexual gratification. Notice that here, too, the purpose of the looking is relevant. It would not necessarily be wrong for a heterosexual male police officer to install and monitor a camera in a women's shower room in order to nab a murderer, if there were no other way of catching the criminal. (In particular, there would have to be no practicable way of having the camera be monitored by, say, a heterosexual woman.)

But now consider a continuum of voyeurism, starting with peeping into the shower room for sexual gratification at one extreme. As the next step, imagine the heterosexual male wearing eyeglasses that process infrared light in a way that enables the formation of clear and accurate images of what people look like under their clothes.[13] There seems to be no significant difference between a heterosexual male's peeking into the shower room for sexual gratification, and his looking through such glasses at women in a crowd, for the same purpose.

For the third step in our continuum, let us suppose that glasses only process visible light, just as our eyes do. These glasses do not see through clothes. However, the glasses have a sophisticated computational apparatus that, from the way clothes lie and move on a person, are able to reconstruct the exact shape of the person wearing the clothes, and present this image to the wearer. There does not seem to be a significant moral difference between analyzing infrared light to form the image and analyzing the movements of clothes to form the image.

As the fourth step, let us imagine a sculptor who, through much experience, has learned how to mentally reconstruct the exact shape of the person wearing the clothes. To engage in such reconstruction for the sake of sexual gratification does not seem significantly morally different from wearing glasses that do the reconstruction for one. If the use of the glasses for sexual gratification is wrong, so is the use of the sculptor's specialized experience.

But now, as the fifth step in the continuum, consider an ordinary heterosexual male who is a "mental undresser" of women—who imagines as naked women that he meets clothed, and does so for sexual gratification. He lacks the special skills of the sculptor, but surely he is engaged in the same task of reconstructing the appearance of the naked woman from what can be seen. His reconstructions may well be far off their mark in a way in which the sculptor's aren't, but there does not seem to be a deep moral difference between the two. Indeed, the ordinary mental undresser would presumably aspire to the superior imaginative abilities of the sculptor.

In all cases, there is a sense in which the victim's privacy is violated for sexual purposes. In some cases, the violation is more successful (as in the case of the peeper or the special glasses) and in some it is less so (as in the case of the ordinary mental undresser who can perhaps only envision generic underclothes features). But the intentional use of another for sexual gratification is common to all the cases.

9. SPERM SAMPLE COLLECTION

A theoretically difficult case concerns the use of masturbation in order to collect sperm for analysis leading, hopefully, to fertility treatment. Because the action is not done for the sake of fraudulent or empty pleasure, the best arguments of this chapter fail to apply. Nonetheless, a version of these arguments does give a prima facie consideration against such collection. Sexuality is very important to human life. To feel fraudulent or empty *sexual* pleasure is particularly problematic because the danger of dissociating the physical and the personal in sexuality seems particularly great; that is one of the lessons we can draw from the experience of the Western world in the last fifty years. One would have to have quite a serious reason to court such a danger. Such a reason does not exist in the case of analysis for fertility treatment, for there is an entirely morally unproblematic method of collection. This is the use in intercourse of a modified condom which retains some semen for analysis and lets other semen pass through.

Nonetheless, even though the question is settled in practice by the above considerations, there is a theoretical question. Would deliberately causing ejaculation not for the sake of union, direct furthering of reproduction, or pleasure, but for the sake of remotely furthering reproduction be morally permissible, if there were no alternatives? Answering this question forces us once again to consider the nature of arousal. For a means necessary to the production of ejaculation through masturbation is the causing of arousal. One might reasonably hold that, just as the sexual pleasure of orgasm is a way of perceiving the occurrent good of union, arousal is a way of perceiving the other's fittedness for sexual union with one. To intend arousal except in the context of arousal at someone with whom it would be appropriate to engage in sexual union would be to intend an inappropriate mental state.

But one could imagine a case of masturbation for the collection of sperm where the man is aroused at his spouse, and so the arousal would not be entirely inappropriate. Nonetheless, the arousal would be used for the attainment of a nonunitive climax, and so one would be causing arousal while "cheating" the arousal, i.e., going against the integrity of the embodied person in sexual matters.

10. AROUSAL AND PHYSICAL DISPLAYS OF AFFECTION

A difficult question, which cannot be settled entirely through clear-cut rules, is what physical displays of affection are appropriate for an unmarried couple. We may begin with a conclusion argued for in section 5 above: it is inappropriate to induce arousal outside of a marital context. Through arousal, one sees the other as someone with whom it would be good to have sexual union, and if one is not married to the other, then sex would be inappropriate, and hence so would arousal.

Thus those activities that are aimed at orgasm or at producing arousal in oneself or the other are morally inappropriate in the context of a relationship where sex is morally inappropriate, i.e., in a nonmarital relationship. Arousal is a state of libidinous desire, with a natural directedness at sex, and where sex is morally inappropriate, likewise this directedness at sex is morally inappropriate.

But as for how one can show affection in nonsexual ways, there is a significant, though not decisive, guide in the customs of one's society. For instance, if an act of affection is one that our society considers acceptable in some entirely nonsexual contexts, such as a hug or holding a hand (one may hug a relative and hold a child's hand), then the way is open to using this act to convey affection in a romantic context.

Another category would be acts of affection, such as lip-kissing in Western culture, that tend to be limited to romantic relationships, but where the acts are not intended to arouse, and the culture sees the acts primarily as expressive of affection rather than as methods for arousal or preludes to sex. Such acts might well be permissible, at least when they do not predictably lead to undue arousal.

The point here is not to give precise rules, as much as to offer social perceptions as a fallible guideline. If in one's society to stroke the left ear is always considered a deeply sexual act and a natural prelude to intercourse, then to stroke the left ear while disclaiming the sexual content is risky. For even if one tells oneself and one's beloved that the meaning of this particular touch is not innate to it, one will find it difficult to divorce oneself from the attitudes of one's community. If the community treats an act as sexually meaningful in a particular way, saying that it is not so for oneself runs the danger of being a self-deception. Moreover, since we humans are communal beings, unless we have very good reason to do otherwise, we *should* express ourselves in accordance to the conventions operative around us, not just because others may otherwise misunderstand us nor because we might deceive ourselves, important as these considerations are, but also simply because we are members of our own community and need to live our lives in union with it, to the extent that we can do so without compromising anything of objective value.

We can, also, say that it would be, in practice, a self-deception to engage, in a romantic or sexual context, in the touching of primary sexual organs while claiming to have a negative attitude toward the arousal that is all but certain to follow, as well as any other touching that results in arousal in a fairly direct way. Granted, it can in principle be permissible to engage in actions that one expects but does not intend will result in arousal, such as rescuing attractive naked people from a burning building. The Principle of Double Effect will allow this: the end is good, the arousal or its induction is not intended either as a means or as an end, and the badness of inappropriate arousal is proportionate to the good sought. Since arousal in a nonmarital context is a tendency toward an activity that is not permissible, to engage in activity likely to lead to arousal, one always needs proportionate reason that cannot be better fulfilled without as great a risk of arousal. The mere desire to physically express affection and closeness is not a proportionate reason, since that desire, insofar as it is appropriate outside of a marital context, can be satisfied by holding hands while sitting on a park bench, sharing ice cream, or maybe playing a video game together.

11. WHAT IS SEX?

We are now in a position to ask the question "What is sex?" To define the word "sex" in a way that matches all our uses of the word is difficult. If one is not careful, or if one has lawyers that force one to be *particularly* careful, some acts that most people would count as a form of "sex" will slip away from the definition. For example, if one defines sex in such a way that primary sexual organs need to be involved, then some lesbian acts will not count as sex. On the other hand, if one includes too much, then hand holding or hugging will count as sex.[14]

But there is also a sense in which the question is now moot. For there are, I think, two kinds of reasons why the question "What is sex?" seems to matter in contemporary Western society. The first is that often there is a physical progression in non-marital romantic relationships, from meeting and talking, to holding hands and kissing, to having sex. Having sex, and the kind of sex one is having, are seen as important markers of the status of the relationship. However, just about everything that a reasonable, ordinary person would call "sex" involves intentional arousal and/or orgasm, and we have argued that these are morally wrong except within marriage. There is no need, then, for sex as a marker of the progress of a nonmarital relationship, except in the negative: if any kind of intentional arousal and especially any intentionally induced orgasm occurs, something has gone morally wrong. And within marriage, it is intercourse that consummates conjugal love, and orgasmic activity outside of the context of intercourse is not morally permissible.

A second need for a concept of "sex" comes from the question of infidelity: Just when does an act done with someone other than one's spouse or romantic partner count as "cheating"? But no plausible account of "sex" will answer this question, because it is clear that there are activities which count as infidelity, and which no reasonable, ordinary person would call sex—such as a married person's sitting in a romantic setting with a person to whom he or she is attracted and softly caressing the other's hand.

Nor is it likely that we will be able to define exactly the range of activities that count as infidelity. But we can probably give some sufficient conditions. Any activity done with someone other than one's romantic partner and intended to produce non-marital arousal or orgasm in oneself or another is a case of infidelity. Is masturbation a form of infidelity? Well, I've argued that it is always wrong, even if it is not a form of infidelity, though I think we are apt to consider it a form of infidelity. Gamete-donation activity, where one's gametes would noncoitally unite with those of someone to whom one is not married, might also be infidelity—but I shall argue in chapter 10 that such acts are anyway also wrong even with one's spouse. Likewise, any activity that acts out of or in support of one's own attraction to another or another's attraction to oneself, when that other is not one's romantic partner, is a form of infidelity to the romantic partner.

But if one still wants a definition of sex, perhaps the best answer is to invoke Aristotle's theory of focal meaning. On Aristotle's view, some words have a family of tightly interconnected meanings. Thus, "healthy" means different things as applied to a body, a food item, or a complexion. A healthy body is one that functions well organically. Healthy food is food that contributes to a body's being healthy. And a healthy complexion is a complexion that tends to be indicative of a body's being healthy. There is a central, primary, or focal meaning: a healthy body being one that functions well organically. The other meanings are related to this meaning—in this case, by producing or indicating health in the focal sense.[15] And of course, other relationships to the focal meaning are possible.

We might then say that in the *focal* sense, sex is intercourse. But we can now give several derivative senses. Thus, we might understand "sex" in a broader sense as indicating the whole activity surrounding intercourse—foreplay, intercourse itself, afterplay, and so on. Or we might understand "sex" as indicating any activity that is significantly like intercourse—like intercourse, for instance, in terms of its social role and the intended occurrence of orgasm. We might come up with some other derivative meanings if we wish. But, fortunately, nothing of great importance rides on these derivative definitions.

Likewise, we might understand "cheating" in the focal sense as intercourse with someone other than one's romantic partner, but then accept various derivative senses of the word.

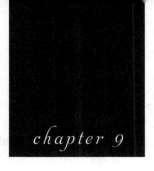

Same-Sex Attraction

1. ORIENTATION

While a majority of people seem to be sexually attracted primarily to members of the opposite sex, some are attracted primarily to people of the same sex and some are roughly equally attracted to people of both sexes. I will use "heterosexual," "homosexual," and "bisexual" to refer, respectively, to these three groups of people. The terms are not meant to be exhaustive and, as I will use them, carry no implication as to sexual behavior or relationships. For instance, one can be a heterosexual and have no sexual relationships, or sexual relationships only with people of the same sex, or sexual relationships only with people of the opposite sex, or, finally, sexual relationships both with people of the same and of the opposite sex.

The three terms are fuzzy. After all, it may be that with physical stimulation and carefully chosen context, any person can be brought to find almost any other person sexually attractive. Or what would we say about the at least logically possible case of a man for whom almost every woman is very attractive, and for whom no man is attractive except for one, but that one man is felt to be more attractive than any woman? Such a person is mainly attracted to women, yet his primary attraction is to a man. Or what would we say of the typical person in a culture where there is a phase in which initial sexual relationships are of the same-sex sort, and are then replaced by opposite-sex relationships?

And what does it mean to be "sexually attracted" to someone? Does it mean to have a tendency to be aroused in their presence? But surely it is possible to find someone sexually attractive without actually being aroused. Does it mean to form the belief that the person is sexually attractive to one? Surely not, since a belief about who is sexually attractive to one may be wrong—for instance, one might confuse admiration of form with sexual attraction. Does it mean to have a noninstrumental desire for a sexual or romantic relationship with the person? Probably not: we can imagine a person who has no sexual attraction to anybody, but who has a noninstrumental desire for a romantic relationship because of a belief, based on the testimony of others, that romantic relationships have noninstrumental value. These and similar questions suggest that there is a cluster of related concepts under the head of "sexual attraction," and any precise definition is likely to be an undesirable shoehorning. But if the concept of sexual attraction is a cluster of concepts, neither are there simply univocal concepts of heterosexuality, homosexuality, and bisexuality.

Fortunately, in the end, little of moral significance will turn on the precise meaning of these terms. Indeed, the main purpose of these brief considerations should, in fact, be a caution not to take the terms very seriously. Nonetheless, for convenience, we will use the terms. But what sexual acts, and with whom, are permissible to one will not in the end depend on whether one is homosexual, heterosexual, bisexual, and so forth, in orientation.

2. EROS AND HOMOSEXUALITY

Homosexuals sometimes experience erotic love for persons of the same sex. The "sometimes" here is not a put-down: we should likewise say that heterosexuals sometimes experience erotic love for persons of the opposite sex. Presumably, just as some heterosexuals have never, in fact, experienced erotic love, some homosexuals have also never experienced it. And since we have seen that sexual activity should be understood as the consummation of erotic love, we need not focus on same-sex attraction apart from erotic love, since it is the love that gives meaning to the attraction.

But on our analysis of erotic love as partly defined by a tendency to sexual union, and of sexual union as partly defined by a biological union of reproductive type as a single organism, the idea of erotic love for persons of the same sex is conceptually problematic. How can there be a tendency to sexual union in the case of a couple who cannot engage in a sexual union, since they are incapable of a reproductive type of act? And how could persons of the same sex, who know how human reproduction works, be desiring a reproductive type of union?

It thus seems that I should have begun this section with the claim that homosexuals *appear* to experience erotic love, to be consistent with the earlier account of erotic love. This idea could then be pushed in two different directions. Liberal readers might push it into a reductio ad absurdum of my account of erotic love: Plainly, they might say, persons of the same sex do experience erotic love, and hence the theory is wrong. Conservative readers might, however, embrace the conclusion and conclude that there can be no erotic love between persons of the same sex.

However, the argument that this book's account of erotic love entails that persons of the same sex cannot have erotic love fails. It is easily possible to have an active tendency toward something that cannot happen. Think of a trapped animal struggling to escape where there is no hope. This can even happen in the case of a human being who *knows* that there is no hope. Likewise, we have seen in chapter 3 that it is possible not to know what one is desiring, so that the argument that homosexuals do not desire a one-body union because they do not see themselves as desiring it fails. If the form of love is determined by the kind of union sought and the aspect under which the beloved is appreciated, it appears quite possible for a same-sex couple to have erotic love—to desire sexual union and to appreciate the other as someone with whom one can enter into such union. Notice that it is not even necessary that the couple be ignorant of what they desire or of the facts of life. They may know that they desire sexual union, without knowing that the sexual union they desire is, necessarily, a union of reproductive type, just as people can knowingly desire water, without knowing that what they desire is, necessarily, H_2O.

The standard parity argument for same-sex marriage, at least as made in the United States, presupposes not just the mere possibility but the actual existence of same-sex erotic love. The question is asked, after all, why people who *love* each other are not allowed to marry each other. And unless the "love" is erotic, the question is an irrelevant one (compare: Why can't siblings who have fraternal love for each other marry each other?). And there is indeed significant evidence for the claim that there is erotic love between persons of the same sex, namely, that many same-sex couples exhibit behaviors very similar to the paradigmatic modes of behavior of opposite-sex couples experiencing erotic love.

Nonetheless, one might object that the love of homosexual couples is not really erotic, but either sui generis or one of the standard nonsexual, nonfamilial loves—friendship being the most plausible example given the way homosexuality is manifested in our society. In the next two sections we examine these two suggestions.

3. IS HOMOEROTIC LOVE A "STANDARD" NONEROTIC FORM OF LOVE?

Perhaps the love that is expressed in the sexual activity of persons of the same sex is not erotic love or some other special kind of love, as in the case of romantic partners of the opposite sex, but simply one of the other "standard" forms of love. At least for the egalitarian forms of same-sex love in our society, the most plausible candidate form would be *friendship*, and so this is the version of the view we will examine. On this view, homosexual love relationships are sexually tinged friendships.

If the friendship hypothesis is correct, we can speculatively make two predictions: (1) sexuality is less important in same-sex love relationships than in opposite-sex love relationships; (2) sexual exclusivity need not be central to same-sex love relationships, since healthy friendships typically do not involve exclusivity. The fact that some of the potential significance of sexuality that is found in opposite-sex love relationships—namely, reproduction and union as one body—simply cannot be found in the same-sex case, makes (1) plausible. The state of sociological research on same-sex relationships is poor, but there is some data supporting (2) in the male case.[1] It could, of course, be that the friendship hypothesis only holds in the male case but not in the female case.

On the friendship view, there are three ways one could approach the sexual aspect of the relationship. First, sexuality might be an aspect of friendly union. Sexuality does not enter into the concept of the union in friendship in general, and hence the aspect would be a contingent one of the friendship qua friendship. Nonetheless, a friendship can be cemented by a variety of activities, and sexual activity might be one of them. After all, one can uncontroversially see how even a married heterosexual couple might engage in intercourse not only as lovers but also as friends—in addition to the joys proper to eros, their sexual activity might well carry the additional meaningfulness that any friendly, good-humored, cooperative activity does.

If this were all there was to same-sex sexuality, however, then prohibitions on same-sex sexual activity should not be quite as problematic to the gay rights community as they are. These prohibitions would be like a prohibition against two people of the same sex cooking together; just as a friendship can be cemented by cooking, so too it can be cemented by sex. The prohibitions would be a hardship and might well be unreasonable if same-sex sexual activity is permissible, but would not hit at anything of great moral significance, in the way in which prohibiting sex to opposite-sex couples is felt to do by those who oppose this prohibition. For even if one cannot cook or have sex together, there are many other ways of cementing a friendship, though for particular pairs of individuals, cooking or sex might be the optimal way of expressing the particular friendship.

In chapter 4, I argued that the force with which prohibitions on same-sex sexual activity are opposed by large segments of our society suggests that sex has a deep significance. This significance seems to point to sex in same-sex love being more than just one of many ways of cementing a friendship, though in section 5 of this chapter I shall argue that any such use of sex is morally inappropriate (in that it misconstrues the beloved and misconstrues the relationship, by creating the illusion of the union proper to erotic love).

Second, sexuality might be irrelevant to the friendship. In this case, the sexuality is not an expression of love, since our operating assumption was that the form of love involved is friendship. But this takes away a central meaning of sexuality. Moreover, the arguments in section 5 below will apply, and so on both this and the previous view, sexual activity will be morally inappropriate in same-sex love relationships.

Third, the sexuality might be a *distortion* of friendship. A man I know has argued for this on the grounds of his personal experience. On theological grounds, he is convinced that same-sex sexual activity is morally inappropriate. However, he found that the desires he had in regard to other men were fulfilled when he was able to engage in deep and chaste friendship with them. Now, granted, one can feel that a desire is fulfilled when it is not. But generally when a desire is not really fulfilled, it returns. A lasting feeling of a desire's fulfillment would at least be some evidence in favor of the claim that the desire was fulfilled. This suggests that, at least for this man, the love really was of a friendly rather than erotic sort, fulfilled in the way friendships are.

Nonetheless, it appears that at least sometimes there is an exclusivity present in same-sex love relationships that, in the case of friendship, would be a distortion of the relationship into cliquishness, as C. S. Lewis has noted. In cases where this exclusivity is an important part of the love, the friendship hypothesis does not seem to apply. It would, on the other hand, be surprising if the friendship hypothesis did not apply to *some* cases, just as it probably sometimes does in heterosexual cases. (Think of the "friends with benefits" relationship.)

4. IS HOMOEROTIC LOVE SUI GENERIS?

In a paper presented at Georgetown University in the spring of 2005, the theologian James Alison has sketched a very interesting argument for the possible permissibility of same-sex sexual relations. My reconstruction of the argument is as follows. Human nature is good, though distorted due to sin and the Fall. These distortions cannot create a new kind of desire ex nihilo: they can only distort an existing desire. Thus, every kind of human desire is either good in itself, or else a distortion of a good desire. Same-sex sexual desire is either sui generis or a distortion of opposite-sex sexual desire. It might turn out—Alison thinks this is a question for science—that it is not in fact a distortion of opposite-sex sexual desire. If that turns out to be correct, same-sex sexual desire will be sui generis, and then it will be good in itself (at least unless further distorted). Thus, to judge same-sex sexual activity wrong requires one to prejudge the scientific question whether same-sex sexual desire is a distortion of opposite-sex sexual desire.

To make this into a positive argument for the permissibility of same-sex sexual activity, one would have to positively show not only that same-sex desire is not a distortion of opposite-sex desire, but also that it is not a distortion of some *other* kind of desire, such as the desires of friendship, a case we considered in the previous section. Moreover, the claim that the judgment as to what is a distortion of what should be a scientific one is questionable. The judgment concerns a *normative* question, and modern science does not answer normative questions as such.

It is not at all clear what kind of a scientific discovery could settle the question. Suppose, for instance, we discover that same-sex sexual desire correlates with one chemical in one part of the brain, while opposite-sex sexual desire correlates with a very different chemical in another part of the brain. Would this show that one is not a distortion of the other? Surely not. For what defines a desire is not the chemicals that correlate with it, but the *content* of the desire. Take, for instance, the experience of the thirst for knowledge. It correlates with certain kinds of electrochemical activity in our brains. But it could also exist in the brain of an alien whose central nervous system is run on very different principles from ours and hence in the absence of the same electrochemical activity. It is quite possible for conceptually very similar mental states to correlate with or be manifested by very different brain structures.

The question whether one desire is a distortion of another seems to be about the content and object of desire. Psychological rather than neurological data seems more relevant. But empirical psychology does not seem up to the task—we have no idea what kinds of experiments would settle questions about what is a distortion of what. Science can tell us what is most prevalent, but cannot tell us what is normal (and the two are different—cf. section 4 of chapter 5). It seems, then, that conceptual data is key, and this is the province of philosophical analysis.

On the conceptual side, one might argue that same-sex sexual desire does not seem to motivate the couple to vaginal-penile intercourse but to other sexual acts, and hence is a different kind of desire from heterosexual desire. Yet many of these "other sexual acts" are ones in which some heterosexual couples engage, and it is plausible that in the heterosexual case these acts do not fulfill some sui generis desire, but at most fulfill a variant or distortion of the desire for sexual union, while at least some same-sex sexual acts, such as the use of a dildo by a lesbian couple, mirror heterosexual intercourse.

Note, too, that we can condemn greed, selfishness, laziness, and dishonesty without engaging in the kind of scientific examination of the underlying desires that Alison's argument would require one to. Nonetheless, the question whether same-sex sexual desire could be sui generis remains. If it were, then the corresponding love would also be sui generis. This might endanger the argument for same-sex marriage, unless this love could be argued to be relevantly similar to erotic love.

However, it does seem plausible that one *could* feel sexual desire for someone of the same sex, in the same sense of "sexual desire" as heterosexuals normally experience it. It is, for instance, easy to imagine a heterosexual man feeling bona fide sexual desire toward someone whom he erroneously believes to be a woman. It is possible that for a particularly homophobic man this desire would turn to disgust or self-loathing upon finding out that the object of the desire is a man. But it also seems possible that the desire might remain, and not be significantly changed either in its biological underpinnings or in its manifestation. This makes it quite probable that at least *some* cases of same-sex sexual desire are the same kind of thing as opposite-sex sexual desire.

There may, of course, be cases of sui generis desire between particular pairs of people. We cannot really rule out this possibility, whether for same- or opposite-sex couples. But such desire would not be sexual desire, except by equivocation. It would be a desire that would call for its own analysis. It could even be a desire that points toward a desirable union. But then the union would not be a sexual one, since if it were a sexual one, this would be a case of sexual desire.

5. THE MORALITY OF SAME-SEX SEXUAL ACTIVITY

Could it be, however, that there is a sui generis desire that might direct *some* same-sex couples to a union mediated by orgasmic sexual acts, a union other than the one-body union of heterosexual desire? Perhaps it would be a somewhat less significant union, but still a significant one. Or could it even be that some couples who have genuine sexual desire opt for the lesser kind of union, realizing that the full sexual union is not actually possible for them?

I have argued in the previous chapter that it is wrong to intentionally induce orgasm outside of the context of penile-vaginal intercourse, because to do so would be to create an illusion of a sexual union in the absence of such union. In the same-sex case, it would create an illusion of a deep union in the absence of the *possibility* of such union, an illusion that would rest on a misunderstanding of the realities involved. Not only is it that sexual union has not yet taken place together with this person, but there *cannot* be sexual union with this person.

But there is an even more serious problem in the same-sex case. In feeling united sexually with someone—and sexual pleasure is one way of having such a feeling—one is affectively treating the other person as someone with whom such union is possible. Indeed, the feeling of sexual pleasure and union is both a kind of completion of the union of erotic love, and something that calls out for erotic love by presenting the other person as erotically lovable. When these feelings are manifested toward someone with whom such union is impossible, and impossible not just due to a disability on the part of either or both (in that case, we could still say that the other is someone with whom *normally* one could unite sexually), one is affectively misconstruing the other person's nature—treating the other as in a relevant way able to be united with one, when the other is not.

The Old Testament condemned the man who slept with a man "as with a woman" (Lev. 20:13). We see here that this description is not inapt, since the feeling of sexual pleasure makes the man appreciate the other as someone with whom he is sexually uniting, but if the argument of this book is correct, he can, in principle, only sexually unite with a woman, and hence the other man is in a sense treated as a woman.

At this point, it is worth briefly and sketchily summarizing the line of argument in this book that leads to the rejection of same-sex sexual acts. We began early in the book with the idea that different kinds of love involve different kinds of consummatory union. We saw that intercourse of a sort that involves united biological reproductive striving is a distinct kind of consummatory union, and it is the union proper to romantic love, a basic form of human love. Thus, same-sex sexual activity is not the consummatory union proper to romantic love. But, nonetheless, same-sex sexual activity feels like a consummation of romantic love. However, one ought not make oneself or another have the experience of consummation of a basic form of human love.

6. TRAGIC LOVE AND A DIGRESSION ON SEXUAL REASSIGNMENT SURGERY

One may call a love that *cannot* reach its consummation "tragic." There are different kinds of tragic love. In one sense, the most tragic is where the "cannot" has the strongest sense, that of metaphysical impossibility. In that way, an intellectual friendship with a statue would be maximally tragic, since it is logically impossible to have an intellectual exchange with something mindless. In another sense, the most tragic is where the "cannot" has a weak sense, that of practical impossibility, as practical impossibility makes the impossibility of consummation more galling. A third aspect of tragedy is when the lover is unaware of the impossibility, as when one believes a statue to be a person, or woos someone secretly engaged to someone else.

Same-sex eros falls closer to the metaphysical impossibility side of the tragedy. It is impossible to unite sexually with someone not of the opposite sex. Here I want to consider the question whether this is a surmountable impossibility or an insurmountable one—namely, whether a sex-change operation could succeed in such a sense as to render someone sexually uniteable with one. If the answer is negative, this strengthens the impossibility of the completion of same-sex eros.

What defines sexual organs is their directedness toward reproduction. A penis, for instance, is not just a clump of erectile tissue, and a vagina is not just the wall of a cavity. Bodily organs are defined by their biological functions. This does not mean that, for a couple to mate, the penis and vagina need be capable of succeeding at reproduction. But the organs need to be capable of *trying* to reproduce. Now if a genetic male or female has organs expressive of the genetic sex, the organs grow because of the genes, and arguably receive their function from the organic identity of the whole—they act on behalf of the whole. For the organs to be what they are, the whole must be directing them toward reproduction. Moreover, the organs need to be appropriately connected to the rest of the body's functioning. A muscular wall of a cavity is only a *vagina* if the cavity is one that is supposed to be directed at the rest of the female reproductive system, or at least at where that system should be. A surgically created artificial "vagina" in a biological male is no more a vagina than the ear canal is, since it does not have that normative role.

Even if the *whole* of the reproductive system were transplanted, including, say, a penis, testicles, and prostate, or a vagina, clitoris, cervix, uterus, fallopian tubes, and ovaries, these organs would not have the same meaning, because surely they would not be directed toward their purposes by the whole organism. A normally functioning, genetically male human body presumably does not direct anything toward its own pregnancy and a normally-functioning, genetically female human body presumably does not direct anything toward making another person pregnant. Hormones would not help, because they would still be an *extrinsic* directing rather than an intrinsic one. Moreover, if Casey, genetically a woman, receives a transplant of Fred's reproductive system, then even if it can be argued that the system would be directed toward human reproduction, it would arguably not be directed toward reproducing *Casey* but toward reproducing Fred, since the genetic material therein derives from Fred.

It may be that if it were possible to change the genetic identity of the whole body, the person would become capable of the sexual union indicated by the newly modified body. But it is not clear that a person could survive a change of an entire chromosome throughout the body. Even if clinical death did not result, it is unclear whether the resulting human being would be *the same person* after such a momentous change. In any case, such a transformation is, at least at present, medically impossible.

Moreover, a homosexual person does not typically wish the beloved to change into being of the opposite sex, even though that would be the only way for them to be united, since then the person would no longer be of the same sex. It is a tragedy that the only way for the love to be consummated would be for one of the persons to change sex, which is at least currently impossible in the relevant sense, and even if that were done, it would probably not be what the lovers want. An additional tragedy is that sometimes the same-sex lovers believe that they *have* united in a way that consummates the love, when, in fact, they have not.

Love calls on us correctly to adjust the relationship to the reality of the other person. Same-sex eros is a love that has failed to be adjusted in this way. This failure may be nonculpable, just as a woman may, inappropriately, have eros for a man without knowing the man to be her brother (a serious danger in an age of sperm donation). Yet something has gone wrong, and to act sexually on this mistaken love is morally wrong, even when nonculpable.

One could claim that even though the love is incapable of fulfillment, it is *appropriate*. After all, some tragic loves can be appropriate. A man who has lost his sexual organs in an industrial accident can quite appropriately retain a romantic love for his wife, a love that is tragic for not being capable of being consummated.

But there is a difference between the case of the accidentally castrated man and the same-sex case, which we may get at by looking at a different pair of cases. Martha has a deep longing to engage in intellectual conversation with Francine, but Francine has suffered a brain injury that makes such conversation impossible. Martha's love needs to adapt to some degree: now she needs to seek the forms of union with Francine that are still possible. But perhaps it is quite appropriate for her also to continue to love Francine with a suffering love that seeks the intellectual communion that is no longer possible. But the case of Alfred, who has a love of intellectual companionship for his goldfish Goldie, is different. Alfred should *not* continue to love Goldie with a suffering love that seeks intellectual communion. Rather, he should love his goldfish with a love appropriate to animals. Why? Perhaps because Alfred's love mistakes the kind of being Goldie is, while Martha's love does not mistake the kind of being Francine is. Francine is a being with whom intellectual conversation would *normally* be possible, but is not under the unfortunate circumstances. On the other hand, goldfish normally cannot engage in intellectual communion.

This suggests that the kind of love that is appropriate to a pair of individuals depends on the kinds of union of which these individuals would *normally* be capable. Or, perhaps better, we might distinguish between natural, artificial, and supernatural kinds of love. Natural kinds of love are loves like fraternal, erotic, filial, and perhaps friendly,[2] in that they are based on relationships and aspects of human beings that simply follow from human nature. It is in the nature of humans to have siblings, to mate, to generate, and to cooperate. Artificial kinds of love follow upon relationships and aspects of human beings that we have created. Thus, there may be a special kind of love between scientists cooperating in the field. Such scientific cooperation is not a part of human nature as such, though it can be explained as a development based on various aspects of human nature.

On the other hand, supernatural kinds of love are tied to relationships and aspects of human beings of which humans are normally incapable, but to which they can be raised by grace. The love between fellow believers in Christ is like this, faith being a supernatural gift of God.

Now, natural loves seek a union that is possible by nature, a union that is normally possible for the individuals. If, then, a union is normally impossible to a pair of individuals, it is not appropriate for them to have a *natural* love of a sort that calls for this kind of union. In the natural loves, one loves the other as someone with whom one can *naturally* have the relevant kind of real union (in Aquinas's sense of "real union"—see section 6 of chapter 2). The love of intellectual communion is, in fact, a quite natural love. We are rational animals, and shared intellectual exploration is quite normal for us. However, to engage in this natural love with a goldfish, at least when the union is actually impossible,[3] is not to be faithful to the kind of love. Being tragic is not something normal in the case of an appropriate instance of natural love, as normally an appropriate instance of natural love can be consummated.

Even if it were possible to make a person receive the sexual organs of the opposite sex, so that the functioning of these organs were genuinely directed toward the person's reproduction, this would not be a normal state. Whether erotic love would be appropriate in such a case is a question for further investigation; I suspect that because erotic love is natural, the answer is negative. However, in any case, a mere fictional possibility of such reception is not enough to make erotic love appropriate. Indeed, erotic love appreciates the other as biologically embodied, and appreciating the other in respect of an *outré* nonnatural possibility—the possibility of being united in fictional circumstances—is not enough to ground erotic love. Thus, same-sex erotic love is not only tragic but inappropriate—it could, at best, attain union by the other's body being radically and artificially changed in precisely those respects that are most relevant to eros. And an inappropriate love is morally inappropriate, since having appropriate love is central to morality.

Nonetheless, it is possible for a morally mistaken relationship to be a source of personal growth and an arena for the exercise of virtue. It is hard to deny, for instance, that the siblings who love each other erotically while not knowing that they are siblings might grow in various ways, enter into a marital relationship they believe to be a valid marriage, and exercise many marital virtues. Nonetheless, the sexual activity within the relationship is wrong, and the relationship as a whole is a distortion of the one that they would have had if they succeeded in following love's call to make the relationship correspond to reality. This failure of theirs may be completely innocent, but it is nonetheless a failure. Innocent failures are just another instance of the fallenness of our world.

Moreover, the couple is *harmed* by the immoral relationship, because one is always less well off for doing something morally wrong, even if one is entirely nonculpable. In the case of incest we can well imagine that if the couple discovered the fact of their incest, they would see their happiness over the past years as in significant part a tragic sham. Their erotic attraction might not immediately disappear—indeed, might never disappear—and it might be a source of suffering and tragic love for years to come. But even if one of them should discover the facts only after the death of the other, pain would no doubt result. If a friend of theirs knew that their relationship was incestuous but did not tell them, the couple would rightly have a claim against the friend—they could rightly complain that the friend harmed them by allowing them to continue in this relationship.

7. WHAT SHOULD ONE DO?

If the above arguments succeed, then same-sex sexual activity directed at orgasm is morally wrong, since in orgasm the couple feels a union that is, in fact, absent. I have also argued that genuinely erotic love can exist between persons of the same sex. Nonetheless, this love is mistaken on its own terms, since it is of the essence of erotic love to seek a sexual union as one body, and two persons of the same sex lack the biological complementarity that would make such a union possible. Erotic love is a love that should exist only between a man and a woman. Thus the love has failed to adapt to the realities of the situation.

Such a failure may, of course, be quite inculpable. But what if a homosexual person finds himself or herself in this position of erotic love for someone of the same sex and becomes convinced by these or other considerations that there is a central distortion or mistake in the form of love? What is the agent morally expected to do about this tragic situation? Could the agent continue in the relationship, reasoning that it was wrong to have entered it, but it would cause too much emotional hurt, to self and especially other, to terminate it?

The answer here is surely negative. To continue to act out of the distorted or mistaken aspects of love is to fail to act out of love's more basic call to adapt to the situation. One has come to understand, say, that the union that previously seemed attainable and appropriate was not attainable, that sexual activity would only give an illusion of attainment, and that the love does not fit the situation. As soon as one understands this, love's basic adaptability requires one to strive to change the form of love. Moreover, love is expressed in action, and is in part constituted by acts of will or dispositions to acts of will. To act and will as if one had a more appropriate form of love already, and to refrain from acting according to the inappropriate form of love, is already to have that more appropriate form of love, at least in part.

At the same time, the genuine commitments of love must be fulfilled. If one has unconditionally committed oneself to love the other person for life, that commitment must be fulfilled, albeit with a new form of love. Circumstances may be such that this commitment will have to be fulfilled at a distance—for instance, if it turns out to be impossible to explain one's reasons for discontinuing the erotic aspects of the relationship to the other. But one can love at a distance—one can appreciate the good of someone, and will good to the person, having a readiness to act overtly should overt action become possible. And as for the question of what new form the love should take, this is one of those ethical questions to which there is no general answer. We can say in general that the love should not be erotic. But which exact form it should take, whether that of intellectual or emotional or spiritual friendship, or collegiality, or conviviality, or something completely different, surely depends on details of the individual situation.

One might worry that love at a distance is content-free. But the sexual abstinence *itself* is now an aspect of the love—one abstains because one now appreciates the other for who the other *really* is, someone with whom one can unite only nonsexually. The abstinence, thus, is an aspect of respect and appreciation, though of course the other may not see it this way. And if one has any commitments incompatible with chastity, then these commitments are not morally binding, since one cannot be morally bound to do something wrong. Finally, if one is a theist, there is one further way to express love at a distance. One can *pray* for the other, with pathos and intensity, with fasting and self-denial, with great persistence. Insofar as one is doing this, one is living a suffering love.

Still, it may be that the commitment to the other was not unconditional. It could be that the love's commitment was implicitly conditional on the other being the sort of person with whom it would be possible to unite sexually. If so, then there is no duty arising from this commitment to maintain the special nonsexual aspects of the love. However, since in any case there is a general duty to love every human being, love needs to remain.

There is an objection that could be made. Suppose that as a contingent psychological fact, the obligations of one's love cannot be lived out apart from a sexual relationship. Perhaps one finds it psychologically impossible to both abstain and to love. What should take precedence? Here the great variety of forms of love can help: surely some appropriate form of love will be possible, at least with God's grace. In love, one ought not to treat someone as what the person is not. One needs to adopt a form of love that treats the other in an appropriate manner.

Now, one may object, all of this seems greatly unfair, especially to someone who was not culpable for getting into the relationship.

After all, heterosexuals are not called to any such sacrifices, the objection goes.

Three things can be said in reply. First, it is indeed true that moral duties are not always apportioned in what we think of as a "fair" way. Each parent has a duty to care for her children. But some parents' children are disabled, and the duties are thus more onerous. Some parents find that the other parent is unhelpful. That is unfair, but they need to make up for the slacker. Some people find themselves in circumstances where keeping their commitments requires moral heroism, while others seem to glide through life without such a case. That is what life in a fallen world is like.

Second, a Christian response can go beyond these harsh facts, since Christians hold that there is loving providence behind them. How providence works is mysterious, but it is plausible that providence makes what seem to be unfair circumstances actually be fair, perhaps by lavishing more grace on those of whom more is required—which grace makes possible the greater rewards that come from accepting this grace and rising to the occasion. Abraham was asked to leave his native land and later to sacrifice his son, while David was asked no such thing. But Abraham was given the graces needed for these actions, and now he is the father of faith.

Third, similar trials can happen in opposite-sex relationships. A heterosexual Christian might marry, divorce, and remarry, not realizing that the unconditionality and exclusivity of the initial marital commitments made the divorce and one's subsequent remarriage a mere legal fiction. At this point, the Christian is obliged, out of fidelity to his or her spouse from the first marriage, to cease from the sexual aspects of the new relationship, since the new relationship is objectively adulterous (see chapter 6). There may be no culpability, but setting things right can be just as difficult when there is no culpability as when there is. It may, after all, be quite impossible to go back to the first spouse—the first spouse may not wish to have one—but nonetheless one's commitment to unconditionality and sexual fidelity is binding.

It can indeed be difficult to set things right when one has done wrong, even inculpably so. One can acquire onerous obligations through no fault of one's own. One can even find oneself with onerous obligations that one literally did nothing to earn—say, when one needs to take care of a severely disabled sibling because one's parents have died. Nonetheless, there are corresponding moral rewards.

A different kind of difficulty of the moral prohibition on same-sex sexual activity is with the obligations incumbent on a homosexual person who has not entered into a relationship. Such a person is morally obliged to refrain from sexual activity and to try to keep from developing a love that misapprehends the reality of the situation. It may well be that understanding the meaning of love, and realizing the availability of other forms of love than eros, such as deep friendship, would be helpful here. But ultimately, the Christian insists, it is all grace.

One may, of course, ask various practical questions. Is it morally acceptable to have a deep friendship with someone of the same sex when one is attracted to this person, for instance? Is it acceptable to kiss, hold hands, hug, and so forth? For a lot of these questions, it is not possible to give answers that are both precise and universally applicable (for instance, in some cultures, same-sex kissing is a standard greeting ritual). Similar practical questions come up in opposite-sex cases, as we saw in section 10 of the previous chapter. The question of how to express affection and whether it is acceptable to have a deep friendship with someone to whom one is attracted sexually, when marriage and hence sex are not options, is a general one, applicable to persons of all sexual orientations. It is questions like this that are the *really* difficult questions of morality.

Where it is a question of clear-cut negative duties, such as the duty not to have sex with someone to whom one is not married, the difficulty is in doing one's duty, not in figuring out what to do. But when it is a question of how to act positively, what sort of friendship to enter into, and how to express the friendship, typically there is no general formula. We can at most list some of the salient factors in such a decision that will need to be balanced: the likelihood of oneself being tempted and of tempting the other, the expected intellectual, moral, emotional, material, and spiritual gains to self and other from the relationship, the history, if any, of the relationship, other preexisting obligations, social expectations, and customs, whether the beloved is being led on or deceived, perceptions of others, and so on. Such lists of salient factors are never exhaustive, and the devil is in the details. That is why the Christian tradition of both the West and the East emphasizes the importance of spiritual advisors who know one well.

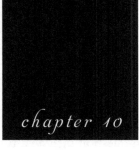

chapter 10

Reproduction and Technology

1. INTRODUCTION

Without the use of special methods, human beings reproduce in two different ways. Our primary way is to reproduce sexually through intercourse, but we also have a less common mode of asexual reproduction through the twinning of an embryo. The causes of the latter are not yet known, but it occurs only in the first fourteen days after fertilization, prior to implantation—the embryo either splits in two or else a new one buds from the old one. Since reproduction by twinning is not subject to our will, it can be omitted in much of the discussion, however.

I have argued that it is morally wrong to engage in orgasmic activity apart from mating, which is the activity that is directed biologically at (perhaps among other things) reproduction. The question now is whether it is morally acceptable to deliberately reproduce in a way that does not involve sexual intercourse. If the answer is positive, then reproductive technologies that work in the context of intercourse, for instance by improving sperm migration, might be acceptable, but other technologies will not be. Earlier in the book, we have seen that it is wrong, and in a certain sense even impossible, to have the unitive aspect of sex without the procreative. The question now is whether it is wrong to have the reproductive aspect without the unitive.

The technologies in question include artificial insemination and in vitro fertilization. One can both ask the general question whether any such technologies are acceptable and also consider special moral questions raised by particular technologies. For instance, in the next section, I shall argue specifically that sperm donation is wrong because of the detached and anonymous way it is practiced.

Likewise, if embryos are persons, then in vitro fertilization at least as currently practiced in the United States tends to result in the production of a significant number of children whose maturation one does not plan on supporting past the embryonic stage. Since it is a basic human duty to nurture children into adulthood, the production of children who, in one's plan, will remain in a freezer for the rest of their lives—or, worse, be killed or used for medical experiments—is surely wrong.

Moreover, most fertility treatments require the couple's persistence in the treatment over a significant period of time, and anecdotal evidence suggests that such treatments can lead a couple to have negative feelings about sexuality.

But we can have a case of reproduction, outside the context of intercourse, where no such special issues come up as with in vitro fertilization or sperm donation. Suppose that a husband has a blockage in the urethra that cannot be repaired, and so fertilization is done by surgically moving sperm from his testicles to his wife's uterus outside the context of intercourse. The husband fully intends to exercise his parental duties, and the wife intends that any resulting embryos should implant and be brought to maturity. Observe that the goal in the action is good—the existence of a new human being and the couple's joint opportunity for loving the new human being. But good goals are not enough—for a right action the means need to be acceptable, too.

It would seem quite consistent with the rest of this book to argue that the significance of intercourse is its connection to reproduction, but reproduction has an innate value independent of intercourse, thereby making it acceptable to seek reproduction apart from inter-course, but not intercourse apart from some connection to reproduction. I shall argue that there are coherent objections, however, which militate against this position. In examining this question, we will also have to sharpen our understanding of the unitive aspect of intercourse.

2. GAMETE DONATION

In this section, I will argue that at least most cases of sperm and egg donation in Western countries are wrong. I think *all* cases are wrong, but this argument does not show it. The argument will be stronger in some cases than in others. Let me begin with the observation that some of the most basic positive human duties are those that flow from the parent-child relationship: the duty of children to respect their parents and take care of them in their times of need (especially old age), and the duty of parents to care for and educate their children morally, religiously, and academically.

For my argument, I only need the duty of parents to children. It is a controversial question whether this duty exists always, or only in the case where the parenthood resulted in a consensual way. But the argument only needs the duty in the case of consensual parenthood.

Now, it is not merely the duty of the parents to bring it about that the children are cared for and appropriately educated morally, religiously, and academically. Rather, it is the duty of the parents to care for and educate the child—i.e., to do it *themselves*. In caring for and educating the child, parents will make use of the help of others, including that of family members, friends, and professionals. How much the parents can rely on the help of others before they have failed in their duty of caring for and educating the child will depend on the circumstances.

There are thus two aspects of the parental duty: (a) caring for and educating, and (b) ensuring that the child is cared for and educated. In other words, there is the aspect of parental activity and the aspect of results. These two aspects need to be balanced prudently, and, moreover, balanced with other duties the parents may have; how they are balanced will depend on particular circumstances. In no cases will it be desirable and rarely will it be possible for the parents directly to care for and educate the child in all respects with the help of no one else. Moral education, for instance, requires contact with virtuous people of a significant variety of different characters, not just the parents. Academic education should typically include education in subjects in which the parents lack competency. The need to work to earn money to provide for the child can force the parents to delegate a significant degree of care to a third party.

Here is an observation worth making. In most couples, there will be specialization. Thus, the mother might be working long hours to earn the money needed to diaper, feed, clothe, and house the child, while the father might be changing the diapers, feeding, clothing, and otherwise taking care of the child for most of the day. It might seem that in such cases, each parent will be neglecting an aspect of the parental responsibility to *himself or herself* care for and educate the child. But we can respond to this by noting that parents should be friends of each other, and bringing in an idea from Aristotle's *Nicomachean Ethics*. Aristotle considers what value there is in having good friends. He observes that friends share a life, a friend is "another self," and one can be active through one's friend's activity: what the friend does virtuously is something that accrues to oneself.[1]

We do act vicariously through our close friends, in such a way that we can say, "*We* did it." If the parents are friends of one another, then each fulfills his or her responsibilities also through the other. After all, insofar as they are friends, each strives to make it possible for the other to act, and they act cooperatively. Thus, there is a real sense in which the father who stayed home with the child can say: "*We* earned the money," and the mother who was away from home can say: "*We* fed the child." (Of course, such statements can be somewhat indecent when the burdens are particularly unequal: it is somewhat indecent for the father to say "We gave birth," and the common locution "We are pregnant" can be criticized, too.) If this is right, then it is also preferable that the parents cooperate closely with, and even be friends with, the professionals who help them in the care of and education of their children.

It is not possible to give precise and general rules about when exactly it is permissible for parents to "outsource" a part of their parental activity. These things must be decided in prudence by the couple. However, we can say that completely handing over the care and education of one's child to a person one does not know very well would *not* be a fulfillment of one's parental responsibilities. In tragic circumstances where one is unable to fulfill one's parental responsibilities by providing oneself for the child's needs, handing over the child for adoption is the best way to do what one can for the child. But it is not the case that by handing the child over to the care of another one has *fulfilled* one's parental responsibilities. It is clear that, at least as long as one's child is a child, one has parental responsibilities—one has not *fulfilled* them in the sense in which one might fulfill a promise and thus be done with it. Rather, the case of adoption is a case where, through tragic circumstances, one was unable to fulfill one's responsibilities, and so one did the best one could in terms of partial fulfillment, and if one was not responsible for one's inability to fulfill the responsibilities, doing one's best here makes one not be culpable for the failure.

It would plainly be wrong to court the kinds of tragic circumstances that make one need to give one's child over to be raised by another. In general, barring a proportionately serious reason, we should not consent to circumstances where we will not be fulfilling a serious personal responsibility. In fact, barring a proportionately serious reason, we should not even consent to circumstances where there is a high likelihood of our failing to fulfill a serious personal responsibility (see also section 7 of chapter 6). If we have duties to care for others, such as children, a spouse, or parents, we have a duty not to engage in extremely dangerous activities such as skating on thin ice, barring proportionately serious reasons. Of course, proportionately serious reasons might arise. One might need to literally skate on thin ice in order to save someone's life, though then one should do so in a way that minimizes the danger of nonfulfillment of responsibilities. (One should ideally have paid up one's life insurance, and one should move on the ice in a way that minimizes danger of death.)

But now consider a case of gamete donation. Only in rare cases will the donor have *any* participation in the care and education of the child, even a participation through friendship with those caring for and educating the child. In the typical case, there will be no participation at all. In sperm donation, the donor generally does not even know *who* is the recipient of the gametes, at best only having read or heard the screening criteria. Were the sperm donor somehow to find out who received the donation and show up, years later, asking to participate substantially in the care and education of his child, the chance of his offer being accepted is slim.

Therefore, the gamete donor gives up the fulfillment of parental responsibilities toward the child. At least in Western countries, donors typically do not find themselves in tragic circumstances that provide them with a proportionately serious reason to undergo the donation procedure. We can imagine a case of someone donating gametes to avoid family starvation. But in Western countries, this is not typically the way it happens because, first, *actual* starvation is rare due to social services, and, second, recipients have a preference for donors with a good education, hoping that this indicates "good genes," whereas persons in grinding poverty tend to be less well-educated.

Typical cases of gamete donation, thus, involve consenting to have a child toward whom one does not plan to fulfill one's parental responsibilities. This is wrong, at least if there are no tragic economic circumstances compelling the donor. (And if the arguments in the succeeding sections are right, it is wrong even then.)

I now turn to consider four objections. The first is that mere genetic derivation is insufficient for parental responsibility, even if this genetic derivation is consensual. The idea behind this objection is that mere genetic derivation is of little moral significance. One might strengthen this by noting that consensual genetic derivation is not *necessary* for parental responsibility, since adoptive parents have parental responsibility, and then one might ask why consensual genetic derivation should be thought sufficient.

One difficulty with this objection is that it is difficult to spell out what one can put in the place of genetic derivation as the condition for parental responsibility. It would not be plausible, for instance, to require one, for the acquisition of parental responsibility, to engage in some kind of overt act of responsibility assumption beyond the physical acts involved in genetic derivation. After all, one could well count as a negligent parent even if one never overtly assumed responsibility for any of one's reproductive actions.

A second difficulty with the objection to our argument is that if genetic derivation is not sufficient for parental responsibility, there is a problem in justifying the clearly appropriate practice of requiring child support payments from fathers who had no relation to the child besides having sex with the mother.

It might, though, be argued that the duty of making child support payments is not grounded in *parental* responsibility, but simply in some more general duty, such as the duty to alleviate hardships one has caused. In this case, one has caused a hardship to the child by bringing it about that the child is raised in difficult circumstances, and so one has the duty to alleviate the hardship. But now note that if *this* is what the duty to make child support payments is grounded in, then anybody else who makes a similar causal contribution to the hardships of another has a similar duty. Suppose, for instance, that a counselor advised Susie to go ahead and have sex with her husband Fred. Susie did this, she got pregnant, and the circumstances were difficult. The counselor made a causal contribution to the hardships suffered by the child, but surely is not liable for child support in the same way that a father is.

Observe that in order to acquire the duty of child support, one need not even act in a way that makes it particularly *probable* that a child will come into existence. After all, if contraception is correctly used, the probability that one's acts will lead to the existence of a child will be slim. But no matter how small the probability that the father's acts will lead to the existence of the child, we take it that there is a duty of child support. Suppose that methods of contraception were used by the father that ensured that the chance of conception would be extremely small: for instance, the father had a vasectomy, *and* used a condom with an extremely effective spermicide, *and* ensured that the mother was on the pill. Nonetheless, very unlikely events do, in fact, happen. As a society, we hold the father to have a duty of child support, even if the father acted in a way that, say, resulted only in a one in a million chance of conception. On the other hand, the counselor's advice might have had a rather higher chance of resulting in conception, since there was, let us suppose, a high chance of the couple acting on it, and the counselor might know that the couple's method of contraception was an oral contraceptive, without addition of the vasectomy, the condom, or the spermicide.

It could be that child support is just a matter of positive law, akin to strict liability in torts, not grounded in some prior moral duty. But I think it fits better with our intuitions to suppose that the basic duty of child support is grounded in a moral duty to care for one's children, and positive law simply determines some of the details of this duty.

Perhaps, though, this moral duty is acquired through intercourse and only through intercourse, and hence not through organ donation. This would lead to the absurd conclusion that if a contracepting couple had penile-vaginal intercourse and pregnancy resulted, then child support would be owed, but if the contracepting couple decided to inject the woman with the man's sperm just because they thought it would be kinky, then child support would not be owed.

There is a final difficulty with the idea that mere genetic derivation, even if consensual, is of low moral significance. For this idea is in tension with one of the main reasons why a woman might make use of sperm donation instead of adopting a child, namely, that she thinks that *her* biological parenthood is important.

A second objection to the argument against gamete donation is that there is no duty to care for and educate children, but only a duty to ensure that one's children are cared for and educated. But the gamete donor can be confident, the objection continues, that the couples that the clinic allows to receive the donation will be selected in such a way that they will provide loving homes for the children, where the children will be cared for and educated, if a sufficiently reputable clinic is involved.

One response to be made is simply to insist that the duty is to care for and educate, not just to ensure care and education. But there is a second response possible in *many* cases of gamete donation, which response works in just about all cases where the donation is made to a clinic rather than to a couple that one knows. Let us suppose for the sake of the argument that the duty is just to ensure care and education. But now let me suppose that my reader has children, or at least can imagine having children, and put my response in the form of the question: What percentage of couples in your country would you actually trust to care for and educate your children?

You might reasonably have some confidence that an average couple would physically care for your children well, would not abuse the children, and so on. But what percentage of couples, even ones selected by a clinic's social worker based on socioeconomic, educational, and relationship criteria, would you trust to provide your child with the kind of moral, religious (if any), and academic education that you think the child should receive? This is a particularly pressing question in a diverse society. For instance, in the United States, no religious group constitutes the majority of the population. Thus, if you live in the United States, then no matter what your religious affiliation (counting lack of religion as an affiliation), the likelihood that a recipient couple will provide the child with the kind of religious education (if any) of which you approve is less than fifty percent. But given the centrality to life of religion, getting religious education right (and of course some may think this means not providing any religious education and simply letting the child choose, and some may think this means providing an atheistic education) is an important part of parental responsibilities. Hence, if you live in the United States, you should think that the couple chosen by the clinic will more likely not provide the right kind of religious upbringing for your child.

Once one adds moral and academic education to the mix, you will surely have to think the likelihood to be slim that a couple chosen by the clinic will provide the right kind of education for your child, except perhaps if you happen to live in a rather monolithic society and agree with the monolithically accepted views and approach to parenting. Thus, in typical cases in Western countries, you should *not* think that even the results-aspect of the parental responsibilities will be fulfilled by the recipient couple.

The third objection (made by a commenter on my blog)[2] is that it is possible for, say, a sperm donor to be released from parental responsibilities by the prospective mother. After all, parents do have significant authority over their children, and so perhaps this authority extends to relieving the other parent of responsibility.

But this is mistaken. It is not possible for one parent simply to *relieve* the other of responsibility, since the responsibility is not owed to the parent but to the child. At most one can talk of *transfer* of responsibility, either transfer to the parent who remains responsible and who now has double the responsibility, or transfer to a third party.

So now the question is whether it is possible for the mother to transfer the father's responsibility to herself (I shall, for linguistic simplicity, stick to the sperm donation case) or to someone else, in such a way that the father no longer has parental responsibility. Here, I think, the answer is negative.

Suppose Bob and Martha are a married couple with five children. Bob becomes an abusive alcoholic, and Martha, who is sober and responsible, kicks him out, saying that he no longer has any responsibilities toward the children, and that Martha will take much better care of them alone than with Bob. If it is possible to transfer responsibility, this would seem to be a paradigmatic case where such transfer is appropriate. But let me continue with the story. A month later, Bob joins Alcoholics Anonymous, and for the next two years or so he is sober. On the other hand, over these two years, Martha herself turns more and more to alcohol. She loses her job. She refuses to buy clothes and food for the children, so as to have money for drink. Finally, she becomes physically abusive. The children knock on Bob's door, begging for help. Bob, however, tells them that he has no parental responsibilities toward them as these were transferred to Martha. Of course, he has the normal human responsibilities for fellow human beings, and so he will do what he would for any set of five children in these circumstances: he will call Social Services on their behalf, and let them wait in his living room until Social Services arrives to take charge of them.

Leaving aside the legal aspects of the case, it is clear that Bob is neglecting his parental responsibility. Martha's effort to relieve him from his responsibilities did not, in fact, remove his special parental responsibility. At most, it gave him reason not to attempt to fulfill this responsibility during the time period when she was more sober than he.

One could, of course, say that when Martha began to neglect her parental responsibility, the transferred responsibility bounced back to Bob. But that seems a poor way to analyze the situation. After all, responsibility isn't some kind of magical fluid that flows between people. Rather, there are facts about what duties one has and to whom. And it is clear from the case that even after Martha kicked Bob out, Bob continued to have the conditional duty to ensure that the children should be cared for if Martha failed to care for them successfully. But this responsibility is one that Bob had *all along*, in virtue of his parental responsibility for the children. Therefore, at least a part of Bob's parental responsibilities remained despite Martha's alleged transfer.

If this is right, then even if a transfer of parental responsibility is possible, such a transfer can only be partial. One *still* has the responsibility to ensure the care and education of the child *if* no one else is caring and educating the child appropriately. But if this is right, then gamete donors have a problem. For they are not relieved of the responsibility to ensure that the child is appropriately cared for and educated, though in typical cases this is a responsibility which they are not in a position to fulfill. Moreover, if my response to the second objection was correct, gamete donors living in a diverse society have reason to think that the child is, more likely than not, being *inappropriately* educated.

A further, and perhaps deeper, problem plagues the parental responsibility transfer hypothesis once we recall that we need to *ourselves* care for the child. The parental responsibility transfer only has a hope of success when the subject to whom the responsibility has been transferred is successfully fulfilling the transferred responsibility. But parental responsibility makes essential reference to the particular, individual parents. It is not just my responsibility to ensure that my children are cared for; it is my responsibility that *I* care for and educate my children, and no one but I can fulfill this responsibility. By ensuring that someone else cares for and educates my children, the responsibility that my children be cared for is perhaps fulfilled. But the second responsibility is not, since another's care is not my care, except, as we saw, in cases of continuing friendship or other close cooperation. But these cases are not what happens in typical instances of gamete donation. A stranger cannot do *my* caring for and educating of my children, for then it is not *my* caring and educating, but the stranger's.

In fact, I suspect that parental responsibility also involves an individual responsibility to ensure that *both* parents be appropriately caring for and educating the child. A part of fulfilling this responsibility is striving to ensure that the other parent is a suitable caregiver and educator, holding the other accountable as needed. If the mother were able to transfer the father's responsibility onto herself or onto another, then she would be bringing it about that *she* no longer has the responsibility to ensure that *the father* appropriately care for and educate the child. But it does not seem likely that she can relieve herself of such a responsibility.

For a fourth objection to the argument against gamete donation, let us suppose the objector grants in light of the above that gamete donation ought not be engaged in except for a grave and proportionate reason, given the nonfulfillment of the donor's responsibilities. But two grave and proportionate reasons are available: (a) the donor enables a recipient couple (the argument is stronger in the case where there is a couple on the receiving end) to enjoy the goods of parenthood, and (b) the donor's actions lead to the existence of a new and unique human being, an existence that the donor has reason to hope will be a happy one.

I will first argue that the first reason is inappropriate on its own, and then that they are not proportionate together, either. With regard to enabling the goods of parenthood, consider the following story of the generous hosts. The generous hosts have a small infant. A childless couple visits their home during a party. The hosts know little about the couple except that the couple was recently certified fit to be adoptive parents by a local social worker. The couple admires their infant with evident longing and suffering in their faces. The hosts confer, and say: "If you like her so much, you can have her." It seems clear that something has gone wrong here. To give over one's child to another simply because it will make the other happy is surely wrong. First, it is incompatible with the dignity of one's child to be given to another to allow the other to enjoy personal fulfillment. The deed rather resembles the case of cultural conventions that dictate that the host give a guest any possessions that the guest admires and treats the child as a possession. Second, one ought not be generous in this way at the cost of having significant unfulfilled parental responsibilities. Such reasons of generosity are not commensurate with the duty to avoid putting oneself in a position of significant unfulfilled parental responsibility.

Next, consider the case of what one might call "the irresponsible couple." Both members of this couple know that they are incapable of taking good care of their children. But nonetheless they engage in sexual relations, without bothering to take any care to avoid conception, whether through contraception or periodic abstinence. They reason that if they should conceive, they will just give the child up for adoption—there are always couples waiting to adopt in their society, we may suppose—and a new and unique human being will come into an existence that one has reason to hope will be a happy one, while a childless couple will be able to experience the joys of parenthood. There is something deeply wrong in the couple's behavior. The problem seems to be that the couple is violating strong reasons grounded in responsibility, in favor of reasons grounded in something like generosity or beneficence. The two are putting themselves in a position where they will be unable to live out the love they will owe to their own children, one of the most important natural loves. But if (a) and (b) justify gamete donation, they also justify the activity of the irresponsible couple. Hence, (a) and (b) do not justify gamete donation.

The four objections to the argument thus fail. Barring a better objection, we need to conclude that most cases of gamete donation in Western countries are wrong, even without considering general questions about assisted methods of reproduction. They are wrong in much the way in which, barring tragic circumstances, it would be wrong for a man and a woman to sign a contract (for whatever reason, whether of generosity or financial advantage) with a clinic to hand over the child resulting from their first pregnancy for adoption by a couple of the clinic's choice.

3. UNITY AND PROCREATION

Sexual union receives its unitive significance from the fact that it is a reproductive-type union—a union of such a sort that the couple's activity includes all the intentional actions that would normally be needed for procreation. I have argued that it is wrong to engage in sex outside of a marital relationship, because that would produce an illusion of full interpersonal union while the union lacked the same fullness. It is wrong to have the pleasure of union without the union itself. Moreover, a willingness to unite sexually outside of marriage (e.g., before marriage) makes one experience sex as less than the most thoroughgoing union possible.

Now, noncoital techniques of reproduction do not make two parents into a single biological organism, because they do not involve the mutual cooperative striving of their bodies on a biological level. Except in cloning and other forms of asexual reproduction, there certainly can be much voluntary cooperative striving—sperm is collected in some way or other with the man's cooperation, the woman becomes pregnant voluntarily, and so on. In coital reproduction, however, the central elements of the cooperative striving typically involve processes that are either instinctive or outside of direct voluntary control, and hence there is another, biological or animal, level to the union.

We are rational *animals,* and coital reproduction emphasizes the animal aspects. Thus, typically, ejaculation does not happen as a result of a positive act of will—it is elicited by means of the sexual excitation that happens through the joint activity of the couple. With training a man can perhaps control ejaculation. But the primary sort of control, even there, is probably not so much ejaculation-on-demand as an ability to "hold back," a phrase that in itself suggests that in the typical case the process is not directly voluntary. Likewise, on the side of the woman, providing tactile stimulation by means of the vagina to elicit ejaculation is typically not directly voluntary, though allowing penetration needs to be voluntary, nor is the acceptance of the seminal fluid into the reproductive system and the partial control of its flow by means of the cervix directly voluntary. Rather, the couple wills the process as a whole, and their organic systems take care of much of it.

But the issue here is not so much the voluntary versus the nonvoluntary. After all, we know that through training many bodily functions which are normally nonvoluntary can be controlled. We could imagine a man and a woman who control almost every aspect of their sexual intercourse, and surely sexual union for them would not be wrong. Rather, the nonvoluntariness here is a way of bringing out the fact that the processes are strongly biologically natural, in the sense that they are processes to which biological human nature specifically impels us. They are not merely natural in the sense in which everything we do rationally that is not contrary to nature is natural, for we do many things rationally to which we are not specifically impelled by biological nature, like read books or dance waltzes. But the processes are strongly biologically natural in the way in which eating or breathing or blood circulation are. Observe that eating *as such* is strongly biologically natural, but eating beef is not, at least not *as eating of beef*—nothing in our nature gives us a biological directedness toward the eating of beef specifically.

It is the fact that coital reproductive processes are strongly biologically natural in their essentials that makes coital reproduction have the one-flesh unitive significance it does. There is nothing morally problematic, of course, in engaging in some processes that are not strongly biologically natural, at least as long as they are not positively unnatural. Writing and reading this book is not strongly biologically natural. Nor is there anything innately inferior in a process that is not strongly biologically natural. Indeed, the Christian tradition has tended to elevate some spiritual activities over the merely biologically natural. But those processes that are not strongly biologically natural nonetheless lack the meaning that comes from the embodiment in our biological nature. And activities done in common that are not strongly biologically natural fail to constitute a union as a single biological organism—they are, thus, in that respect less unitive.

The couple's activity in voluntary noncoital reproduction is not strongly biologically natural.[3] Thus, the union to which the activity gives rise is not the thoroughgoing union as one organism that is the consummation of romantic love. Now the reason coitus gives rise to sexual union lies in the reproductive directedness of coitus. If voluntary noncoital reproduction were morally permissible, then a couple could achieve the union that romantic love seeks in one set of acts, namely intercourse, while achieving the goal which gives meaning to those acts through a very different act, namely noncoital reproduction.

The first thing to note about such an option is that it would weaken the felt connection between intercourse and reproduction for the couple. What made intercourse the appropriate consummation for romantic love was the great significance of the end toward which the bodies were united in striving. But noncoital forms of reproduction render coitus less significant since coitus is no longer the only morally available way to reproduce voluntarily. In weakening the connection between intercourse and reproduction, intercourse is made less significant to the couple. Moreover, insofar as intercourse is the consummation of romantic love, romantic love itself is made less significant, in the way that premarital sex weakens the significance of marriage from its status as being the only morally acceptable venue for sexual activity (as it was argued to be in chapter 6). Moreover, the couple that has intercourse regularly but that reproduces noncoitally would likely come to see intercourse in terms of something other than a reproductive striving, and this would further decrease the felt significance of intercourse. This decrease would be qualitative, not merely quantitative.

Now a qualitative decrease in the felt significance of intercourse has to come along with one of three things. Either the couple would downgrade the level of union for which their romantic love strives, or they would no longer see love's union as consummated in intercourse, or they would recognize a gap between feeling and reality in intercourse. The first two outcomes are clearly undesirable. The third is less problematic, but since feelings are an important secondary aspect of sexual union, a gap between feeling and reality in intercourse would be a definitely negative outcome.

But one might instead argue that love's union is not consummated in an instant, but by a whole series of acts, including acts of interpersonal interaction, acts of intercourse, as well as, possibly, acts of noncoital reproduction. Thus, the objection goes, the couple that reproduces noncoitally has decreased the unitive meaning of intercourse in their lives but they have reintroduced this significance elsewhere, namely, in their noncoital reproductive activity.

However, the response appears incorrect. For intercourse is still sufficient for their one-flesh union, assuming emotional, intellectual, and spiritual closeness as well as the relevant commitments, without any of the noncoital reproductive activity. A married infertile couple who does not engage in noncoital reproductive activity can still have the consummation of union in romantic love—they become one organism, and can be united emotionally, intellectually, and spiritually in an appropriately committed way.

While romantic love has a directedness toward children, and while sexual union is defined in terms of the reproductive teleology of the sexual act, nonetheless a thoroughgoing union can be achieved apart from having children. Children are a good that we intend for our romantic beloved, but union comes from the common seeking of this good, not the common *achievement* of the good. The people working together to get a candidate elected are united by their common striving, and are no less united if their candidate is not elected.

Having children together makes possible many unitive activities, such as bathing the child, discussing schooling options, or being worried together when the child is ill. But not having children of one's own also makes possible many unitive activities, such as trying to have or adopt a child, or devoting more of the couple's time to common prayer, study, and charitable activity directed beyond the confines of the family. While romantic love makes one desire for the other the goods particularly appropriate to romantic love, and this involves the goods of reproduction and education of children, something is not lacking from love's *union* when these striven-for goods are absent.

However, the infertile couple that has intercourse regularly but reproduces noncoitally may say that if they had not engaged in, say, in vitro fertilization, they would not be seriously striving for reproduction, and hence they would be lacking in the *striving* that is unitive. They might argue that the infertile couple for whom noncoital reproduction is not technically or economically possible unites fully in intercourse, but an infertile couple for whom noncoital reproduction *is* technically and economically feasible would not be fully united if they limited themselves to acts of intercourse which, in their case, are sterile. Now one might question here the economic feasibility of noncoital reproduction for *any* couple concerned about social justice, given the high costs of the medical procedures involved, money that might be better spent providing basic care to people in parts of the world where basic care is lacking. But let us put that concern to the side, important as it is.

Instead, we can simply respond that an infertile couple that refrains from in vitro fertilization for *moral* reasons is not any less serious about reproductive striving than the couple that reproduces noncoitally: both are doing all that they believe to be morally possible. We need to recognize constraints beyond those of technical and economic feasibility.

Moreover, the view that love's union is achieved for the infertile couple only when they *both* have intercourse *and* engage in all the feasible reproductive technologies—or maybe all the feasible *morally permissible* reproductive technologies—is one that may preclude any notion of a consummation where at least the specifically romantic aspects of the union are *fulfilled*. The same argument that claimed that the striving was not serious unless noncoital forms of reproduction were tried would imply that as long as more could be attempted in the way of reproduction, one would not be fully serious in the reproductive striving. But there is *always* more that could be attempted. Even if the funds for noncoital reproduction run out, one can fall back on coitus—again and again, without consummation being achieved at any point, because there is always more that can be done for reproduction, since one can always have sex again another day. If it is true that as long as more can be done, consummation has not been achieved, then consummation is never achieved by the infertile couple that never succeeds in having children. And that is surely false. For we should say that they were, in fact, successful at consummation each time they had intercourse (at least assuming no barrier methods of contraception were used).

In fact, the same reasoning would imply that whether the couple is fertile or not, they have not achieved love's union until they *succeeded* in reproducing. But why stop there? The same kind of "real seriousness of striving" argument applies just as well no matter how many children the couple has. Thus, the view implies that there is more and more union the more times the couple has sex, since this shows a greater seriousness in reproductive-mindedness. This does not seem right, and would lead to a serious distortion of marital sexuality.

Maybe, though, all that is needed for the fullness of cooperative union at a given time is that one have done all that one reasonably could *by that time*. But then a newlywed couple could count as having consummated their marriage as soon as they have exchanged their vows, since at that time they have done all that they *by that time* reasonably could in the way of cooperative union, if they did not procrastinate their wedding.

Thus we need to reject the idea that the fullness of cooperative union requires that everything be done for the goal sought. Intercourse serves as the physical aspect of a complete romantic union, and so the couple that opts for noncoital forms of reproduction does indeed devalue the sexual act that consummates romantic love for *all* couples, fertile or not. In fact, the significance of an activity decreases the more approaches are pursued for those ends from which the activity gains its significance (there is no special significance in eating quiche insofar as there are many other foods on which we can live; but if one could only live on quiche, eating quiche would be more significant).

But the loss of significance is not just on the side of intercourse. John Paul II wrote about children "crowning" the marital union.[4] Now a crown symbolizes but does not *make* a monarch. The union can lead to children, and the children are then a natural sign of it. But, on the present view, it is the acts that strive for children that make the union. Hence, the children are a fruit of the union, rather than the union itself. One way to see this is to take a case where the husband dies shortly after intercourse, but before successful fertilization. The union is fruitful, reproductively complete. But nonetheless the future children are not a part of the erotic union, since the commitments that are partially constitutive of romantic union end with death. For all of the child's life, the child will be a symbol and crown of that union, a crown that survives the death of the monarch and is not buried with the monarch (in this metaphor, "the monarch" is the romantic union, not the husband).

Observe, finally, that if noncoital reproduction were morally licit, then children would no longer be a sign of marital union in the same way. Counting noncoital reproduction as morally illicit, we can say that every child brought into existence in a morally licit manner symbolizes the erotic union from which the child comes. This gives another significance to the life of a child—the child lives as the fruit of love's union. But in severing the link between reproduction and coitus, one is removing this symbolism, since now it becomes morally possible for a child to come from something other than marital union.

4. MAKING AND BREEDING PEOPLE

There is something odd about the phrase "making people." We do not think of either human or animal reproduction as a case of "making." While God *made* (*'asah*) and *created* (*bara'*) human beings in his own image (e.g., Gen. 1:26–27, Gen. 9:6), Adam did not make a child: he *had a child* (*vayoled*) after his image (Gen. 5:3). There is, I think, a feeling that we are apt to have that there is something problematic in any action described as "making people." Likewise, people seem to be repelled by the idea of breeding people.

Robert George and Gerard Bradley have argued that sexual intercourse may only be engaged in to consummate the unitive marital good.[5] To have sex for pleasure *or* for reproduction is wrong. Of course, one may have sex to fulfill the marital good and further intend to get pleasure or reproduction out of it. But the marital good is the primary object of one's activity. I will now consider an argument for George and Bradley's position that having sex just in order to reproduce is wrong.[6] To examine this argument, we first need to look at the reasons one might have for procreation.

There seem to be two primary types of reasons for having a child. Let us suppose the child will be Sophie. The two kinds of reasons are: (1) the value of Sophie herself; (2) goods that Sophie's existence makes possible. The goods that Sophie's existence makes possible are of different sorts, and the "makes possible" functions differently in different cases. There are goods that are partially constituted by Sophie's existence, such as the existence of the next generation or the existence of yet another human person. There are goods that Sophie may *cause*, such as her parents' delight in looking at her, a tax break for her parents, or the clients' satisfaction from her later work as, say, a lawyer. And there are goods for which Sophie's existence is a precondition, either logical, as in the case of the moral good accruing to the parents from making sacrifices for Sophie's sake, or causal, as when Sophie's behavior presents the parents with an opportunity for patience.

Now the value of *Sophie* herself could not have been a reason for procreating. For it was not known that *Sophie* would arise from procreation, and the value of an individual cannot be grasped in abstraction from that individual. The value of Sophie herself is not something in respect of which Sophie is fungible. Moreover, even talking of "the good of that individual, whoever he or she may be, who will result from our having sex" does not make sense until it is settled that this individual *will* exist, and that is precisely the question. To make decisions on the grounds of the value of the particular individual makes sense only once it has been decided that the individual will exist.

Of course, the couple could intend the good of a new human being existing, the good of a child of theirs existing, the good of *having* a child, and so on. But none of these is the value of Sophie herself, as all of these goods would still be present had the reproductive activity resulted in the existence of another human being, say, Bob or Jennifer. (Of course, the name is not the issue—the value of Sophie is not the same as the good that someone with the *name* "Sophie" exists.) If we say that an individual *x* is fungible with respect to a good *G* providing that good *G* could have been equally well promoted by a different individual, then we have to say that Sophie is fungible with respect to all of these goods.

God in deciding to create a human being would arguably know the identity of that human being who would arise from the decision, and thus could create a human being for that human being's own sake, for the sake of a good in which the individual is not fungible. But we are not in that divine situation. The view that there is some peculiar good in each existing individual, precisely as that individual, is somewhat controversial. But it fits well with the lack of fungibility in love relationships and helps explain why God chose to create such imperfect creatures as we are—he chose us because of the peculiar good that we *ourselves* instantiate, that no one but we can instantiate, even though in all other respects persons other than ourselves, it seems, could be better.

Now it is plausible that we should avoid treating people as interchangeable. Yet, it seems, in the act of procreation we cannot but treat the person most intimately concerned, the resulting child, as interchangeable. For it seems we can only intend the goods of the second type, the goods in respect of which the individual is fungible. Now, it might be argued that there is nothing wrong in general with treating someone as interchangeable. After all, there is nothing wrong with calling up a helpdesk saying: "Could you send me someone who knows about WiFi configuration?"

But while it is acceptable to intend to *meet* someone under the description "someone who knows about WiFi configuration," to intend to *procreate* someone under this description is more problematic, and not just because WiFi technology may be out of date by the time the person matures. We saw in section 4 of chapter 8 that in sexual cases we are bound by a higher standard in respect of using people than in most nonsexual cases. Likewise, in respect of procreation it seems we are bound by that higher standard. The reasons for procreating someone are a kind of judgment on the value of the person's *existence* rather than on the value of the person's *presence*, as in the case of the call to the helpdesk.

When we make an artifact for a purpose, that purpose helps define its essence. If we work a block of wood into something with the sole intention of eating on it, it is therefore a table, even if it is not very good at performing the functions of a table. The resulting item exists for the sake of its ability to support eating. To procreate because of the goods that the child instantiates, but in respect of which the child is fungible, is to treat the child as an artifact, as something *made,* which exists for the sake of reasons defined by us. The fact that not all of the reasons are as utilitarian as getting WiFi configured does not greatly affect the argument. The maker's intention can define a portrait into either a work of art or a tool for law enforcement (think of a Wanted poster) or both. If the maker defines it into a work of art, then that is what it is. Then, the purpose of the object is to *be* a work of art, rather than to fulfill some utilitarian function. Likewise, if the parents' purpose is to bring it about that another human being exists, or that they have at least two children, or that they have an opportunity for lavishing love, then the parents are, it seems, defining the purpose of the child, and thus treating the child as an artifact. Indeed, is it not somewhat offensive to exist solely in order that there be one more person existing or to provide an opportunity for someone else to love one?

On Kant's view, human beings are ends in themselves, and so to attempt to define the value of their existence by creating them for a particular purpose seems to be morally reprehensible. On a theistic view, however, human beings are *God's* creatures, and to attempt to define their value is to trespass on God's prerogative. We may know that *one* of the values of people is to be human beings. But, arguably, the primary reason God creates a person is because of the particular value of *that* person, and God may have various particular reasons, including the particular vocation he has for that person, for creating a person of a particular sort. It does not infringe on the dignity of a human being to have God set one's purposes in existence, but it does for a human being to do it.

One might object that there is nothing wrong with generating a human being for a purpose it is natural for human beings to subserve. It is natural for human beings to be rational, and so it would be no objectionable imposition to impose rationality on someone in creating them for the sake of the existence of another rational being. However, while it is no undue burden to be made in order to be rational, it may still be the case that it is not our right to make someone to be rational, since we are not the ones deciding on the functions of human beings. Even if our choice in fact matches the nature of the human being, we are overstepping our bounds in having a purpose for the existence of another human being. Further, all such purposes are ones in respect to which the human being is fungible, and hence do not touch the central value of the person as an individual. Note, too, the excessive weight of responsibility on a child procreated solely to fulfill her parents' intentions.

If this is right, then while procreative sexual activity is morally acceptable, the primary purpose should be something other than procreation itself. This condition can be satisfied if, for instance, the purpose of sex is to engage in reproductive-*type* activity, say, because one recognizes the value of that activity. There is probably nothing morally objectionable in acting so that procreation should be a *part* of one's reason for the action, or even in modifying the action so that it might be done in a way that is more likely to result in procreation. For then insofar as one has a further good reason, beyond procreation, for sex, the resulting child does not exist *solely* for the sake of fulfilling her parents' intentions for her.

Now, one might object that surely it is better for a couple (a) to procreate a child solely to allow the couple the joys of having a child than (b) to procreate a child solely to satisfy their sexual passion or even to unite sexually. But this objection rests on an equivocation. For on the view being defended in this section, option (a) is only objectionable as a reason when we read "solely to allow" as modifying "a child," implying that this is the *child's* purpose in existing, but in (b) "solely to satisfy . . . or . . . to unite" is read as modifying "to procreate"— it is not the child's existence that unites sexually on the relevant reading of (b), and hence *the child* is not being used for the sake of union.

The view defended in this section seems to go against the common intuition that it is better to be a *wanted* child, to be generated *on purpose*. That intuition, however, equivocates between "wanted" and "generated on purpose." Many things are wanted once they exist, but we did not intend their existence. Moreover, in talking of a child "generated on purpose," one must distinguish generating the particular individual on purpose from generating someone-or-other on purpose. But it is impossible to generate the particular child on purpose since we cannot grasp the child in his or her particularity prior to generation, while if we are talking of generating someone-or-other on purpose, then that treats the child as fungible.

William E. May has argued that there is even a deep theological reason why the making of a child is wrong.[7] Just as Christ is "begotten, not made," so too, our children should be "begotten, not made." One might object that all human beings are *made*, in the sense of being created by God. But presumably, May's analogy is between the Trinitarian relationship between the Father and the Son and the relationship between the parents and the child. That the child is made *by God* does not harm this analogy.

An obvious objection is that it would follow from the view being defended that clearly innocent actions are wrong. The royals who procreate in order to ensure the political stability of their people and the peasants who make a baby in order to have help on the farm are both doing wrong. Yet we have the intuition that at least the peasants are not doing anything immoral.

I think, though, there is a way of seeing the intentions of the royals and the peasants that allows one to hold on to the idea that sex merely for reproduction is wrong, and yet allow a large role to be played by the reproductive hopes. Conjugal sex is innately good, being a consummation of sexual love. A married couple always has a good reason to have sex. At the same time, the couple may have reasons *not* to have sex—reasons that function as "defeaters" for their general reason to have sex. For instance, having sex may be inconvenient on a given occasion, or the couple may be tired from too much diplomacy or plowing, or there may be a fear of the pains of childbirth, and so on. But the value of political stability or of help on the farm can then defeat these defeaters: sex may be inconvenient, but considerations of this inconvenience are overridden by considerations of the benefits brought by the child. The goods in respect of which the child is fungible, then, need not be the main goods aimed at in the sexual act.

The couple can still be having sex primarily because sex is good. But the goods that the child provides enter into their deliberation as defeaters to defeaters, as overriding reasons not to have sex.

In fact, I think we *should* be concerned that purely reproductive sex might make the couple feel like they are engaging in something clinical rather than "making love," and might lead to a negative attitude toward sexuality. Leiblum quotes a husband who claimed to share his wife's desire for a baby, but who said that he was beginning "to feel like a machine! I never have a right to develop a headache or just plain be disinterested if she thinks she's ovulating," even though earlier, their sex life was "terrific."[8] Anecdotal data indicates that such feelings are not uncommon. We could take them as an indicator that there is something wrong with purely reproductive sex. At the same time, modest majorities of both female and male patients (more on the female side) with fertility issues agree that "the childlessness" has brought them closer together, that it has strengthened their relationship.[9] And while sexual dysfunction is prevalent among both male and female partners in infertile couples, the dysfunction still only occurs in a minority of cases.[10] Thus, the argument against purely reproductive sex based on the anecdotal data about negative attitudes toward sexuality, while suggestive, is not conclusive.

But now it is worth adding the following argument. Start by observing that it is wrong to engage in sexual union except with a spouse. Thus, the couple must be aware that each is having sex *with a spouse,* and if this conjugality is not in some way a part of their perception of the act, then their mental state need not differ intrinsically from that of an adulterous couple. Thus it is morally problematic for the couple to have *only* reproduction in mind, since then conjugality is not in mind.

We can deepen this line of thought as follows. In intercourse, the couple does indeed unite biologically. We have argued earlier that biological union is only appropriate in the context of a *personal* union. The personal union is effected in and through the biological union. It is not sufficient for interpersonal union that each member of a cooperative community have the same intention—that could happen by coincidence. Rather, it seems, each needs to have the intention, at least in part, because the whole does—only then is it a *shared* intention, rather than a case of accidental agreement. To unite in intention, the couple needs to intend reproductive cooperation not just because it is reproductive but also because it is cooperative.[11]

The couple that makes love in order to reproduce needs to be reproducing *as a part of the conjugal good,* on the present argument. It is not that the child is a *means* to a conjugal good, since that would be treating the child instrumentally. It is not even that the existence of the child is a *part* of the conjugal good, since then the act would be an attempt to define the child's value in a way dependent on the parents' conjugal good, rather than as an independent value, an end in itself or a creature whose ends can only be set by God. Rather, it is the *act* of reproducing that needs to be a part of the conjugal good.

But this seems to create a tension for the view that I have defended earlier in the book that what constitutes the unitiveness of intercourse at least in part is the reproductive striving. For if intercourse has its value because it is a joint reproductive striving, then likewise the jointly taken actions of the couple in a case of in vitro fertilization (IVF) treatment should be unitive in the same way. If we want to make it an extreme case, we can assume that the spouses are both medical technicians and perform the whole procedure cooperatively. And we could imagine a couple that engages in IVF treatment not just to reproduce, but in order to unite through their cooperative activity. A close analogy between this and intercourse, however, is psychologically implausible. While married couples often have intercourse even if they are not hoping to reproduce, it is hard to realistically imagine a couple that would engage in IVF for the sake of the unitive good, without hoping to reproduce.

Moreover, the *biological* unitiveness of intercourse is constituted by a joint biological striving, a striving that is strongly biologically natural in the sense of the preceding section. In the case of IVF, the striving is all at the voluntary level, and no biological drive is engaged. The activity is not strongly natural, and the two persons are not joined as one flesh. Furthermore, in the case of IVF the value of the cooperation itself does not seem to be as significant an aspect of the act as the cooperation is in the case of intercourse. These considerations, however, only show that in the case of joint IVF striving, the value of the union is *less* than in the case of intercourse.

Furthermore, if someone insists that the medical technician couple are seeking the good of cooperating in IVF, and not primarily engaging in an attempt at procreation, we might try to argue that it appears wrong to reproduce for a *minor* reason. Just as it is disproportionate to do something that unintentionally leads to a great evil for the sake of a minor good, so too, it is disproportionate to do something that unintentionally leads to a great good merely for the sake of a minor good. Imagine a couple that reproduced, whether naturally or by IVF, primarily in order to win a prize in a frivolous contest (say, a contest for the first birth in a new year or for having sex on all and only prime numbered days of the month for a year). Just as it is contrary to the dignity of a person to be brought into existence for a purpose not defined by God, so too, it seems contrary to one's dignity to be brought into existence because one's parents had sex for a trivial reason. The good of marital union wrought by intercourse is a highly nontrivial reason—it is the consummation of love's union of two lives into one. But the union in IVF-based cooperation does not seem to have the kind of significant value that the good of marital union has. In fact, the union in IVF-based cooperation seems to be valuable almost entirely as a means to the value of the resulting child—if the couple could just press a button and conception were to magically occur, without any complex IVF machinery, then that would be preferable.

Above, I have argued that it is wrong to do actions aimed solely at procreation. But what about *helping* procreation? For surely it would not be wrong for a medical professional to induce ovulation to increase the chance of conception from an act of intercourse. Yet it seems that in such an act one is aiming solely at procreation.

But that is an oversimplification. We can charitably assume that a medical professional's intention is not just to increase the population of the world, but to help a couple suffering from a fertility problem. The professional is acting in part on behalf of the couple, and hence their intention is in part normative for the professional. Now the couple should be intending not just that there be another person, but that their marital union be fruitful. The good that is willed is still tied to the marital act. Of course, the child is desired and intended as well, but the child is not the sole object of the action. For if the activity of intercourse is valuable and its biological end is valuable, then there is a great value for intercourse to be biologically successful, and it is this with which the professional helps. Consequently, even in the act of enhancing the fertility of a sexual act, the focus is not just on the child.

Procreation, thus, seems paradoxical. It results in the existence of a being that has individual dignity. If the above arguments are sound, then because this individual dignity is the central value of that being, it is wrong to aim to produce the being for another reason. Many outcomes are too evil for it ever to be right to intend them. The outcome of procreation seems in a sense too good for it to be right for us to intend it directly, at least for any reason but that good which the child's individual existence will have, a good on which we cannot base our decisions without presupposing the decision to procreate.

Procreation is, in a sense, all about the child. But because we cannot grasp the child as an individual in the decision to procreate, the procreative act cannot focus solely on the child. Making persons is not for the likes of us. On this argument, the way we can permissibly reproduce is by doing something of great independent value, namely uniting maritally, that provides God with the occasion for making persons.

There is, however, a powerful theistic rejoinder to the above arguments. As an initial attempt at formulating it, note that it seems permissible for God to treat us as instruments of his loving will. Can we not, therefore, reproduce, even with IVF, in order to provide a child so that God might treat the child as an instrument of his loving will?

But things are not so easy. If I procreate so that the child might be an instrument of God's will, then *I* have a purpose for the child, namely, that the child should fulfill God's will. Thus, it seems the child is *my* (constitutive) instrument to God's having an instrument for his loving will.

A better version of the theistic rejoinder might be that the couple does not actually intend the child as an instrument of God's will, but intends their act of reproduction as a fulfillment of God's will. This is, in fact, quite reasonable in the case of intercourse, since quite possibly God does command married couples to engage in marital union, barring their having good reason to the contrary—the Christian tradition does closely tie marriage with reproduction. Perhaps, then, we could say that, likewise, God wants couples to engage in IVF. But here we have an evidential problem. While God does say in scripture to human beings, "Be fruitful and multiply" (Gen. 1:22, 9:1, 7), it is surely not the case that this must be fulfilled by everyone, at all costs. An argument would be needed to show that God also wants reproduction from those couples who can reproduce only by IVF. It is not clear what grounds we would have for supposing such a divine command or desire, and it is presumptuous to say that one is acting in order to fulfill the will of God if one does not have good reason to suppose that one is acting to fulfill the will of God.

5. GIFT

William E. May has argued that a child should be seen as a gift rather than the object of a reproductive action.[12] Presumably, the idea here is that the child is a gift of God to the child herself, to the parents, and to the world. This attitude is relatively easy to attain in the case of intercourse—the intercourse is good, and the child is a gift superadded by God to this good—and one can also treat the child as a gift a fortiori in the case of twinning where there is no voluntary input by us at all. But, May thinks the child is not treated as a gift in the case of voluntary noncoital reproduction.

There is a Jewish joke in which a prospective host gives a friend whom he has invited a series of odd directions for getting to the party, such as that he will push open the door of the building with his knee, press the elevator button with his shoulder, ring the doorbell with his elbow, and so on. The prospective guest asks why it must all be done in this strange way, and the host responds: "Well, aren't your hands going to be full?" The joke is funny precisely because gifts, much less a hands-filling multiplicity of them, are not something at which a host should directly aim. They are not something we should *expect* in the normative sense in which one expects people to do their job, and even to hint that one is expecting a gift can be a breach of etiquette. One may, of course, take steps to ensure that *if* one is to receive a gift, it not be something deleterious to one. If every Christmas, one has received from a friend a fruitcake made with nuts to which one is allergic, one might mention the allergy to the giver before the next Christmas, but the challenge in doing so is to do it in such a way as not to indicate an expectation of the gift. However at least in Western cultures (and presumably May's gift analogy is an analogy to the gift-as-understood-in-Western-culture), we are expected not to expect gifts, and we even have social rituals of feigned surprise and abortive refusal ("You shouldn't have!") to drum the point home.

It is perhaps possible, too, that when strapped for resources, one might act in such a way as to maximize the probability of receiving gifts. Thus an impoverished couple getting married might invite a rich aunt. At the same time, it would be crass to invite the aunt *solely* for the purpose of getting a gift from her. There must, from the couple's point of view, be a value in the aunt's attendance, independent of the gift that one hopes (but does not in the normative sense expect) she will give, a value that should be sufficient to make inviting her worthwhile, though the hope of a gift may also enter into consideration by defeating some reasons against inviting her (say, the expected cost of entertaining another guest).

One might argue that in reproductive intercourse, it is not difficult to keep in mind this aspect of the child as a gift, for several reasons. The connection between intercourse and the child is mediated by many causal steps that occur outside of our direct control, and the chance of successful conception appears not to exceed about one half on the most fertile of days.[13] Intercourse has a value in itself, and most married couples at least sometimes—perhaps most or all the time— engage in intercourse without positively planning to have a child. Moreover, reproduction through intercourse is a process that has a certain mystery, as the process is not one we humans have designed. When humans engage in intercourse, even with reproduction in mind, the details of the process, such as that the mucus should preserve sperm and release it at staggered intervals, are not of human making, and the people involved typically do not even think of them.

In the case of IVF and other reproductive technologies, it seems contingently and psychologically much easier to think of the child as a human artifact, as something one has made, something one has *obtained*, rather than a gift of God. This is particularly true if the embryos were preselected for specific characteristics, such as hardiness, but even without any such preselection it seems easy to think of the child as a product of technology. It is easy to dismiss this kind of an argument as merely based on contingent features of human character that need not be present in every case, saying: "Others may fall into the trap of feeling in such-and-such a way, but I can make sure that I don't." But arguments based on contingencies of human feeling should not be dismissed out of hand, and the resilience of our feelings should not be underestimated.

However, let us probe further. Is it simply that IVF *feels* like a making rather than a receiving of a gift, or are there ways in which IVF *treats* the process as one of making rather than receiving? Let me begin with one central aspect in which in *both* IVF and reproductive intercourse the child can be argued to be a gift. On traditional Christian views, human beings are composed of a physical body and a nonphysical soul. Biological processes do not cause the existence of immaterial objects—and hence the soul—which is what makes us distinctively human, is not produced by *either* IVF *or* reproductive intercourse. It is quite possible, thus, to think of the soul as a gift in both cases. It is true that it is a gift for which we might provide the occasion, as when the pouring of water and recital of a text provides the occasion for the grace of baptism, but that does not render it any less a gift.

Assuming that souls are immaterial, we can say that every human being is still in a crucial sense a gift, even if the human being is produced by IVF. Furthermore, many Christian theologians have held that every action of ours is one with which God in some way cooperates, since all our power is a mere participation in divine power. God is then still intimately involved in the production of a child through IVF. But even if *objectively* the child is still, through and through, a gift, there is the question whether the child is being *treated* by the human agents as something other than a gift. Now, considerations of soul do make it possible to say that one treats the child's spiritual or mental nature as a gift in IVF, but the *whole* human person needs to be treated as a gift. Insofar as IVF makes it easy to treat the *body* as a mere product of our manufacturing, it could contribute to a gnostic way of thinking of the soul as the only bearer of transcendent value in human beings.

But does IVF treat the child's body as a mere product, or does it simply make it easy to think about it in this way? As with intercourse, IVF does not have a very high rate of reproductive success. For simplicity, let us suppose the two rates are on par. Reproduction through intercourse does involve a greater number of steps beyond our control, and the more a process is under our control, the more the outcome of the process is something that we have produced. This does not, however, point to an *innate* difference between intercourse and IVF. There is some evidence that, with training, various previously involuntary activities can be controlled voluntarily. Suppose that it were possible for a woman and man to minutely control their reproductive processes, and they did so. Surely this would not make reproductive intercourse wrong, as long as the control did not change the nature of the act. Conversely, we could imagine an IVF-like procedure where some kind of a randomization phase is inserted in the process—say, a coin is tossed by a machine and a sperm is only allowed to go through if the coin lands heads—which decreases the probability of conception, and this randomization surely would not significantly change the moral nature of the procedure.

At the same time, the fact that we would consider it rather odd if someone wanted a randomization phase to be inserted in IVF does suggest that we judge IVF by the efficiency criteria with which we judge manufacturing processes. We do not find it similarly odd if a couple has intercourse in a position that is somewhat less likely to result in conception, even if they would, in fact, like to have a child.

The fact that the intrinsic value of engaging in IVF-style processes is low or even negative (IVF is not only a great hassle, but may take a significant emotional toll on the couple; there is also the issue, which we are bracketing here, of left-over embryos) does show a significant difference between IVF and intercourse. As we saw, the concept of a gift is such that it is crass to invite the rich aunt to the wedding unless there is an independent value in her attendance. Otherwise, one is not inviting the aunt but the gift, and in a real sense the gift is something that one has given to oneself by means of inviting the aunt.

At the same time, one can come up with outlandish scenarios where there is an independent, intrinsic or extrinsic, value in IVF. Thus, the painfulness of the extraction of ova might be taken on as an ascetical practice. Or perhaps the government could offer tax incentives for engaging in IVF in a country facing the danger of depopulation. In such a case, one could indeed engage in IVF while accepting the child as a bonus, a gift. But to invade the integrity of the body with medical procedures for the sake of tax incentives or ascetical practice seems at least a little problematic.

Consider next the already noted difference between IVF and reproductive intercourse, that reproductive intercourse is not a process we have designed. In engaging in a process that is designed by nature or by someone else, it is easier to accept the outcome of that process as a gift. An eccentric inventor uncle leaves us his apartment, telling us to first rub the mirror, then pull up the carpet and lift a floorboard, and then to plug the kettle in. Upon doing all this, suddenly, the chandelier descends and on top of it is a large ingot of gold. The ingot is a gift rather than something we have obtained. But if we ourselves set up a process for extracting an ingot of gold from the uncle's apartment, then our possession of the gold is being treated less as a gift, even if obtained with the uncle's permission.

The arguments in this section rest on the assumption that a child *should* be treated as a gift. This assumption can be questioned, of course. One way to back up the assumption is to return to the arguments of the previous section that we should not be setting the purpose of a child. When we obtain something for ourselves, we obtain it for a purpose. But in the case of a gift, especially a gift from God, the purposing is on the side of the giver. Indeed, children not infrequently get gifts from parents where the parents have a hidden educational purpose for the gift.

Furthermore, it is a particularly momentous and God-like thing to procreate. Human beings are, after all, made in the image and likeness of God. A failure to treat the child as a gift may be a case of idolatry—of putting oneself or a technician in the place of God. Humility is needed in the process, and guarding this humility may have great value.

Now, granted, such arguments may not sound very plausible to a couple that is deeply distressed by the inability to have a child. But at the same time, the couple may need to examine whether their own distress may not be in part due to treating a child as something other than a gift. One thing, after all, that is distinctive in receiving a gift is that if nothing is given, there is no ground for resentment. There may, of course, be a disappointment and a frustrated hope, but there should be no frustrated *expectation*. If the rich aunt does not give one a gift, and one is frustrated in expectation, exclaiming, "Why did we bother putting up with her?" then one did not treat what one hoped to obtain as a gift, but as one's due. A part of the attitude of receptivity to a gift is a willingness to accept the situation if a gift is not given.[14] But of course this is easier said than done, and in practice it can be difficult to draw the line between a feeling of frustrated hope and one of frustrated expectation.

6. CHILDREN AS THE FRUIT OF MARRIAGE

It is fairly plausible that we should have children only as the fruit of marriage. Suppose we accept this intuition, still widely held in our society, and universally accepted in Christian history. One could take this claim to say merely that two people should have a child together only if they are married. This by itself rules out the use of the gametes of someone to whom one isn't married. However, one might also take the claim more strongly as saying that the origination of the children should be tied to the marital relationship itself, rather than the marital relationship being a mere morally necessary condition for procreation. The stronger claim is, of course, more controversial. But I think it is still plausible.

If we take the claim in this stronger way, then it becomes plausible that children should flow from the act that consummates a marriage, namely, unitive marital intercourse. It is a directedness at unitive intercourse that makes a love erotic in nature, and the life of marriage is the life of consummated eros. Marriage is, thus, defined in terms of unitive intercourse. When procreation flows from intercourse, then we can say that the child is truly the fruit of marriage.

The obvious objection is that marriage is not just sex. Marriage includes mutual self-giving of a nonsexual nature, a sharing of ideas, burdens, feelings, and goods of all sorts. And children produced by means other than intercourse can be the fruit of this loving sharing. Indeed, perhaps love is needed to motivate a couple to undertake the emotional and financially costly noncoital reproductive procedure. The argument in the previous paragraph showed that *if* procreation flowed from marital unitive intercourse, then it was a fruit of marriage. But it did not show that this was true *only* if it flowed from marital unitive intercourse.

However, note that all of the substantive nonsexual aspects of giving and sharing are ones that can permissibly occur outside of marriage. It is, indeed, possible to have a couple who are unmarried but cohabit in a committed nonsexual relationship for life, sharing ideas, burdens, goods, and feelings. Indeed, it may be that the Eastern Christian rite of brother-making (*adelphopoiêsis*)[15] was precisely aimed at such a relationship. Procreation originating in these giving and sharing aspects of marriage, while still being a genuine fruit of the relationship, is not a fruit of that aspect of marriage that distinguishes marriage from other loving relationships. It flows from the marital relationship, but from it insofar as it is a committed and loving relationship, and not insofar as it is a *marital* relationship.

It is only coital reproduction that can make the child the fruit of marriage as a whole, both the fruit of that which distinguishes marriage from other relationships, and of the loving and sharing aspects of the relationship that ought to be present in marriage. These loving and sharing aspects can exist outside of marriage, but are still expressed in intercourse, since intercourse expresses the union of love. If we thus have a strong intuition that children should be the fruit of marriage, then we should conclude that we should reproduce only coitally.

7. IDOLATRY, HUMILITY, AND SACRAMENT

In procreating, we are about as God-like as we can be. But, as C. S. Lewis has forcefully argued,[16] it is when we are most God-like that we face the greatest danger of idolatry. It is then that we need humility most. A plausible way to inculcate this humility in oneself is to procreate by a method designed not by ourselves but by our Creator (or by nature).

With technological advances, we can do many things "our way," in many ways improving on nontechnological ways of proceeding. That is quite natural, since we are, by nature, intelligent beings, though it is not "strongly natural" in the terminology of section 3 above. Among our actions are some that have a particularly deep theological significance. In these actions, we express our humility before the Creator by doing them in a way that, *in its essentials,* does not vary, and in doing the actions in this particular way, we emphasize that the religious goods involved transcend our power, and we are mere cooperators with God. For instance, while with technological advances one might synthesize water for baptism out of the hydrogen and oxygen in the air, it is essential that it be *water* that one has synthesized. It would not do to use an antimicrobial alcohol-based gel in baptism on the grounds that the gel is an even better symbol than water of baptismal purification. Even when water is unavailable, gel should not be used—in such a case, the spiritual ends should instead be achieved by spiritual means in "baptism of desire," where the sincere desire for baptism suffices.

Procreation is not a sacrament in the sense of a bestowal of an extraordinary grace. What is bestowed in procreation is "ordinary" human life. But the "ordinary" here is only ordinary in the sense of "routine" and "natural" to humans. A king's business is indeed ordinary to the king, though, in a different sense, being a king is by no means ordinary. It is only in the sense in which the king's business is ordinary to the king that being human is ordinary to a human. Human life is the life of an image of God, and the procreation of such a life has eternal consequences. Those actions that are sacraments in the technical sense involve something that goes over and beyond human nature. But human nature is itself a sacrament, a *mysterium,* in a less technical sense. And for Christians, procreation is also the living out of a sacrament in the technical sense, namely matrimony. Marriage has been defined in the Christian tradition partly in terms of a certain kind of willingness, or at least lack of unwillingness, to have children together, and procreation is a way of living out the sacramental mystery of marriage. Therefore, it is plausible that procreation should be limited to a particular, divinely sanctioned form of action, passed down from past times, namely intercourse.

It might be objected that the core of the procreative "sacrament" is not intercourse but the attempted meeting between a sperm and an egg. This would rule out cloning, but would not rule out IVF if the couple's own genetic material were to be used. However, this objection is not particularly plausible. In sacramental-type actions, the core action is something visible that manifests an invisible reality. If the true core of our participation in the procreative mystery were found in the attempted meeting of sperm and egg, then for centuries, no one was able to see this core. It is intercourse that is the overt action, and so it is intercourse, not a hidden meeting between sperm and egg, that is a sacramental type of action.

This argument is based on an analogy between procreation and the sacraments in the technical sense. There are, however, two important disanalogies. First, sacraments like baptism have more of the nature of *public* acts, while intercourse is a paradigmatically private act. Second, sacraments do not succeed—are not *valid*—if the core actions are not done, so that if one baptizes with antimicrobial gel, the candidate does not thereby come to be baptized, while IVF can succeed. Third, sacraments always succeed when the core action is done, while intercourse can fail to reproduce.

The first of these disanalogies is easy to dismiss. For in fact two sacraments are not *intrinsically* public. In the Catholic and Orthodox Churches, penance is usually implemented in the context of private confession, though it used to involve public confession in the early Church. Actually, the preferred Roman Catholic practice now seems to involve a public service followed by private confession, which closely mirrors the way a public wedding is followed by private union. Moreover, in the early Church, the Eucharist was celebrated privately, with the nonbaptized not being allowed to witness it. And the Eucharist is a close analogy to intercourse, since the Eucharist effects our bodily union with Christ through our eating his body, a union that is fruitful in grace leading to deeper love.

The second and third disanalogies are significant. A sacrament, it seems, succeeds if and only if the core action is done, while one can procreate without intercourse and have intercourse without procreating. Nonetheless, it is precisely because success is actually possible without the core action of intercourse that the danger of feeling that procreation is something *we* do, rather than something *God* does in cooperation with us is pressing, though the fact that IVF does not always succeed decreases the danger somewhat. The disanalogies do weaken the argument, but do not destroy it.

Our argument does not require that one accept a full Catholic or Orthodox sacramental theology, though such a theology strengthens it. In fact, this argument can, to some degree, be run on the basis of mere theism. All it requires is a recognition of the sacredness in procreation and an agreement that the Catholic and Orthodox sacramental theologies embody truths about the way sacred actions function in people's lives. The argument makes it plausible that there are significant limits on how we should procreate, if we are to treat ourselves as mere participators in something sacred rather than primary agents.

8. CONCLUSIONS

Several arguments make it very plausible, on different sets of assumptions, that we should engage in procreation only coitally. Some of these arguments are theological in nature, though one involves a Kantian worry about turning people into products.

The arguments do leave open a question about when an act of procreation ceases to be coital. It seems that helping sperm get to the ovum by removing obstructions does not render the reproductive act noncoital. Rather, the removal of obstructions is simply a way of helping the coition to be fruitful. But what if the husband and wife have intercourse, and then the sperm ejaculated in intercourse is extracted, and joined with the woman's ovum, either in vitro or in the fallopian tube?

There are difficult questions here, which I will not settle. But the principle is that a given reproductive intervention is only permissible when it can be seen as a way of helping the coition to be fruitful, so that the child remains a fruit of the marital act. Whether a particular intervention can be seen as a way of helping coition to be fruitful is a matter for further investigation.

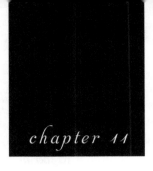

Celibacy

There is one final major topic, of which I shall treat only very briefly. The Christian tradition has generally held that celibacy is superior to marriage, but that marriage is itself good (this is particularly clear in Augustine's treatise *On the Excellence of Marriage*).[1] The tradition has generally held that not everyone is called to or capable of celibacy. An analysis of celibacy could easily take a book, but in this chapter I simply respond to one moral question: Can celibacy be good, and if so, what sort of a good?

It is challenging to see why exactly celibacy should be a good. Technically, celibacy is merely the absence of marriage. (That the absence of sex should come along with absence of marriage is taken for granted by the Christian tradition.) Celibacy is thus defined as the absence of a particular good, and a good central to the human species, at that. Permanent celibacy seems not very different in this way from permanent abstinence from speech (not even the Trappists practiced that, since they would still pray and confess their sins), a way of denying something central to being human.

A view that celibacy *as such* is a great good would be hard to defend. I would suggest that the Christian tradition, at its best, was talking not about celibacy as such, but about celibacy entered into for particular reasons—"for the sake of the kingdom of heaven" (Matt. 19:12). The celibacy that the Christian tradition praised was not just a lack of a good, but the *sacrifice* of a good. Death is the cessation of life and life is a good, but to *sacrifice* one's life for another's sake is a yet greater good than to preserve one's life. The notion of sacrifice implies that something is being given up *for something else*. Celibacy should, thus, probably be seen in the context of other ascetical practices.

But at the same time, there is a deeper sense in celibacy within the Christian tradition than just that of yet another ascetical sacrifice. Sexuality is about reproduction and union. Becoming united with another human being as much as is humanly possible does not preclude union with God. Indeed, we also love God through loving our neighbor. But at least for most of us, there can be a tension. In marriage, one commits much of one's energy to a deep union with a spouse, and then one unites to God in and through one's matrimonial identity. In the writings of the mystics, however, we find that a more straightforward and direct kind of union with God is also possible, which, it is not unreasonable to suppose, might be impeded by the energies expended on union with a spouse—we are finite beings, after all.

Moreover, celibacy enables one to give more of oneself to a wider variety of strangers. For even though one can be united with God in and through one's marital relationships, this identity does ensure that we can give less of ourselves to people outside of our family circle, since marriage gives rise to strong particular duties to spouse and children.

Marital love gives us an example of the intensity, though not of the form, of love that a Christian should have for God and for neighbor. But marital love has an exclusivity in it, and the celibate may be freer to have an intense, inclusive love of others. It is no surprise that many Christian spiritual writers warn the celibate against the danger of "particular friendships."[2] The danger is not so much that these might lead one into unchastity, but that they might interfere with that purity of intense, inclusive love for others that celibacy, when embraced for the right reasons, can promote. Of course it need hardly be said that in a particular case it is possible to be celibate, even for the right reasons, and have much less of that intense, inclusive love of others than many a married person. But celibacy is valuable by making *possible* an intensity of inclusive love, even if not all celibate persons live this out.

In section 8 of chapter 6, I suggested that virtues needed for a normal part of human life are moral excellences for every human being, even if this human being does not expect to live out that aspect of life. If I am right about this, then marital virtues are also virtues that the celibate person needs to have. The kind of willingness to give oneself completely to another that characterizes marriage needs to also characterize the celibate person's life, even if the giving does not take the same physical form.

Thus, just as a hatred for one's fellows is among the worst of reasons to become a hermit, so too, a difficulty in developing the virtues needed for marriage is not a good reason to commit to celibacy. For even if one remains celibate, one will need to develop such virtues in order to live a fully human life. But while celibacy may make the development of some virtues easier, such as the virtues of a deep life of contemplative silence, it may also make the development of the virtues needed for marriage more difficult, since it is easier to deceive oneself and others that one has a virtue when one is exercising it less overtly. Thus, it is easier for poor rather than rich misers to believe that they have a generous spirit, because it is easy for the poor misers to deceive themselves that they would be generously sharing *if only they could*.

Marriage is the normal state for human beings. To commit to abstain from marriage is, thus, a significant gesture, a gesture that can signify the living out on earth of the heavenly life that Christ has made possible by making the Kingdom of God be among us. This gesture needs to be made not from an unwillingness to make the sacrifices marriage involves, but from a willingness to live the spirit of fruitful marital self-giving in a wider way.

Notes

Chapter 1. Introduction

Unless noted otherwise, all biblical translations are from *The Holy Bible: Revised Standard Version, Catholic Edition* (Oxford: Oxford University Press, 2004).

1. Wojtyła, *Love and Responsibility;* John Paul II, *Man and Woman He Created Them.*

2. Krosik et al., *Human Sexuality.*

3. Particularly important representatives of the line of thought that this book stands in continuity with include: Wojtyła, *Love and Responsibility;* John Paul II, *Man and Woman He Created Them;* Grisez, *The Way of the Lord Jesus,* vol. 2; Finnis, "Law, Morality, and 'Sexual Orientation'"; Lee and George, *Body-Self Dualism.*

Chapter 2. Love and Its Forms

1. It has been suggested that the Gospel writers only quote the first verse of Psalm 22, meaning to indicate that Christ recited the whole psalm, and hence the feeling of abandonment expressed by the verse is not to be attributed to Christ, given that the psalm as a whole progresses to divine triumph. This is implausible. First of all, in both Mark's and Matthew's versions, the bystanders misunderstood the *Elahi* of Christ's Aramaic cry as Christ's calling upon Elijah, *Eliyahu.* If the rest of the psalm were recited,

the mistake would be less likely. Second, while the cry almost surely is a quotation of Psalm 22, it is a quotation of it in Aramaic rather than Hebrew. It seems more consonant with subsequent Jewish practice that a full text would have been memorized in the liturgical language of Hebrew rather than in the Aramaic vernacular. The use of the vernacular suggests a cry from the heart. Finally, the main theological reason adduced for supposing that Christ did not feel the stark abandonment indicated by the text is the unbroken union of the man Jesus with God, both through the Incarnation and, at least in Catholic theology, through a constant beatific vision. But there is no reason to suppose that such a union would be incompatible with a *feeling* of abandonment. Perceptual illusion seems compatible with the Incarnation, and emotive illusion could be so as well.

2. Kierkegaard, *Journals and Papers*, vol. 3, #2423.

3. E.g., Romans 13:8–10 and Galatians 5:14.

4. Augustine, "Homilies on the First Epistle of John," Homily 7.

5. Nygren, *Agapê and Eros*.

6. Aristotle, *Nicomachean Ethics*, VIII.7.

7. Cicero, "On Friendship," section 20.

8. Benedict XVI, *Deus Caritas Est*, section 31.

9. Ibid.

10. Lewis, *The Four Loves*, 123.

11. Nozick, *The Examined Life*, 80.

12. Ibid., 68–69.

13. Cf. Thomas Aquinas's statement in *Summa Theologica*, II-II.23.1. reply 2 that in loving a person, one loves those connected with the person.

14. On the order of charity, see Aquinas, *Summa Theologica*, II-II.31.3.

15. In the end, I actually think that for mountain climbing to be good, it must be an exercise of love, perhaps love for the created world around me, or maybe of well-ordered self-love (I am grateful to an anonymous reader for the latter suggestion).

16. Aquinas, *Summa Theologica*, I-II.28.1–2.

17. Augustine, *The Trinity*.

18. Thomas Aquinas, *Summa Contra Gentiles*, 1.91.

19. Augustine, *The Trinity*, X.

20. Aristotle, *Nicomachean Ethics*, IX.9.

21. Cf. Aquinas, *Summa Theologica*, I-II.28.3.

22. Aquinas, *Summa Theologica*, I-II.28.2.

23. Emily Glass has suggested to me that nonetheless a *lifetime* of living with someone may be something greater than giving up one's life for this person. This is why I am comparing the giving up of one's life to an individual one of the consummatory acts.

24. Aristotle, *Nicomachean Ethics*, IX.3.

25. Kierkegaard, *Journals and Papers*, vol. 3, #3608.

26. Ibid., vol. 4, #4752.

27. "No, a Holy Scripture requires 'faith,' and for this very reason there must be disagreement so that the choice of faith can take place or that faith becomes a choice and the possibility of offense gives tension to faith" (ibid., vol. 4, #3860).

28. Here it may help to distinguish a moral right to count on someone's doing something from an epistemic right to expect something will happen (I am grateful to Emily Glass for a comment leading to this distinction). I have an epistemic right to think that the moon will rise around 8:04 p.m. tonight—that is, after all, what the astronomy software on my PDA says. But I have a moral right to count on a friend's keeping a promise, in the sense that I not only have the right to expect *that* she will keep the promise, but I have a right to expect the keeping of the promise *of her*, and to hold her responsible should she fail.

29. Kierkegaard talks of "the absolute resting in a conviction" (Journals and Papers, vol. 3, #3608).

30. The Council writes that "those who have accepted the faith under the guidance of the church can never have any just cause for changing this faith or for calling it into question." Tanner, *Decrees of the Ecumenical Councils*, vol. 2, 808.

Chapter 3. Desire

1. A search for the phrase on Google (May 2012) resulted in 1,890,000 hits.

2. This absurd view of sexual desire (there need be nothing sexual about enjoying the comfort of contact with a cat—or a baby, for that matter—curled up on one's lap) is defended by Goldman, "Plain Sex."

3. This is the central thesis of Scruton, *Sexual Desire*.

4. Lewis, *The Four Loves*, 94–95.

Chapter 4. The Meaningfulness of Sexuality

1. Frankfurt, *The Reasons of Love*, 3–32.

2. Ibid., 90n3.

3. As I write about stamp collecting, I keep at the back of my mind Krzysztof Kieslowski's delightful film *Decalogue X*.

4. Aristotle, *Nicomachean Ethics*, I.1.

5. Frankfurt, *The Reasons of Love*, 23–28.

6. Cf. Parfit, *Reasons and Persons*, chap. 8.

7. Goldman, "Plain Sex."

8. Marcus Aurelius, *Meditations* 6.13, quoted in Hadot, *Philosophy as a Way of Life*, 185.

9. An exception is jurisdictions where parental permission allows for underage persons to marry, and where the resulting marital sex is legally permitted—however, I think there is something deeply inappropriate about allowing those who are not capable on their own of giving valid consent to marry, since marriage involves a first-person commitment.

10. Plato, *Republic*, 331c.

11. Palmer, "'Hi, My Name Isn't Justice, Honey,' and Shame on Lockyer."

12. Orthodox Judaism waives the requirements of kashrut in cases where life is in danger, except in circumstances of persecution where strict observance is required. Thus, the circumstances in question would have to be ones of persecution.

13. Of course anybody who accepts the psychological harm account will admit that there are also other causes of harm present, and those would not be removed by the attitude changes. However, since *ex hypothesi* these other harms are not the primary cause of the badness, although removal of the psychological attitudes would not remove all harm from rape, we can plausibly say that on this hypothesis total harm would be mitigated as much as by preventing many occurrences of rape.

14. Cf. May, "Four Mischievous Theories of Sex," 199.

15. Solomon, "Sexual Paradigms."

16. The Christian tradition is unanimous that there are angels, but it is not unanimous on the question of whether they are embodied.

17. The failure of the idea that romantic love is the conjunction of love and sexual attraction is emblematic of the way conjunctive definitions typically fail—for what is needed, typically, is not just a conjunction, but an *interplay* of the factors.

18. This is a variant of the point made about the good by Geach, "Good and Evil."

19. It could, for instance, be that sticking a finger in someone's ear is a medical procedure that consummates a physician-patient relationship.

Chapter 5. One Flesh, One Body

1. Genesis 2 is a Yahwist text, and the Yahwist is indeed very much concerned with sexual relationships: for instance, he gives us a version of the Hagar and Ishmael story, the story of Isaac finding his wife and later pretending she is his sister, and the tale of Jacob, Leah, and Rachel.

2. We may ask the philosophical question whether the soul can survive the death of the body. The Christian tradition uniformly answers in the positive. But at the same time, it seems right to say that the person survives the death of the body in a highly truncated way, and hence a resurrection of the body is needed.

3. For instance, in the case of Matthew 16:26, this includes the Revised Standard Version, New Revised Standard Version, New American Bible, and New Jerusalem Bible. Notably, the New International Version has "soul."

4. Nozick, *Anarchy, State and Utopia*, 42–45.

5. One who wishes to try for something a step more literal, might try to build on the social-person approach of J. Lee, *Is "Social Justice" Justice?*

6. If there is a further metaphysical fact about being one body, then we do not really know whether the geep is one body or not.

7. Long, *Veterinary Genetics and Reproductive Physiology*, 33–34.

8. This mirrors how Edwin Muir, "Annunciation," describes marriage as a "liberty / Where each asks from each / What each most wants to give / And each awakes in each / What else would never be." *Collected Poems*, 117.

9. See Bollinger et al., "Biofilms in the Large Bowel."

10. There are different ways of trying to reduce the concept of proper function to non-normative facts of natural selection. Thus, Wright, *Teleological Explanations,* says that a feature F has G as its proper goal, provided that F exists *because* it tends to produce G. In evolutionary cases, this would mean that some system has a particular goal if the system was evolutionarily selected *because of* its tending to achieve that goal. This would reduce the question of a proper goal or function to the non-normative question of why some feature F exists. On this view, eyes do tend to produce visual representations, and we have eyes *because* they produce visual representations—it is because eyes produce visual representations that the genes coding for them were selected for. But a version of the evil scientist scenario also shows that this reduction fails. We could imagine everybody who lacks some genetic defect being killed by the evil scientist. Then, in the next generation, we would have to say that the defect was not a defect at all—it had the function of protecting people from the killer. (Cf. Plantinga, *Warrant and Proper Function,* 199–211.) Valiant attempts have been made to fix up Wright's account. For instance, Bedau, "Where Is the Good in Teleology?" added conditions about the goodness of the function, while Robert Koons, *Realism Regained,* 145, tried to add the condition that the function has to contribute to the harmony or homeostasis of the organism (in personal communication, Koons has backed away from this account). Neither approach works, since the proper function of something could be evil (e.g., a dirty bomb) or destructive to the organism (e.g., a self-destruct gene, or perhaps a reproductive

process that results in the parent organism being destroyed and more than one child organism resulting—that might be the right way to understand ameba reproduction). The prospects for a reduction of the claim that cooperation is normal to non-normative facts about natural selection are bleak.

11. This of course is an adaptation of Thomas Aquinas's celebrated refinement of the unequivocal-equivocal distinction for the sake of saving theological language.

12. Ratsch, "Design, Chance and Theistic Evolution."

13. There are some philosophical difficulties with reconciling the notion of divine design with random evolution, but these could be taken care of either by positing occasional direct divine intervention in the evolutionary process and thus denying that the evolutionary processes count as random, or by weakening one's picture of the explanatory claims made by standard evolutionary theories. See Pruss, "How Not to Reconcile the Creation of Human Beings with Evolution" and "A New Way to Reconcile Creation with Current Evolutionary Science."

14. This last example is used by Aristotle, *Physics,* II.8.

15. The first two secondary "first principles of natural law" specify that it is good for humans to live and to reproduce. It is clear from *Summa Theologica* I-II.94.2 that this is true of nonhuman animals as well.

16. If normalcy were defined by the mean instead of the median, this would be logically possible, but because the mean weight would seem to me likely to be skewed upward of the median (a typical adult can survive being 150 pounds overweight but not being 150 pounds underweight), it is unlikely to happen in the case of weight.

17. Most of these ideas about physicians come from James Lennox, in conversation.

18. Some scholars have questioned the Pauline authorship of Ephesians. But in any case, Ephesians clearly explores Pauline themes.

19. Augustine, *The Trinity,* XII.2.

20. The Eastern Orthodox distinguish the divine *energeia* from the divine essence. I do not think the question whether the distinction is appropriate affects the present argument.

21. Andrea Dworkin, in *Intercourse,* chap. 7, argues that heterosexual intercourse is expressive of the subjugation of women. Her argument is twofold. The first is that our patriarchal culture assigns this meaning to intercourse. At least to a Christian, this argument should not be persuasive, because it is essential to Christianity that, by divine grace, the Christian community is capable of being a culture of love that resists unjust outside influences. Of course, in practice, Christian communities do not always fulfill this capability, but grace justifies an optimism about the possibility of doing so, and hence of giving sexual intercourse—since this is something that

Christianity holds to be morally permissible—a positive meaning. The philosophically more daring part of Dworkin's argument is that the subjugation of women is intrinsically a part of the meaning of penile-vaginal intercourse in virtue of the physically invasive character of this, a meaning that is present regardless of whether the parties involved consciously recognize it. However, this argument appears to depend too much on culturally accepted ways of describing the sexual act, including terminology such as "penetration." As has been pointed out by another author, heterosexual intercourse can also be conceptualized in such a way that the mechanics are not seen as having sexist implications: parallel to "penetration" one can, for instance, talk of "enveloping," implying an active role for the woman. Newton and Einstein teach us that the question of what is in motion and what is not is a merely relative one. The question of whose muscles are somewhat more active is not a merely relative one, but does not seem of much moral significance. The crucial worry, though, is not with regard to activity/passivity, but with regard to the allegedly invasive nature of the act. However, there, too, it is largely a matter of conceptualization. We do not think of the joey's hiding in its mother's pouch as an *invasion*. There is no threat or violence implied either by the joey's entry or by the kangaroo mother's envelopment. A moral principle that prohibits the entry of one person's body parts inside another person would make many medical procedures normally thought unproblematic, such as heart surgery, morally unacceptable. And one might ask, perhaps only somewhat frivolously, if it is wrong to shake hands with a person who has large hands that would entirely surround one's hand in the handshake. But the obvious objection to Dworkin is that, as she realized, the universal following of her morality in the days before artificial insemination would have led to the extinction of the human race. And certainly at least a theist who thinks that God intended us to reproduce cannot accept that.

22. Goldman, "Plain Sex."

23. For what limited worth this may have in regard to human beings, it should be noted that this has been confirmed in male fruitflies by Partridge and Farquhar, "Sexual Activity Reduces Lifespan of Male Fruitflies."

24. Smart and Williams, *Utilitarianism: For and Against,* 25.

25. Aristotle, *Nicomachean Ethics,* X.4.

26. Cf. the view of emotions as concern-based construals in Roberts, *Emotions: An Essay in Aid of Moral Psychology.*

27. See Solomon, "Sexual Paradigms."

28. Grewen et al., "Effects of Partner Support."

29. This thought experiment in this context is due to a speaker at the Cardinal Newman Lecture Series at the Pittsburgh Oratory, probably in the late 1990s. Unfortunately, my memory does not suffice to let me be completely certain as to the identity of the speaker.

30. Dworkin, *Intercourse*, 133.

31. Cf. the argument for altruism of Nagel, *The Possibility of Altruism*.

32. Suarez and Pacey, "Sperm Transport in the Human Female Reproductive Tract," 26.

33. Wildt et al., "Sperm Transport in the Human Female Genital Tract," 658.

34. Ibid., 664.

35. See Suarez and Pacey, "Sperm Transport in the Human Female Reproductive Tract," 28, and references therein.

36. R. Levin, "The Physiology of Sexual Arousal in the Human Female," 409.

37. Arguably, a pre-implantation embryo can be described as reproducing asexually when it twins.

38. John of Damascus, *Exposition of the Orthodox Faith*, part I.

39. In the Capilano Suspension Bridge experiment, male subjects were more likely to call back a pretty female experimenter when they met her on a high, swaying suspension bridge than on a solid lower bridge: Dutton and Aron, "Some Evidence for Heightened Sexual Attraction under Conditions of High Anxiety." The two-factor theory of emotion holds that when we are in the throes of a physiological arousal, we seek for a cognitive interpretation, and the emotion is the combination of the interpretation and the arousal. The classic work here is Schachter and Singer, "Cognitive, Social, and Physiological Determinants of Emotional State." Their work, as well as that of Dutton and Aron, shows that a theory on which emotion is entirely constituted by a physiological reaction is highly implausible. One needs either to take it that emotion includes a physiological state, plus something not introspectible in the same way that the physiological state is, or else to follow Schachter and Singer in taking emotion to be an interpreted physiological reaction. The latter option does not seem to allow one to say that one is mistaken in what emotion one is having, except in cases of gross inappropriateness of emotion to reaction, since one's interpretation is significantly definitive of the emotion. However, I think, a more natural way of interpreting the experimental data is that we simply have a case of the misidentification of an emotion.

40. Stocker, "The Schizophrenia of Modern Ethical Theories."

41. Apparently there have been tribes where the connection between reproduction and intercourse was not known. Some may still be around nowadays. And even in our society, there apparently are adults unaware of the connection.

42. Current Catholic canon law requires that the consummating act be the *kind* of act that can result in reproduction, and this is taken by some to exclude the use of condoms which change the nature of the act: Beal,

Coriden, and Green, *New Commentary on the Code of Canon Law*, 1364. Oral contraceptives do not appear to change the nature of what the couple is doing *while having sex*, or at least not in the same way.

43. Ibid., 1284–86.

44. It was once speculated that Cowper's fluid secreted during coitus interruptus would carry sperm and thus be capable of leading to fertilization. If true, this might strengthen that argument somewhat, by making the secretion of Cowper's fluid be analogous to ejaculation, though it would still seem to be the case that Cowper's fluid is secreted for lubrication rather than fertilization. In any case, current microscopic evidence suggests that Cowper's fluid does not contain sperm: see Zukerman, Weiss, and Orvieto, "Does Preejaculatory Penile Secretion Originating from Cowper's Gland Contain Sperm?"

45. Grisez et al., "Every Marital Act Ought to be Open to New Life."

46. Nagel, "Sexual Perversion."

47. For a discussion, see R. Levin, "The Physiology of Sexual Arousal in the Human Female."

Chapter 6. Union, Commitment, and Marriage

1. Matthew 22:30 says that there is no marrying or giving in marriage (*oute gamousin oute gamizontai*), and that those in heaven are like the angels. The context is a response to the question of to whom a woman would be married in heaven, if she had a series of husbands. For the response to be a good one, it must be understood as implying not only that there is no acquiring new marriages once one is in heaven, but that the old ones are dissolved as well.

2. Jesus' saying that there is no marriage in heaven (Matt. 22:30) is given precisely in response to a question about the heavenly marital status of someone who had been married and widowed a number of times.

3. Cf. Punzo, *Reflective Naturalism*.

4. Nonhuman animals seem to be blessed with a richer set of instincts than we are, and it may be that they can cooperate with less of a mental component.

5. If my heart is transplanted into you, then it seems right to say that my heart, a part whose function was to promote *my* life, has ceased to exist, and you came to have a heart made out of what used to be my heart.

6. Punzo, *Reflective Naturalism*.

7. The question of the moral evaluation of the actions of nonresponsible agents, such as that of the insane, is difficult and beyond the scope of

this book. I think a good heuristic for figuring out what action is right or wrong for a nonresponsible agent is to ask what would be right for a responsible agent to do. Thus, I would say that it would be *wrong* for an insane person to kill an innocent person, since that is the sort of action that it would be clearly wrong for a sane person to do, but the insane person is not *culpable* for this wrong. There are also complications with partial responsibility.

8. For details, see Beal, Coriden, and Green, *New Commentary on the Code of Canon Law*, 1334–35.

9. Ibid., 1352–55.

10. Meyendorff, *Marriage: An Orthodox Perspective*, 15.

11. See Kaczor, "Marital Acts without Marital Vows: Social Justice and Premarital Sex."

12. See, for instance, Manski et al., "Alternative Estimates of the Effect of Family Structure during Adolescence on High School Graduation."

13. Osborne, Manning, and Smock, "Married and Cohabiting Parents' Relationship Stability."

14. Conception probabilities depend on the day of the reproductive cycle relative to ovulation. My rough calculation of the overall conception probability was made by summing up the day-by-day conception probabilities, and dividing by a fixed cycle length of 29.1. This is not entirely accurate given that actual cycle length varies, but should be close. The day-by-day conception probabilities and the average cycle length are taken from B. Colombo et al., "Cervical Mucus Symptom and Daily Fecundability." It is also worth noting that sexual desire of women in long-term committed sexual relationships (and only those women) is higher on cycle days on which the probability of conception is higher, according to Pillsworth, Haselton, and Buss, "Ovulatory Shifts in Female Sexual Desire." Thus, in the case of unmarried women in long-term committed relationships, assuming the likelihood of intercourse increases with desire, the actual conception probability will presumably be higher than 5 percent (note also that in the work of Colombo et al. the day-by-day conception probability peaks at 42.9 percent).

15. Kost et al., "Estimates of Contraceptive Failure from the 2002 National Survey of Family Growth."

16. Glasier, "Implantable Contraceptives for Women."

17. This is one of the hypotheses to explain why an increase in out-of-wedlock births accompanied the availability of contraception and abortion in the United States given by Akerlof, Yellen, and Katz, "An Analysis of Out-of-Wedlock Childbearing in the United States."

18. For a historical discussion, see Jones, *The Soul of the Embryo*.

19. For the Greek, see Lake, *The Apostolic Fathers*, vol. 1, 310–12. The translation here is mainly mine.

20. See Olson, *The Human Animal*. For defenses of arguments against abortion and discussion of opposed arguments, see Napier, *Persons, Moral Worth, and Embryos*.

21. This is noted in the (different) argument against premarital sex in Punzo, *Reflective Naturalism*.

22. Meyendorff, *Marriage: An Orthodox Perspective*, 15.

23. See John Paul II, *Man and Woman He Created Them*.

24. Wittgenstein, *Philosophical Investigations*, 178.

25. R. R. Bollinger et al., "Biofilms in the Large Bowel."

26. In the case of a suicide in order to avoid physical pain—as in euthanasia—Kant points out another kind of internal self-contradiction. Physical pain is a survival mechanism. But in such a suicide, this survival mechanism becomes twisted into a motivator for self-destruction.

27. Punzo, *Reflective Naturalism*.

28. Children may not be able to make the commitment yet, but if they are psychologically normal, they can simply wait until they become more mature.

29. Punzo, *Reflective Naturalism*.

30. Aquinas, *Summa Theologica*, II-II.154.2.

31. Ibid.

32. On the bonobos, see Roughgarden, *Evolution's Rainbow*, 149–50.

33. The exact relation between laws of physics and the natures of entities is a difficult question that we do not need to settle here.

34. Note that although the two laws fit the observed data very similarly, the difference between the two laws is one we cannot ignore as irrelevant. One law predicts that y is always proportional to x and the other predicts that for large values of x, y is approximately proportional to the square of x.

35. This divine-command approach to generalizing from for-the-most-part prohibitions to complete prohibitions comes from a remark of Stephen Evans in conversation.

36. For instance, perhaps I could make a promise I cannot escape from to a person who is about to fall into a coma for the rest of his life, since while in a coma he cannot release me.

37. Arguably, one can only promise something to someone who has a sufficient interest in one's maintenance of the promise. Thus, I cannot promise you to be kind to my wife, unless you have an interest in my being kind to her, say, because you are a friend of hers.

38. Epstein, *Marriage Laws in the Bible and the Talmud*, 14–15, finds the innovation so startling that he decides that "adultery" is not to be understood literally here.

39. Some manuscripts make 19:9 closer to 5:32, however.

40. Jurgens, *Faith of the Early Fathers*, vol. 1, 141.

41. Ibid., vol. 2, 178.

42. Ibid., vol. 1, 268.

43. Ibid., vols. 1–3.

44. In his Montanist period, Tertullian would likely prohibit the remarriage of women divorced on account of the husband's adultery, given that in *Monogamy* he even prohibits the remarriage of widows. See Tertullian, *Treatises on Marriage and Remarriage*, 89–90.

45. Jurgens, *Faith of the Early Fathers*, vol. 2, 185.

46. Lake, *The Apostolic Fathers*, vol. 2, 79.

47. Jurgens, *Faith of the Early Fathers*, vol. 1, 212.

48. Ibid., vol. 1, 253.

49. In his letter to Amandus, Jerome states that remarriage is forbidden to women, no matter how unfaithful the husband (ibid., vol. 2, 185). If we combine that with his principle of equality in sexual matters, it follows that husbands are also absolutely forbidden from remarriage.

50. Ibid., vol. 2, 7–8.

51. Thus, Origen (ibid., vol. 1, 212), the Council of Elvira (ibid., vol. 1, 253), probably St. Basil (ibid., vol. 2, 7–8), St. Jerome (see n. 49 above), and St. Augustine (ibid., vol. 3, 132–33).

52. Lake, *The Apostolic Fathers*, vol. 2, 79.

53. Tigay, *The JPS Torah Commentary: Deuteronomy*, 221.

54. Ibid.

55. Granted, the move to make adultery a sin against the woman *was* radical. But by itself it would not have been a radical *tightening* of existing rules, but simply a different way of understanding the sinfulness of an act that the Jewish community would have rejected for other reasons.

56. Epstein, *Marriage Laws in the Bible and the Talmud*, 174.

57. Ibid., 246.

58. The hypothesis of a scribal as opposed to authorial gloss would have no evidential basis as far as I know.

59. *The Book of Common Prayer.*

60. Karant-Nunn and Wiesner-Hanks, *Luther on Women*, 117.

61. Cf. the remark of St. Jerome's that we do not allow men what we do not allow women: Jurgens, *Faith of the Early Fathers*, vol. 2, 185.

62. I am grateful to Ron Belgau for this last argument.

63. In much later rabbinical practice, the public shaming (removal of a shoe and being spat on) became the preferred resolution, and indeed stopped being considered shameful.

64. I am grateful to Amy Pruss for this point.

65. Epstein, *Marriage Laws in the Bible and the Talmud*, 11.

66. E. Levin, *Sex and Society in the World of the Orthodox Slavs, 900–1700*, 163; especially see the references in 163n7.

67. It seems that some scribes may have found the blunt *opheilê* too sexually explicit, and so many later manuscripts talk about *opheilê eunoia*, the "due benevolence" (to use the King James translation)!

68. Cf. Wojtyła, *Love and Responsibility*, 66–69.

69. Aristotle, *Nicomachean Ethics*, IX.4.

70. *The Book of Common Prayer*.

71. One might marry one's commanding officer. But such mixing of relationships is unlikely to be advisable.

72. Aquinas, *The Catechetical Instructions of St. Thomas Aquinas*.

73. Cf. Beal, Coriden, and Green, *New Commentary on the Code of Canon Law*, 1378–84.

Chapter 7. Contraception and Natural Family Planning

1. I will not discuss this particular case further. One might ask whether there isn't something wrong with failing to take such medication in cases where the medication is cheap and easily available, and one is abnormally infertile (a twenty-year-old who is infertile is abnormally so, but a 110-year-old is not abnormally infertile), since it seems to be a good thing to repair bodily abnormalities. The answer is not completely clear.

2. The latter example is due to an anonymous reader.

3. Aristotle, *Nicomachean Ethics*, IX.3.

4. Love always comes with a tendency to union, but perhaps sometimes this tendency is experienced not as a desire but as a purely voluntary striving.

5. In practice, it appears that psychological attitudes do affect fertility. But they do not do so in any simple volitional way such that the choice to reproduce causes reproduction. Rather, what appears to be the case is that stress can reduce fertility. For a review of the literature, see Nakamura, Sheps, and Arck, "Stress and Reproductive Failure."

6. Things might be different in respect of spiritual desires induced by the Holy Spirit. Whether they are or not depends on deep questions on the interplay between grace and free will.

7. Lake, *The Apostolic Fathers*, vol. 1, 376–77. I changed Lake's translation of "gives birth" to the contextually appropriate "conceives."

8. Ibid. I changed Lake's "because of uncleanliness" and "unclean" to "through impurity" and "impure," respectively.

9. Ibid., vol. 1, 375.

10. Jurgens, *The Faith of the Early Fathers*, vol. 1, 173; J.-P. Migne, *Patrologiae Cursus Completus, Series Graeca*, vol. 16/3, col. 3387.

11. Noonan, *Contraception*, 94.

12. If so, then Hippolytus would very much like the argument of Grisez et al., "Every Marital Act Ought to Be Open to New Life."

13. For a detailed discussion of the history, see Noonan, *Contraception*.

14. This is in his commentary on the story of Onan. See Luther, *Lectures on Genesis, Chapters 38–44*.

15. Noonan, *Contraception*, 353.

16. E.g., Sarna, *The JPS Torah Commentary: Genesis*, 267.

17. Lake, *The Apostolic Fathers*, vol. 1, 310–13, with the translation of the abortion and infanticide clauses modified to follow the Greek more closely.

18. Migne, *Patrologiae Cursus Completus, Series Graeca*, vol. 16/3, col. 3387.

19. According to the Torah, touching a dead body incurs ritual impurity. But it is not *immoral* to incur ritual impurity. And, in any case, the purely ritual rules do not apply to Christians in the same way.

20. There are specific rules about treatment of some animals, but there are no rules that would say that causing needless pain to one's cat is wrong.

21. Augustine, *The Trinity*, XII.2.

22. Grisez et al., "Every Marital Act Ought to Be Open to New Life." A recent defense of and elaboration of this line of argument is given by Masek, "Treating Humanity as an Inviolable End."

23. Grisez et al., "Every Marital Act Ought to Be Open to New Life," 371.

24. The main Christian body officially opposed to positive contraception is the Catholic Church. This opposition is found in the context of the encyclical *Humanae Vitae*, which can reasonably be read as concerned with the consensual marital case. Nuns in danger of rape have had contraceptive decisions left to their individual conscience, and current U.S. Catholic medical ethics guidelines in the United States permit the use of emergency birth control (EBC) in cases of rape providing that it has been checked that the woman is not yet pregnant: United States Conference of Catholic Bishops, *Ethical and Religious Directives for Catholic Health Care Services*, directive 36.

25. Grisez et al., "Every Marital Act Ought to Be Open to New Life," 390.

26. For one fairly recent discussion, see Cavanaugh, *Double-Effect Reasoning*. For a controversial modification of the traditional version of PDE (the differences do not matter for the purposes of this book), see Pruss, "Accomplishment of Plans."

27. The original version of this example involved a human agent rather than a robot. A reader objected that in this case one's intention could be to prevent the intrinsic wrong of cloning (assuming cloning is wrong). But a

nonconscious robot does no wrong, and I set up the example to assume that no one programmed the robot to do this. Perhaps the robot's activity is the unfortunate outcome of an experiment in random programming.

28. This holds even though one might not always know which one, as in cases of terrorists who set a bomb to go off at a later time.

29. Corvino, "Homosexuality," 137, uses the example of the mouth as an organ that has many uses. However, it is better to run this argument in the case of an organ like a kidney, whose purpose is well-defined. The mouth is already a multipurpose organ, and so it would be less of a surprise to find that some action is a purpose of it.

30. Grisez et al., "Every Marital Act Ought to Be Open to New Life."

31. For the most recent work in this direction, see Beckwith, *Defending Life;* George and Tollefsen, *Embryo;* and the essays in Napier, *Persons, Moral Worth, and Embryos.*

32. Milsom and Korver, "Ovulation Incidence with Oral Contraceptives: A Literature Review."

33. Larimore and Stanford, "Postfertilization Effects of Oral Contraceptives and Their Relationship to Informed Consent."

34. See the discussion in Wildt et al., "Sperm Transport in the Human Female Genital Tract," 661.

35. For a review of the evidence, see Larimore and Stanford, "Postfertilization Effects of Oral Contraceptives and Their Relationship to Informed Consent," 127–30.

36. Larimore and Stanford, "Ectopic Pregnancy with Oral Contraceptive Use Has Been Overlooked," based on data in Coste et al., "Risk Factors for Ectopic Pregnancy," and Thorburn et al., "Background Factors of Ectopic Pregnancy."

37. Stanford and Mikolajczyk, "Mechanisms of Action of Intrauterine Devices."

38. Germano and Jennings, "New Approaches to Fertility Awareness–Based Methods."

39. Stryder, "'Natural Family Planning.'"

40. Frank-Herrmann et al., "The Effectiveness of a Fertility Awareness–Based Method to Avoid Pregnancy in Relation to a Couple's Sexual Behaviour during the Fertile Time."

41. For a discussion of reasons for having sex on fertile days, see Sinai et al., "Fertility Awareness–Based Methods of Family Planning."

42. Glasier, "Implantable Contraceptives for Women."

43. Ibid.

44. In fact, in most cases, the days of heaviest flow are infertile, *except* when this is not a genuine menstrual period but "breakthrough bleeding."

However, in practice, it is not easy to recognize the difference without Natural Family Planning methods.

45. Noonan, *Contraception*, 120.

46. The source is the Supplement to the *Summa*, written by a disciple of Thomas's based on Thomas's ideas: Aquinas, *Summa Theologica*, Supplement 64.3.

47. Latz, *The Rhythm of Sterility and Fertility in Women*, 106.

48. Ibid., 34–41.

49. Pius XI, *Casti Connubii*, section 59.

50. John Paul II, *Familiaris Consortio*, section 32.

51. Pontifical Council for the Family, *Vademecum for Confessors Concerning Some Aspects of the Morality of Conjugal Life*.

52. The Catholic Church holds that when the Catholic Church as a whole believes something in a definitive way, this is infallible. It is clear that in the past the Church (both by the Catholic definition, and by Protestant definitions) as a whole believed in a definitive way that contraception is wrong. It is not completely clear that the teaching on the permissibility of periodic abstinence, though it appears quite universally accepted, is accepted with the same definitiveness.

53. Readers interested in decision theory will recall Good's Theorem here: Good, "On the Principle of Total Evidence."

54. Indeed, the contrary may sometimes be true, in that the earlier abstinence may make for greater sperm availability during the acts in which they actually engage.

55. And even if it were found that there is some strange effect, such as that thinking about fertility makes one less fertile, the question should not really be whether fertility is affected in this way, but whether it is *intentionally* affected.

56. If not, then the case is like that of a married woman who used an oral contraceptive and then changed her mind, wishing she hadn't used the contraceptive. In such a case, I would argue, she did wrong in taking the contraceptive, since she intended to engage in contracepted sex, but she did not do wrong in engaging in sex after she changed her mind, because there no longer was a contraceptive intention in her mind; there was no assent of will to her act of contraception at the time of the sexual act. For the same reason, it is permissible for a person who undergoes a sterilization and then has a change of heart to engage in marital intercourse even without reversing the sterilization (e.g., because the reversal is impossible or is too expensive).

57. Wilson, "The Practice of Natural Family Planning Versus the Use of Artificial Birth Control."

58. Newman, *A Letter Addressed to His Grace the Duke of Norfolk*, 75.

59. Newman, *Sermons Preached on Various Occasions,* 67.

60. Newman, *Essay on the Development of Christian Doctrine.*

61. For instance, those regimens discussed by Germano and Jennings, "New Approaches to Fertility Awareness–Based Methods."

62. On the face of it, a similar position is held by rabbinical Judaism, which also prohibits coitus interruptus and the condom but allows some other forms of contraception. But the similarity is deceptive. Rabbinical Judaism prohibits male-centered contraception on the grounds that it involves an immoral spilling of seed and that it is contrary to the man's duty of procreation, while allowing female-centered contraception, explicitly including barrier methods, at least when it is medically necessary, since the woman is not seen as having seed that can be wasted and since the duty of procreation is believed to fall only on men. Thus, the grounds of the prohibition are different and the practical distinction falls differently: the position of the above-mentioned Christian theologians would commit them, unlike the rabbis, to condemning the diaphragm.

63. The joke as I came across it continues with the judge sentencing the arm to jail, and the man then removing his arm—which turns out to have been prosthetic. If in the case of a prosthesis we recognize what is done with it as done by the person, a fortiori we should recognize this in the case of a nonprosthetic limb.

64. Reid uses this as an argument for a natural language. Reid, *Inquiry into the Human Mind on the Principles of Common Sense,* 51.

65. Personal communication (May 2009).

66. Huber et al., "Non-contraceptive Benefits of Oral Contraceptives."

67. Nakamura, Sheps, and Arck, "Stress and Reproductive Failure."

68. One imagines that it would be possible to stop transmission in the other direction with some creative use of technology, such as a condom-like device with a one-way valve or *maybe* even a condom with a sufficiently small puncture, sufficient to allow one-way transmission of semen. This is a matter for scientific research.

69. Rhonheimer, "The Truth about Condoms."

70. Ibid.

71. Grisez et al., "Every Marital Act Ought to Be Open to New Life."

72. Grisez, "Moral Questions on Condoms and Disease Prevention."

73. Trimpop, *The Psychology of Risk Taking Behavior,* chap. 8.

74. Sagberg, Fosser, and Saetermo, "An Investigation of Behavioral Adaptation."

75. Shelton, "Confessions of a Condom Lover," 1947. On the same page, Shelton notes that he is nonetheless someone who has "helped [his] agency [the US Agency for International Development] provide billions" of

condoms. Shelton ends up advocating a strategy where "partner limitation takes center stage," but condoms are a part of the strategy.

76. For some preliminary mathematical modeling leading to heuristics, see Pruss, "Risk Reduction Policies."

77. Cf. McCarthy and Pruss, "Condoms and HIV Transmission."

78. I think this point in this context is due to Mark Murphy, in discussion.

79. In an electronic discussion, someone once compared the use of the condom to shaking hands with the Queen while she is wearing gloves.

80. Cf. Beal, Coriden, and Green, *New Commentary on the Code of Canon Law*, 1364.

81. Cf. Akerlof, Yellen, and Katz, "An Analysis of Out-of-Wedlock Childbearing in the United States."

Chapter 8. Sexual Pleasure and Noncoital Sexual Activity

1. Grisez uses the phrase "complete [sexual] satisfaction" to describe orgasm (*The Way of the Lord Jesus*, vol. 2, 645). The English word "satisfaction," however, is ambiguous between the actual satisfaction of a need or desire and a feeling of such satisfaction. Since sexual desire is a desire for a union with the other person, and orgasm can occur apart from that union, it is better to talk of orgasm as a *feeling* of complete sexual satisfaction.

2. I also think that nothing hangs on the fact that the commander was the one who set the bomb. Even if it were a subordinate who did so, with the commander's fingerprint being needed to defuse it, using the commander's finger for this purpose would still seem appropriate.

3. For an excellent discussion of lying, see Garcia, "Lies and the Vices of Deception." Moreover, the sorts of cases that are widely, though I believe incorrectly, taken to justify lying to evildoers do not appear to justify cases of self-induction of solitary sexual pleasure—the self-deception is not a way of tricking an evil part of the body into doing what it should be doing.

4. This could perhaps even happen in a case where the couple is not morally permitted to have sex at the moment, for instance because some pressing duty does not give them the time for it, or perhaps because the couple needs to abstain (this could either be a part of long-term or periodic abstinence) because of the imprudence of conceiving at this time. For in those cases, what the arousal is aimed at, sex with this person here and now, a person here and now experienced as a spouse, is not intrinsically wrong, though the sex is wrong because of extrinsic considerations, such as those of prudence.

5. Here, one might ask whether it is permissible for a married couple to be aroused at each other in a context where they do not experience each other as spouses. Since the experience of the other as a spouse—the experience of the other in the context of the marital relationship—suffuses so much of one's thinking, this would have to be a case where the members of the couple feel some kind of dissociation. And this dissociation would, I think, make sex problematic.

6. An excessive fixation on how one's spouse *used to look* is at least unhealthy. It is an interesting question whether it is appropriate to be aroused by how one's spouse used to look. At least we can say that there would be something creepy about becoming aroused at pictures of one's spouse that significantly predate one's relationship.

7. Scruton, *Sexual Desire,* chap. 10.

8. Dworkin, "Pornography Happens to Women."

9. Paul, *Pornified,* 72–106.

10. See ibid., as well as Wolf, "The Porn Myth."

11. See St. Thomas on the sin of morose delectation: Aquinas, *Summa Theologica,* I-II.74.6.

12. This is most obviously true on libertarian accounts of free will, and forms the centerpiece of the famous free will defense of Plantinga, *The Nature of Necessity.* But surprisingly, this could also be true on compatibilist accounts on which one acts freely provided that, roughly speaking, one knows what one is doing, one is not constrained, and one's action flows from one's character. For the fantasizer can fantasize about people freely acting in ways that are in fact contrary to their character, while on the compatibilist notion of freedom, God cannot make a person freely act contrary to character, except by first changing the person's character; moreover, not all imaginable divinely produced changes in a person's character need be compatible with the person's freedom (divine brainwashing would be contrary to a person's freedom just as much as being brainwashed by a fellow human).

13. This is not science fiction. Apparently, infrared-sensitive cameras are capable of seeing through some clothes made of artificial fibers.

14. Hugs that satisfy a desire for physical contact count as sex according to the definition of Goldman, "Plain Sex."

15. Cf. Aristotle, *Metaphysics,* XI.3.

Chapter 9. Same-Sex Attraction

1. Adam, "Relationship Innovation in Male Couples"; Yip, "Gay Male Christian Couples and Sexual Exclusivity."

2. Lewis, *The Four Loves*, holds that friendship is "artificial," but he may be using the term in a subtly different way from the present use.

3. What if, by a miracle, Goldie became capable of thought and speech? It can be argued that if this happened, then Goldie the Goldfish would have ceased to exist, replaced by a goldfish-like person, and so it would no longer be a love for *Goldie*. Alternately, perhaps a *supernatural* love matching Goldie's miraculous state would become possible?

Chapter 10. Reproduction and Technology

1. Aristotle, *Nicomachean Ethics*, IX.9.

2. "Tim" posting on AlexanderPruss.blogspot.com on June 5, 2008.

3. One form of noncoital reproduction that may in a sense be strongly natural is twinning. We do not understand enough scientifically about the causes of twinning or have enough of a philosophical understanding of its metaphysics (we do not know answers to questions like: "In twinning, is one individual replaced by two new ones, the old perishing, or does the old individual survive in some sense as both, or does the old survive as precisely one of the new ones?") to know whether twinning is strongly natural. But nonetheless, if it is strongly natural, it is strongly natural only to a very young embryo. One could not infer that cloning ourselves is strongly natural. Nor would it be strongly natural for us to clone an embryo, since while the twinning might be strongly natural, our act of *inducing* twinning would not be. It might be strongly natural for the embryo to clone itself, but the embryo seems to lack the conceptual skills to do so voluntarily anyway, so the question is moot. And besides this, it is clear that asexual reproduction is not intrinsically biologically unitive, precisely because it is *a*sexual. There might be a cooperative union between a person being cloned and a doctor, but this union is not essential to the act of cloning, since cloning, unlike sexual reproduction, can be done alone, assuming one has the requisite technical skills.

4. John Paul II, *Familiaris Consortio*, section 14.

5. George and Bradley, "Marriage and the Liberal Imagination."

6. For a version of this argument, see May, "Begetting vs. Making Babies."

7. Ibid.

8. Leiblum, "Infertility."

9. Schmidt et al., "Does Infertility Cause Marital Benefit?"

10. Nelson et al., "Prevalence and Predictors of Sexual Problems, Relationship Stress, and Depression in Female Partners of Infertile Couples"; A. W. Shindel et al., "Sexual Function and Quality of Life in the Male Partner of Infertile Couples."

11. This account of a cooperative community is largely taken from Wojtyła, *Osoba i Czyn* [*The Acting Person*], chap. 7.

12. May, "Begetting vs. Making Babies."

13. Cf. Colombo et al., "Cervical Mucus Symptom and Daily Fecundability," 172.

14. This is somewhat complicated in cases of promised gifts. We do have a right to expect that people will keep their promises to us. In the case of a promised gift, we can say that the real gratuity is in the promise rather than the delivery.

15. See the report of the Secretary of the Greek Synod Committee on Legal and Canonical Matters: Mantzouneas, "Fraternization from a Canonical Perspective."

16. Lewis, *The Four Loves*.

Chapter 11. Celibacy

1. Augustine, *Marriage and Virginity*.

2. Though St. Francis de Sales thinks the warnings against particular friendships apply only in monastic kinds of settings: de Sales, *Introduction to the Devout Life*, 175.

Bibliography

Adam, Barry D. "Relationship Innovation in Male Couples." *Sexualities* 9 (2006): 5–26.

Akerlof, George A., Janet L. Yellen, and Michael L. Katz. "An Analysis of Out-of-Wedlock Childbearing in the United States." *Quarterly Journal of Economics* 111 (1996): 277–317.

Aquinas, Thomas. *The Catechetical Instructions of St. Thomas Aquinas.* Translated by J. B. Collins. New York: Joseph F. Wagner, 1939.

———. *Summa Contra Gentiles.* Vol. 1. Translated by the English Dominican Fathers. New York: Benziger, 1924.

———. *Summa Theologica.* Translated by the Fathers of the English Dominican Province. New York: Benziger 1920.

Aristotle. *Metaphysics.* In *The Complete Works of Aristotle,* vol. 2, edited by J. Barnes, 1552–1728. Princeton: Princeton University Press, 1984.

———. *Nicomachean Ethics.* In *The Complete Works of Aristotle,* vol. 2, edited by J. Barnes, 1729–1867. Princeton: Princeton University Press, 1984.

———. *Physics.* In *The Complete Works of Aristotle,* vol. 1, edited by J. Barnes, 315–446. Princeton: Princeton University Press, 1984.

Augustine of Hippo. "Homilies on the First Epistle of John." Translated by H. Browne. In *Nicene and Post-Nicene Fathers,* edited by P. Schaff, 459–529. Vol. 7. Edinburgh: T&T Clark, 1888.

———. *Marriage and Virginity: The Excellence of Marriage, Holy Virginity, The Excellence of Widowhood, Adulterous Marriages, Continence.* Translated by Ray Kearney. Hyde Park, NY: New City Press, 1999.

———. *The Trinity.* Translated by Edmund Hill, OP. Brooklyn: New City Press, 1991.

Beal, John, James A. Coriden, and Thomas J. Green. *New Commentary on the Code of Canon Law*. New York: Paulist Press, 2000.

Beckwith, Francis J. *Defending Life: A Moral and Legal Case Against Abortion Choice*. Cambridge: Cambridge University Press, 2007.

Bedau, M. "Where Is the Good in Teleology?" *Philosophy and Phenomenological Research* 52 (1992): 781–801.

Benedict XVI. *Deus Caritas Est*. Available at http://www.vatican.va/holy _father/benedict_xvi/encyclicals/documents/hf_ben-xvi_enc _20051225_deus-caritas-est_en.html, 2005.

Bollinger, R. R., A. S. Barbas, E. L. Bush, S. S. Lin, and W. Parker. "Biofilms in the Large Bowel Suggest an Apparent Function of the Human Vermiform Appendix." *Journal of Theoretical Biology* 249 (2007): 826–31.

The Book of Common Prayer and Administration of the Sacraments and Other Rites and Ceremonies of the United Church of England and Ireland. London: Suttaby, 1863.

Cavanaugh, T. A. *Double-Effect Reasoning*. Oxford: Oxford University Press, 2006.

Cicero, Marcus Tullius. "On Friendship." In *Letters of Marcus Tullius Cicero with his Treatises on Friendship and Old Age and Letters of Gaius Plinius Caecilius Secundus*. Translated by E. S. Shuckburgh and W. Melnoth. New York: Collier and Sons, 1909.

Colombo, B., A. Mion, K. Passarin, and B. Scarpa. "Cervical Mucus Symptom and Daily Fecundability: First Results from a New Database." *Statistical Methods in Medical Research* 15 (2006): 161–80.

Corvino, John. "Homosexuality: The Nature and Harm Arguments." In *The Philosophy of Sex: Contemporary Readings,* 4th ed., edited by Alan Soble, 135–46. Lanham, MD: Rowman & Littlefield, 2002.

Coste, J., N. Job-Spira, H. Fernandez, E. Papiernik, and A. Spira. "Risk Factors for Ectopic Pregnancy: A Case-Control Study in France, with Special Focus on Infectious Factors." *American Journal of Epidemiology* 133 (1991): 839–49.

de Sales, Francis. *Introduction to the Devout Life*. Translated by John K. Ryan. New York: Image, 1989.

Dutton, Donald G., and Arthur P. Aron. "Some Evidence for Heightened Sexual Attraction under Conditions of High Anxiety." *Journal of Personality and Social Psychology* 30 (1974): 510–17.

Dworkin, Andrea. *Intercourse*. New York: Free Press, 1997.

———. "Pornography Happens to Women." Speech delivered at conference on Speech, Equality and Harm: Feminist Legal Perspectives on Pornography and Hate Propaganda, University of Chicago Law School, March 6, 1993. Available at http://www.nostatusquo.com/ACLU/ dworkin/PornHappens.html.

Epstein, Louis M. *Marriage Laws in the Bible and the Talmud*. Cambridge, MA: Harvard University Press, 1942.

Finnis, John. "Law, Morality, and 'Sexual Orientation.'" *Notre Dame Law Review* 69 (1994): 1049–76.

Frankfurt, Harry G. *The Reasons of Love*. Princeton: Princeton University Press, 2004.

Frank-Herrmann, P., J. Heil, C. Gnoth, E. Toledo, S. Baur, C. Pyper, E. Jenetzky, T. Strowitzki, and G. Freundl. "The Effectiveness of a Fertility Awareness–Based Method to Avoid Pregnancy in Relation to a Couple's Sexual Behaviour during the Fertile Time: A Prospective Longitudinal Study." *Human Reproduction* 22 (2007): 1310–19.

Garcia, J. L. A. "Lies and the Vices of Deception." *Faith and Philosophy* 15 (1998): 514–37.

Geach, Peter T. "Good and Evil." *Analysis* 17 (1956): 33–42.

George, Robert P., and Gerard V. Bradley. "Marriage and the Liberal Imagination." *Georgetown Law Journal* 84 (1995): 301–20.

George, Robert P., and Christopher Tollefsen. *Embryo: A Defense of Human Life*. New York: Doubleday, 2008.

Germano, Elaine, and Victoria Jennings. "New Approaches to Fertility Awareness–Based Methods: Incorporating the Standard Days and Two-Day Methods into Practice." *Journal of Midwifery and Women's Health* 51 (2006): 471–77.

Glasier, A. "Implantable Contraceptives for Women: Effectiveness, Discontinuation Rates, Return of Fertility, and Outcome of Pregnancies." *Contraception* 65 (2002): 29–37.

Goldman, Alan H. "Plain Sex." *Philosophy and Public Affairs* 6 (1977): 267–87.

Good, I. J. "On the Principle of Total Evidence." *British Journal for the Philosophy of Science* 17 (1967): 319–21.

Grewen, K. M., S. S. Girdler, J. Amico, and K. C. Light. "Effects of Partner Support on Resting Oxytocin, Cortisol, Norepinephrine, and Blood Pressure before and after Warm Partner Contact." *Psychosomatic Medicine* 67 (2005): 531–38.

Grisez, Germain. "Moral Questions on Condoms and Disease Prevention." *National Catholic Bioethics Quarterly* 8 (2008): 471–76.

———. *The Way of the Lord Jesus*. Vol. 2, *Living a Christian Life*. Quincy, IL: Franciscan Press, 1993.

Grisez, Germain, Joseph Boyle, John Finnis, and William E. May. "Every Marital Act Ought to Be Open to New Life: Toward a Clearer Understanding." *The Thomist* 52 (1988): 365–426.

Hadot, Pierre. *Philosophy as a Way of Life*. Malden, MA: Oxford University Press, 1995.

Hardy, Thomas. *Tess of the d'Urbervilles*. Addison-Wesley, 2003.

The Holy Bible: Revised Standard Version, Catholic Edition. Oxford: Oxford University Press, 2004.

Huber, J. C., E.-K. Bentz, J. Ott, and C. B. Tempfer. "Non-contraceptive Benefits of Oral Contraceptives." *Expert Opinion on Pharmacotherapy* 9 (2008): 2317–25.

John of Damascus. *Exposition of the Orthodox Faith*. Translated by H. Browne. In *Nicene and Post-Nicene Fathers*, 2nd ser., edited by Philip Schaff. Vol. 9. Edinburgh: T&T Clark, 1899.

John Paul II. *Familiaris Consortio*. Available at http://www.vatican.va/holy _father/john_paul_ii/apost_exhortations/documents/hf_jp-ii_exh _19811122_familiaris-consortio_en.html, 1981.

———. *Man and Woman He Created Them: A Theology of the Body*. Translated by Michael Waldstein. Boston: Pauline Media, 2006.

Jones, David Albert. *The Soul of the Embryo: An Enquiry into the Status of the Human Embryo in the Christian Tradition*. London: Continuum, 2004.

Jurgens, W. A., ed. and trans. *The Faith of the Early Fathers*. 3 vols. Collegeville, MN: Liturgical Press, 1970–79.

Kaczor, Christopher. "Marital Acts without Marital Vows: Social Justice and Premarital Sex." *Josephinum Journal of Theology* 9 (2002): 310–19.

Karant-Nunn, Susan C., and Merry E. Wiesner-Hanks. *Luther on Women: A Sourcebook*. Cambridge: Cambridge University Press, 2003.

Kierkegaard, Søren. *Journals and Papers*. 7 vols. Edited and translated by H. V. Hong and E. H. Hong. Bloomington: Indiana University Press, 1967.

Koons, Robert C. *Realism Regained: An Exact Theory of Causation, Teleology, and the Mind*. Oxford and New York: Oxford University Press, 2000.

Kost, Kathryn, Susheela Singh, Barbara Vaughan, James Trussell, and Akinrinola Bankole. "Estimates of Contraceptive Failure from the 2002 National Survey of Family Growth." *Contraception* 77 (2008): 10–21.

Krosik, Anthony, et al. *Human Sexuality: New Directions in American Catholic Thought*. New York: Paulist Press, 1977.

Lake, Kirsopp, ed. and trans. *The Apostolic Fathers*. Vol. 1. Cambridge, MA: Harvard University Press, 1985.

———, ed. and trans. *The Apostolic Fathers*. Vol. 2. London: Heinemann, 1913.

Larimore, Walter L., and Joseph B. Stanford. "Ectopic Pregnancy with Oral Contraceptive Use Has Been Overlooked." Letter to the Editor. *British Medical Journal* 12 (200): 450.

———. "Postfertilization Effects of Oral Contraceptives and Their Relationship to Informed Consent." *Archives of Family Medicine* 9 (2000): 126–33.

Latz, Leo J. *The Rhythm of Sterility and Fertility in Women*. Chicago: Latz Foundation, 1934.

Lee, John R. "Is 'Social Justice' Justice? A Thomistic Argument for 'Social Persons' as the Proper Subjects of the Virtue of Social Justice." PhD diss., Baylor University, 2008.

Lee, Patrick, and Robert P. George. *Body-Self Dualism in Contemporary Ethics and Politics*. Cambridge: Cambridge University Press, 2008.

Leiblum, S. R. "Infertility." In *Handbook of Behavioral Medicine for Women*, edited by E. A. Blechman and K. D. Brownell, 116–25. New York: Pergamon, 1988.

Levin, Eve. *Sex and Society in the World of the Orthodox Slavs, 900–1700*. Ithaca: Cornell University Press, 1989.

Levin, Roy J. "The Physiology of Sexual Arousal in the Human Female: A Recreational and Procreational Synthesis." *Archives of Sexual Behavior* 31 (2002): 405–11.

Lewis, C. S. *The Four Loves*. Orlando, FL: Harcourt Brace, 1988.

Long, Susan. *Veterinary Genetics and Reproductive Physiology*. Philadelphia: Elsevier, 2006.

Luther, Martin. *Lectures on Genesis, Chapters 38–44*. Edited by Jaroslav Pelikan. St. Louis: Concordia Publishing House, 1965.

Manski, Charles F., Gary D. Sandefur, Sara McLanahan, and Daniel Powers. "Alternative Estimates of the Effect of Family Structure during Adolescence on High School Graduation." *Journal of the American Statistical Association* 87 (1992): 25–37.

Mantzouneas, Evangelos K. "Fraternization from a Canonical Perspective." Available at http://www.qrd.org/qrd/religion/judeochristian/eastern _orthodox/Church.of.Greece.on.adelphopoiia. 1982 (edited 1994).

Masek, L. "Treating Humanity as an Inviolable End: An Analysis of Contraception and Altered Nuclear Transfer." *Journal of Medicine and Philosophy* 33 (2008): 158–73.

May, William E. "Begetting vs. Making Babies." In *Human Dignity and Reproductive Technology*, edited by Nicholas Lund-Mofese, 81–92. Lanham, MD: University Press of America, 2003.

May, William F. "Four Mischievous Theories of Sex." In *Wing to Wing, Oar to Oar: Readings on Courting and Marrying*, edited by Amy A. Kass and Leon R. Kass, 189–202. Notre Dame, IN: University of Notre Dame Press, 2000.

McCarthy, Anthony, and Alexander R. Pruss. "Condoms and HIV Transmission." In *Fertility & Gender*, edited by Helen Watt. Oxford: Anscombe Bioethics Centre, 2011.

Meyendorff, John. *Marriage: An Orthodox Perspective*. Crestwood, NY: St. Vladimir's Seminary Press, 1975.

Migne, J.-P. *Patrologiae Cursus Completus, Series Graeca.* Vol. 16/3. Paris, 1863.

Milsom, I., and T. Korver. "Ovulation Incidence with Oral Contraceptives: A Literature Review." *Journal of Family Planning and Reproductive Health Care* 34 (2008): 237–46.

Muir, Edwin. "Annunciation." In *Collected Poems,* 117. London: Faber and Faber, 1970.

Nagel, Thomas. *The Possibility of Altruism.* Princeton: Princeton University Press, 1978.

————. "Sexual Perversion." *Journal of Philosophy* 66 (1969): 5–17.

Nakamura, K., S. Sheps, and P. C. Arck. "Stress and Reproductive Failure: Past Notions, Present Insights and Future Directions." *Journal of Assisted Reproduction and Genetics* 25 (2008): 47–62.

Napier, S., ed. *Persons, Moral Worth, and Embryos: A Critical Analysis of Pro-Choice Arguments from Philosophy, Law, and Science.* Dordrecht: Springer, 2011.

Nelson, C. J., A. W. Shindel, C. K. Naughton, M. Ohebshalom, and J. P. Mulhall. "Prevalence and Predictors of Sexual Problems, Relationship Stress, and Depression in Female Partners of Infertile Couples." *Journal of Sexual Medicine* 5 (2008): 1907–14.

Newman, John Henry. *Essay on the Development of Christian Doctrine.* London: Longmans, Green and Co., 1920.

————. *A Letter Addressed to His Grace the Duke of Norfolk on Occasion of Mr. Gladstone's Recent Expostulation.* New York: Catholic Publication Society, 1875.

————. *Sermons Preached on Various Occasions.* New edition. London: Longmans, Green and Co., 1898.

Noonan, John T., Jr. *Contraception: A History of Its Treatment by the Catholic Theologians and Canonists.* Enlarged ed. Cambridge, MA: Belknap Press, 1986.

Nozick, Robert. *Anarchy, State and Utopia.* New York: Basic Books, 1974.

————. *The Examined Life.* New York: Simon and Schuster, 1989.

Nygren, Anders. *Agapê and Eros.* Chicago: University of Chicago Press, 1982.

Olson, Eric T. *The Human Animal: Personal Identity without Psychology.* Oxford: Oxford Unviersity Press, 1999.

Osborne, Cynthia, Wendy D. Manning, and Pamela J. Smock. "Married and Cohabiting Parents' Relationship Stability: A Focus on Race and Ethnicity." *Journal of Marriage and Family* 69 (2007): 1345–66.

Palmer, Tom G. "'Hi, My Name Isn't Justice, Honey,' and Shame on Lockyer." *Los Angeles Times* (June 6, 2001), B11.

Parfit, Derek. *Reasons and Persons.* Oxford: Oxford University Press, 1984.

Partridge, Linda, and Marion Farquhar. "Sexual Activity Reduces Lifespan of Male Fruitflies." *Nature* 294 (1981): 580–82.

Paul, Pamela. *Pornified: How Pornography Is Transforming Our Lives, Our Relationships, and Our Families.* New York: Times Books, 2005.

Pillsworth, E. G., M. G. Haselton, and D. M. Buss. "Ovulatory Shifts in Female Sexual Desire." *Journal of Sex Research* 41 (2004): 55–65.

Pius XI. *Casti Connubii,* Available at http://www.vatican.va/holy_father/pius_xi/encyclicals/documents/hf_p-xi_enc_31121930_casti-connubii_en.html, 1930.

Plantinga, Alvin. *The Nature of Necessity.* Oxford: Oxford University Press, 1974.

———. *Warrant and Proper Function.* Oxford: Oxford University Press, 1993.

Plato. *Republic.* Translated by G. M. A. Grube. Revised by C. D. C. Reeve. Indianapolis: Hackett, 1992.

Pontifical Council for the Family. *Vademecum for Confessors Concerning Some Aspects of the Morality of Conjugal Life.* Available at http://www.vatican.va/roman_curia/pontifical_councils/family/documents/rc_pc_family_doc_12021997_vademecum_en.html, 1997.

Pruss, Alexander R. "The Accomplishment of Plans: A New Version of the Principle of Double Effect." *Philosophical Studies.* Forthcoming.

———. "How Not to Reconcile the Creation of Human Beings with Evolution." *Philosophia Christi* 9 (2007): 145–63.

———. "A New Way to Reconcile Creation with Current Evolutionary Science." *Proceedings of the American Catholic Philosophical Association* 85 (2011): 213–22.

———. "Risk Reduction Policies." Available at http://alexanderpruss.blogspot.com/2010/12/risk-reduction-policies.html, 2010.

Punzo, Vincent. *Reflective Naturalism.* New York: Macmillan, 1969.

Ratsch, Del. "Design, Chance and Theistic Evolution." In *Mere Creation,* edited by William Dembski, 289–312. Downers Grove, IL: InterVarsity Press, 1998.

Reid, Thomas. *Inquiry into the Human Mind on the Principles of Common Sense: A Critical Edition.* Edited by Derek Brookes. University Park: Pennsylvania State University Press, 1997.

Rhonheimer, Martin. "The Truth about Condoms." *The Tablet* (July 10, 2004): 10–11.

Roberts, Robert C. *Emotions: An Essay in Aid of Moral Psychology.* Cambridge: Cambridge University Press, 2003.

Roughgarden, Joan. *Evolution's Rainbow: Diversity, Gender, and Sexuality in Nature and People.* Berkeley: University of California Press, 2004.

Sagberg, Fridulv, Stein Fosser, and Inger-Anne F. Saetermo. "An Investigation of Behavioural Adaptation to Airbags and Antilock Brakes among Taxi Drivers." *Accident Analysis and Prevention* 29 (1997): 293–302.

Sarna, Nahum M. *The JPS Torah Commentary: Genesis*. Philadelphia: Jewish Publication Society, 1989.

Schachter, S., and J. Singer. "Cognitive, Social, and Physiological Determinants of Emotional State." *Psychological Review* 69 (1962): 379–99.

Schmidt, Lone, Bjørn Holstein, Ulla Christensen, and Jacky Boivin. "Does Infertility Cause Marital Benefit? An Epidemiological Study of 2250 Women and Men in Fertility Treatment." *Patient Education and Counseling* 59 (2005): 244–51.

Scruton, Roger. *Sexual Desire: A Philosophical Investigation*. London: Continuum, 2006.

Shelton, James D. "Confessions of a Condom Lover." *The Lancet* 368 (2006): 1947–49.

Shindel, A. W., C. J. Nelson, C. K. Naughton, M. Ohebshalom, and J. P. Mulhall. "Sexual Function and Quality of Life in the Male Partner of Infertile Couples: Prevalence and Correlates of Dysfunction." *Journal of Urology* 179 (2008): 1056–59.

Sinai, Irit, Rebecka Lundgren, Marcos Arévalo, and Victoria Jennings. "Fertility Awareness–Based Methods of Family Planning: Predictors of Correct Use." *International Family Planning Perspectives* 32 (2006): 94–100.

Smart, J. J. C., and Bernard Williams. *Utilitarianism: For and Against*. Cambridge: Cambridge University Press, 1998.

Solomon, Robert C. "Sexual Paradigms." *Journal of Philosophy* 71 (1974): 336–45.

Stanford, Joseph B., and Rafael T. Mikolajczyk. "Mechanisms of Action of Intrauterine Devices: Update and Estimation of Postfertilization Effects." *American Journal of Obstetrics and Gynecology* 187 (2002): 1699–1708.

Stocker, Michael. "The Schizophrenia of Modern Ethical Theories." *Journal of Philosophy* 73 (1990): 453–66.

Stryder, R. E. J. "'Natural Family Planning': Effective Birth Control Supported by the Catholic Church." *British Medical Journal* 307 (1993): 723–26.

Suarez, S. S., and A. A. Pacey. "Sperm Transport in the Human Female Reproductive Tract." *Human Reproduction Update* 12 (2006): 23–37.

Tanner, Norman P., ed. *Decrees of the Ecumenical Councils*. Vol. 2. London: Sheed & Ward, 1990.

Tertullian. *Treatises on Marriage and Remarriage*. Translated by William P. LeSaint. Westminster, MD: Newman Press, 1951.

Thorburn, J., C. Berntsson, M. Philipson, and B. Lindblom. "Background Factors of Ectopic Pregnancy. I. Frequency Distribution in a Case-Control Study." *European Journal of Obstetrics, Gynecology, and Reproductive Biology* 23 (1986): 321–31.

Tigay, Jeffrey H. *The JPS Torah Commentary: Deuteronomy*. Philadelphia: Jewish Publication Society, 2003.

Trimpop, Rüdiger M. *The Psychology of Risk Taking Behavior*. Amsterdam: North-Holland, 1994.

United States Conference of Catholic Bishops. *Ethical and Religious Directives for Catholic Health Care Services*. 5th ed. Available at http://www.usccb.org/about/doctrine/ethical-and-religious-directives, 2009.

Wildt, L., S. Kissler, P. Licht, and W. Becker. "Sperm Transport in the Human Female Genital Tract and Its Modulation by Oxytocin as Assessed by Hysterosalpingoscintigraphy, Hysterotonography, Electrohysterography and Doppler Sonography." *Human Reproduction Update* 4 (1998): 655–66.

Wilson, Mercedes A. "The Practice of Natural Family Planning Versus the Use of Artificial Birth Control: Family, Sexual and Moral Issues." *Catholic Social Scientist Review* 7 (2002). Available at http://cssronline.org/CSSR/Archival/vol_vii.htm.

Wittgenstein, Ludwig. *Philosophical Investigations*. 2nd ed. Translated by G. E. M. Anscombe. Oxford: Blackwell, 1999.

Wojtyła, Karol. *Love and Responsibility*. Translated by H. T. Willets. San Francisco: Ignatius Press, 1993.

———. *Osoba i Czyn oraz Inne Studia Antropologiczne* [*The Acting Person*]. 3rd ed. Cracow: Wydawnictwo Towarzystwa Naukowego Katolickiego Uniwersytetu Lubelskiego, 1985.

Wolf, Naomi. "The Porn Myth." *New York Magazine* (October 20, 2003). Available at http://nymag.com/nymetro/news/trends/n_9437/.

Wright, L. *Teleological Explanations*. Berkeley: University of California Press, 1976.

Yip, Andrew K. T. "Gay Male Christian Couples and Sexual Exclusivity." *Sociology* 31 (1997): 289–306.

Zukerman, Z., D. B. Weiss, and R. Orvieto. "Does Preejaculatory Penile Secretion Originating from Cowper's Gland Contain Sperm?" *Journal of Assisted Reproduction and Genetics* 20 (2003): 157–59.

Index

ALEXANDER R. PRUSS

is associate professor of philosophy at Baylor University. He is the author and co-editor of a number of books, including *The Principle of Sufficient Reason: A Reassessment.*

CPSIA information can be obtained
at www.ICGtesting.com
Printed in the USA
LVHW041101190123
737397LV00007B/259